W. E. Berdel   H. Jürgens   Th. Büchner   J. Ritter
J. Kienast   J. Vormoor (Eds.)

Transplantation in Hematology and Oncology II

Springer-Verlag Berlin Heidelberg GmbH

W. E. Berdel H. Jürgens Th. Büchner
J. Ritter J. Kienast J. Vormoor (Eds.)

Transplantation in Hematology and Oncology II

With contributions by

H.-J. Kolb, C. Annaloro, J. Boos, M. Bornhäuser, D. Bunjes, A. Chybicka, U. Creutzig, P. Dreger, U. Ebener, E. Faber, T. Fietz, B. Fröhlich, S. Grupp, M. Kröger, N. Kröger, T. Lapidot, I.G.H. Lorand-Metze, M. Machaczka, M.F. Martelli, T. Niehues, A. Nolte, G. Rosti, O. Ryzhak, P. Schlegel, U. Schuler, J.L. Schultze, W. Siegert, M. Theobald, X. Thomas, S. Wehner, and A. Zander

Springer

W. E. Berdel, Prof. Dr. med.
Th. Büchner, Prof. Dr. med.
J. Kienast, Prof. Dr. med.
Department of Internal Medicine Hematology/Oncology
University of Münster
Albert-Schweitzer-Straße 33
48129 Münster, Germany

H. Jürgens, Prof. Dr. med.
J. Ritter, Prof. Dr. med.
J. Vormoor, Dr. med.
Department of Pediatrics Hematology/Oncology
University of Münster
Albert-Schweitzer-Straße 33
48129 Münster, Germany

ISBN 978-3-642-62660-9 ISBN 978-3-642-55774-3 (eBook)
DOI 10.1007/978-3-642-55774-3

Library of Congress Cataloging-in-Publication Data. Transplantation in hematology and oncology II/W. E. Berdel ... [et al.], eds. ; with contributions by H.-J. Kolb .. [et al.].p. ; cm. Includes bibliographical references and index. ISBN 3540421556 (hardcover : alk. paper) 1. Cancer -- Immunotherapy. 2. Cell transplantation. 3. Hematopoietic stem cells. 4. Blood--Diseases. I. Berdel, Wolfgang E. [DNML: 1. Cell Transplantation. 2. Hematopoietic Stem Cell Transplantation. 3. Hematologic Diseases--therapy. 4. Hematopoietic Stem Cell Mobilization. 5. Immunotherapy. 6. Neoplasms--therapy. 7. Tissue Transplantation. WO 660 T769742 2002]
RC271.C44 T73 2002 616.99'406--dc21

http://www.springer.de

Originally published by Springer-Verlag Berlin Heidelberg in 2003
Softcover reprint of the hardcover 1st edition 2003

Cover design: *design & production* GmbH, Heidelberg
Typesetting: Goldener Schnitt, Sinzheim
SPIN: 10831005 21/3130 5 4 3 2 1 0 – Printed on acid-free paper

Contents

Preface

Hematopoietic stem cell and immune cell transplantation has continued as a promising therapeutic alternative and a fascinating area of cell biology as well as a field of persistent procedural problems. This explains why substantial parts of basic research on cell growth and differentiation, immune tolerance and antitumor effects, gene transfer, minimal residual disease and supportive care have settled around clinical transplantation in hematology and oncology. This second volume again updates the current role of allogeneic and autologous transplantation in leukemias, lymphomas and solid cancers, including controversial strategies and novel experimental approaches.

In particular, cellular immune therapy, new conditioning strategies, mismatched donor transplantation, updated clinical transplantation, antiangiogenesis and strategies against fungal infections are focused upon. Outstanding representatives of leading groups guarantee first-hand information and indicate how we can work and cooperate more effectively to the benefit of our patients.

The editors are indebted to the *Gesellschaft zur Bekämpfung der Krebskrankheiten Nordrhein-Westfalen* for a substantial support of the publication. They also acknowledge the major contribution of Beate Kosel as coordinator of the editorial work.

Wolfgang E. Berdel
Heribert Jürgens
Thomas Büchner
Jörg Ritter
Joachim Kienast
Josef Vormoor

Cellular Therapy: Targets and Effectors

Adoptive Immunotherapy in Chimeras

H.-J. Kolb, Ch. Schmid, M. Schleuning, O. Stoetzer, X. Chen,
A. Woiciechowski, M. Roskrow, M. Weber, W. Guenther, and G. Ledderose

Clinical Cooperative Group Hematopoietic Cell Transplantation,
Dept. of Medicine III, Klinikum University of Munich – Grosshadern, and
GSF-National Research Center for Environment and Health, Munich, Germany

Experiments in Dogs

Depletion of T-cells from the marrow by treatment with absorbed antithymocyte globulin (ATG) prevents GVHD in DLA-identical littermates and transfusion of donor lymphocytes on days 1 and 2, 21 and 22 induces fatal GVHD. However transfusion on days 61 and 62 dose not produce GVHD and the animals survive. These animals were mixed lymphoid and myeloid chimeras prior to transfusion and they became complete chimeras thereafter [2]. The donors were immunized against tetanus toxoid and the recipients developed antibody titers after DLT that persisted for more than 3 years after booster injections. Transfused and non-transfused animals were immunized against diphtheria toxoid as a new antigen. Transfused dogs developed significantly higher antibody titers than non-transfused dogs.

These experiments indicated that two months after transplantation tolerance is established that allowed the DLT without the risk of GVHD. Moreover residual hematopoietic cells of the host are eliminated without GVHD. Similar results were obtained in a leukemia model in mice [15].

Results of Donor Lymphocyte Transfusions in CML

Three patients with recurrent CML after allogeneic marrow transplantation were treated with DLT in 1988 and 1989 [16], they are still in hematologic and molecular remission of CML. The results were confirmed by others [17–23], the analysis of the results of centers of the European Cooperative Group of Blood and Marrow Transplantation (EBMT) showed best results in cytogenetic and hematologic relapses of CML, intermediate results in transformed phase CML, acute myeloid leukemia (AML) and myelodysplastic syndromes (MDS) and poor results in acute lymphoblastic leukemia (ALL) [4]. Complications of the treatment were GVHD and myelosuppression. Both absence of chimerism [5]and presence of GVHD were adverse factors for a response. In CML the graft-versus-leukemia effect (GVL) correlated with the severity of GVHD, but responses were also seen in patients without GVHD. However GVL was limited to patients with an allogeneic donor, it failed in patients with a monozygotic twin donor. Antigen presentation could be improved by treatment with cytokines. In particular the combination of interferon-α (IFN-α) and GM-CSF improved the expression of HLA class I and II antigens, CD 40 and CD 80 [6]. Preliminary results confirm the beneficial effect of GM-CSF and IFN-α in patients with recurrent CML refractory to donor lymphocytes.

Prevention of GVHD could be achieved by two methods without ablating the GVL effect: depletion CD8-positive T cells from the transfusion [20, 24] and using escalating doses of DLT [21] starting at a dose of 2 x 10^6 lymphocytes per kg. The escalating dose schedule has significantly lowered the risk of GVHD. Patients should be surveyed by regular quantitative RT-PCR for bcr/abl and in case of persisting or recurrent positivity the proposed schedule is a starting dose of 2 x 10^6 lymphocytes per kg from unrelated donors and 1 x 10^7 lymphocytes per kg from an HLA-identical sibling donor. Doses are escalated, if there is no GVHD within 30 days or no response within 60 days.

Results of Donor Lymphocyte Transfusions in AML

The EBMT results indicated inferior responses in patients with recurrent AML after DLT. In patients without chemotherapy induced remission the response rate was 25 per cent with very few patients surviving more than 4 years. Only limited data were available on the FAB subtype and cytogenetic analyses in these patients. With these limitations FAB subtype did not influence the response and a proportion of patients with an unfavorable karyotype did respond to this form of treatment.

Poor antigen presentation and the rapid progression of the disease were considered as the major obstacles for adoptive immunotherapy in recurrent AML. Improvement of antigen presentation and production of cytotoxic T cells against autologous blasts was studied in vitro (Fig. 1). The combination of GM-CSF, IL-4, TNF-α and FLT3-L was particularly effective in inducing dendritic cells from AML blasts [7]. The culture was effective in 77 per cent of patients and included patients with complex karyotypes. Specific cytotoxic T-cells against autologous blasts could be produced in more than 60 per cent of these patients.

We have used low dose cytosine arabinoside as mild chemotherapy for halting progression of the disease. Mobilized blood was transfused as a preparation of stem cell enriched donor lymphocytes and GM-CSF was applied for 14–28 days after transfusion. This way antigen presentation was optimized by induction of dendritic cells from AML blasts and substitution of dendritic cells derived from CD34-positive cells of the graft. The response rate was improved from 25 to 67

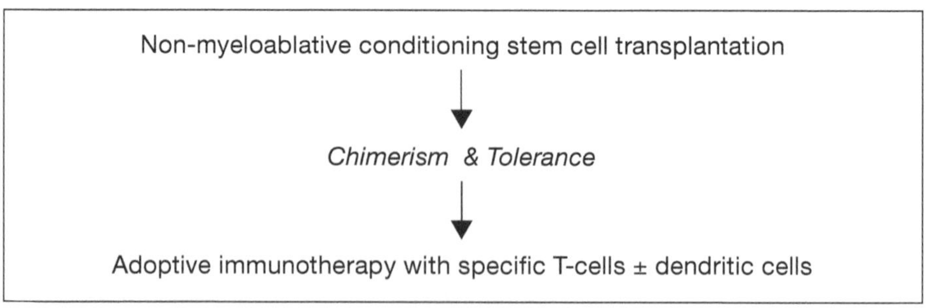

Fig. 1. AML Cells May Develop to Antigen Presenting Cells

per cent and the actuarial probability of survival is 25 per cent at 4 years [8]. However GVHD and extramedullary relapses remain therapeutic problems. In some patients low dose cytosine arabinoside is not effective in halting disease progression and more intensive chemotherapy including anthracyclins is necessary. In these cases severe GVHD may develop following transfusion of mobilized blood cells and treatment with GM-CSF. Moreover GM-CSF may mobilize blasts from the marrow into the blood. In these cases GM-CSF has to be stopped and in case of severe GVHD immunosuppressive treatment with steroids, cyclosporin A and azathioprine or others has to be started. Unfortunately leukemia may recur during immunosuppressive treatment and few therapeutic options remain. Improvement of the results is expected from the immunization of donor cells against minor histocompatibility antigens expressed on hematopoietic progenitor cells [25]. They should not react against other tissues of the patient and thus not produce GVHD. Sensitized donor lymphocytes should be transduced with a suicide gene that kills the cells in case of severe GVHD.

Responses to DLT have been reported for several other diseases like multiple myeloma, chronic lymphatic leukemia and Non-Hodgkin lymphoma of low grade malignancy. Common to these diseases is the slow progression of the disease and their response to IFN-α. At this time it is not known whether mature B-lymphocytes common to all of them are effective in antigen presentation to allogeneic lymphocytes or whether the relevant antigens are presented by other cells of the patient or the graft.

Any conclusions on the treatment of solid tumors with adoptive immunotherapy are premature, but the possibility exists that neoplasia as renal cell cancer, breast cancer and ovarian cancer respond to allogeneic transplants because of an immune graft-versus-tumor effect [26].

Adoptive immunotherapy against viral infections has been successful in the case of Epstein Barr Virus infections (EBV) [27, 28] and cytomegalovirus infections (CMV) [29]. In these cases very few unmodified T cells were effective in the treatment of EBV-associated lymphoma in transplant patients, but severe GVHD was a problem. CD8-positive T-cell clones were effective in preventing CMV disease, but the clones did not survive without the help of CD4-positive T-cells. Lines of T-cells comprising CD8- and CD4-positive cells survived in the transplanted patients and they were reactivated with reactivation of EBV.

Transplantation from HLA-haploidentical family members

The availability of donors has greatly increased in the last decade because of the registries of unrelated donors. However, logistic problems limit the use of second donations from unrelated donors. Therefore regimens for transplantation from family members sharing one HLA-haplotype and differing in 0–3 HLA-antigens (A, B, DR) of the second haplotype are being developed. The combination of marrow on day 0 and CD6-depleted mobilized blood on day 6 has shown promising results on otherwise refractory leukemia [9]. CD6-negative marrow and mobilized blood preparations contain a population of natural suppressor cells that suppress mixed lymphocyte reactions and cytotoxic T cell reactions. Suppression was exhibited by the CD8-positive subset of CD6-negative cells and suppression was abrogated by the depletion of CD8-positive cells and not by the depletion of NK-cells or monocytes. However recurrent immune deficiency and recurrent infections remain problems to be solved. The 2 year actuarial survival is 22 %, the relapse rate 60 %. However infections present therapeutic problems. Future attempts will be directed to transplantation at an earlier stage of the disease and better prevention of infections by improving immune reconstitution.

Outlook for adoptive immunotherapy

Hematopoietic cell transplantation has come a long way from bone marrow transplantation to adoptive immunotherapy in chimeras. However the mechanisms of adoptive immunotherapy in chimeras are still far from being understood. The immunobiology of leukemia, other neoplasia and viral infections has to be studied in human patients. The mechanism of immune tolerance, immune reactivity against normal cells and transfer of immunity can be studied in animal experiments.

Immunization of donor T cells against minor histocompatibility antigens of the recipient is currently studied in the dog. Sensitized cells convert mixed to complete chimerism much faster than naïve T-cells. Tests have been developed to demonstrate cellular immunity to hematopoietic progenitor cells in vitro allowing the definition of minor antigens in the dog [30]. The incidence of severe GVHD after transfusion of sensitized donor lymphocytes into stable chimeras may be 30–50 per cent [31]. The percentage is expected to be higher in human patients, since patients and their donors are exposed to a multiplicity of histocompatibility and viral antigens during their life. Preventive measures against severe GVHD are necessary. Modification of donor lymphocytes with a suicide gene is the most promising way of prevention. T-cells of the donor are infected with a replication-deficient retrovirus carrying the herpes Simplex thymidine kinase gene which can phosphorylate ganciclovir and the resulting nucleotide leads to stop of DNA polymerization during cell division [32]. Current problems of the method are altered immune reactivity of transduced T-cells, immune reaction against the viral protein and rejection of the transduced cells and altered sensitivity of transduced cells to ganciclovir due to splice variants of the gene. We have studied the method in the dog and found a good immune reactivity of transduced canine T-cells in vitro. Transfusion of transduced T-cells into a canine chimera resulted in a complete chimerism and transfer of immunity to tetanus toxoid, but the level of detection of transduced cells was low and only detected by PCR [33].

Adoptive immunotherapy in chimeras is a promising way to the treatment of leukemia and possibly solid neoplasia. In particular the immune reactivity against leukemias and neoplasia otherwise refractory to chemotherapy gives new perspectives in hematology and oncology.

Summary

The use of donor lymphocytes for the treatment of recurrent leukemia has changed the perspectives of hematopoietic stem cell transplantation [1]. The antileukemic principles of myeloablative conditioning have been substituted by adoptive immunotherapy. Experiments in dogs had shown that graft-versus-host tolerance can be induced by depletion of T-cells from the graft and donor lymphocytes could be transfused without graft-versus-host disease (GVHD) later than 60 days after transplantation [2]. In dogs donor lymphocytes converted mixed chimerism into complete chimerism, transferred immunity to tetanus from the donor to the host and improved the response to diphtheria toxoid. Donor lymphocytes eliminated leukemia in patients with recurrent chronic myelogenous leukemia (CML) after allogeneic bone marrow transplantation [3]. The analysis of the results of centers of the European Cooperative Group of Blood and Marrow Transplantation (EBMT) revealed best results in cytogenetic and hematologic relapses of CML, intermediate results in transformed phase CML, acute myeloid leukemia (AML) and myelodysplastic syndromes (MDS) and poor results in acute lymphoblastic leukemia (ALL) [4]. Complications of the treatment were GVHD and myelosuppression. Both absence of chimerism [5]and presence of GVHD were adverse factors for a response. In CML the graft-versus-leukemia effect (GVL) correlated with the severity of GVHD, but responses were also seen in patients without GVHD. However GVL was limited to patients with an allogeneic donor, it failed in patients with a monozygotic twin donor. Antigen presentation could be improved by treatment with cytokines. In particular the combination of interferon-α (IFN-α) and GM-CSF improved the expression of HLA class I and II antigens, CD 40 and CD 80 [6]. Preliminary results confirm the beneficial effect of GM-CSF and IFN-α in patients with recurrent CML refractory to donor lymphocytes.

The possibility of differentiation to dendritic cells as professional antigen presenting cells is common to CML and AML. The leukemic origin of dendritic cells in culture could be shown by FISH analysis showing the characteristic chromosomal aberration. In AML the combination of GM-CSF, IL-4, TNF-α and FLT3-L were particularly effective in inducing dendritic cells from AML blasts [7]. The culture was effective in 70 per cent of patients and included patients with complex karyotypes. In patients with recurrent AML after allogeneic transplantation the success of donor lymphocyte transfusions is limited because of poor antigen presentation of the blasts and rapid progression of the disease. We have used low dose cytosine arabinoside as mild chemotherapy for halting progression of the disease. Mobilized blood was transfused as a preparation of stem cell enriched donor lymphocytes and GM-CSF was applied for 14–28 days after transfusion. This way antigen presentation was optimized by induction of dendritic cells from AML blasts and substitution of dendritic cells from the graft. The response rate was improved from 25 to 67 per cent and the actuarial probability of survival is 25 per cent at 4 years [8]. However GVHD and extramedullary relapses remain therapeutic problems. Improvement of the results is expected from the immunization of donor cells against minor histocompatibility antigens expressed on hematopoietic progenitor cells. Sensitized donor lymphocytes should be transduced with a suicide gene that kills the cells in case of severe GVHD. Experiments in dogs are in progress.

Logistic problems limit the use of second donations from unrelated donors and favor family donors. Therefore regimens for transplantation from HLA-haploidentical family members are being developed. The combination of marrow on day 0 and CD6-depleted mobilized blood on day 6 has shown promising results on otherwise refractory leukemia [9]. CD6-negative marrow and mobilized blood preparations contain a population of natural suppressor cells that suppress mixed lymphocyte reactions and cytotoxic T cell reactions. However recurrent immune deficiency and recurrent infections remain problems to be solved.

The treatment of leukemia and neoplastic diseases has changed during the last decades. Bone marrow transplantation once thought an experimental procedure in selected cases of extremely poor prognosis has become standard treatment for a variety of diseases [10, 11]. The progress of hematopoietic transplantation is related to several areas of improvement: the availability of a donor, the expansion of the source of stem cells, the better diagnosis and treatment of infections, and the use of adoptive immunotherapy and less intensive conditioning regimens. Ten years ago the procedure was limited to minority of patients with a HLA-identical sibling, today more than 80 per cent of patients find a suitable donor in internationally available donor registries. The use of mobilized blood as source of stem cells [12] has improved the availability of donors and the amount of CD34-positive cells as putative stem cells available. Early diagnosis of cytomegalovirus infections and preemptive treatment has decreased the severe complications of CMV disease. The use of donor lymphocytes for the treatment of recurrent or residual leukemia has stimulated the search for less intensive conditioning treatments [13, 14]enabling the provision of transplantation to patients formerly not considered suitable candidates for transplantation. The dilemma between induction of transplantation tolerance by depletion of T cells and the beneficial effect of T cells on residual leukemia has prompted us to investigate in the dog whether the procedure can be separated into two steps: first transplantation of T cell depleted marrow and secondly the transfusion of donor lymphocytes (DLT) for restitution of immunity (Fig.2).

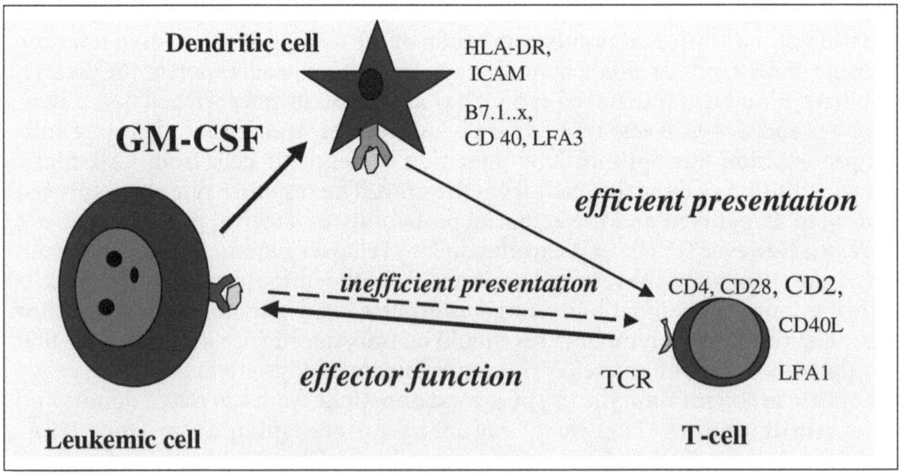

Fig. 2

References

1. Antin JH. Graft-versus-leukemia: no longer an epiphenomenon. Blood 1993; 82:2273–2277.
2. Kolb HJ, Günther W, Schumm M, Holler E, Wilmanns W, Thierfelder S. Adoptive immunotherapy in canine chimeras. Transplantation 1997; 63:430–436.
3. Kolb HJ, Mittermueller J, Clemm C, Ledderose G, Brehm G, Heim M, Wilmanns W. Donor leukocyte transfusions for treatment of recurrent chronic myelogenous leukemia in marrow transplant patients. Blood 1990; 76:2462–2465.
4. Kolb HJ, Schattenberg A, Goldman JM, Hertenstein B, Jacobsen N, Arcese W, Ljungman P, Ferrant A, Verdonck L, Niederwieser D, van Rhee F, Mittermüller J, De Witte T, Holler E, Ansari H. Graft-versus-leukemia effect of donor lymphocyte transfusions in marrow grafted patients. Blood 1995; 86:2041–2050.
5. Schattenberg A, Schaap N, van de Wiel-van Kemenade E, Bar B, Preijers F, Van Der Maazen R, Roovers E, De Witte T. In relapsed patients after lymphocyte depleted bone marrow transplantation the percentage of donor T lymphocytes correlates well with the outcome of donor leukocyte infusion. Leuk Lymphoma 1999; 32(3–4):317–325.
6. Chen X, Regn S, Raffegerst S, Kolb HJ, Roskrow M. Interferon alpha in combination with GM-CSF induces the differentiation of leukaemic antigen-presenting cells that have the capacity to stimulate a specific anti-leukaemic cytotoxic T-cell response from patients with chronic myeloid leukaemia. Br J Haematol 2000; 111(2):596–607.
7. Woiciechowsky A, Regn S, Kolb H-J, Roskrow M. Leukemic dendritic cells generated in the presence of FLT3 ligand have the capacity to stimulate an autologous leukaemia-specific cytotoxic T cell response from patients with acute myeloid leukaemia. Leukemia 15, 246–255. 2001.
8. Schmid C, Lange C, Salat C, Stoetzer O, Ledderose G, Muth A, Schleuning M, Roskrow M, Kolb H-J. Treatment of recurrent acute leukemia after marrow transplantation with donor cells and GM-CSF. Blood 94[10 Suppl 1], 668a–668a. 1999.
9. Kolb H-J, Hoetzl F, Guenther W, Fuehrer M, Schmid C, Ledderose G, Stoetzer O, Bender C, Schleuning M. CD-6 negative blood stem cells facilitating HLA-haploidentical transplantation in the treatment of advanced leukemia. Blood 96[11], 208a–208a. 2000.
10. Goldman JM, Schmitz N, Niethammer D, Gratwohl A, Accreditation Sub-Committee of the EBMT. Allogeneic and autologous transplantation for haematological diseases, solid tumours and immune disorders: current practice in Europe in 1998. Bone Marrow Transplant 1998; 21:1–7.
11. Rizzo JD. 1998 IBMTR/ABMTR Summary Slides on State-of-the-Art in Blood & Marrow Transplantation. ABMTR Newsletter 5[1], 4–10. 1998. Milwaukee WI USA, IBMTR/ABMT Statistical Center, Medical College of Wisconsin.
12. Schmitz N, Linch DC, Dreger P, Goldstone AH, Boogaerts MA, Ferrant A, Demuynck HMS, Link H, Zander A, Barge A, Borkett K. Randomised trial of filgastrim-mobilised peripheral blood progenitor cell transplantation in lymphoma patients. Lancet 1996; 347:353–357.
13. Giralt S, Estey E, Albitar Meal. Engraftment of allogeneic hematopoietic progenitor cells with purine analog-containing chemotherapy: harnessing graft-versus-leukemia without myeloablative therapy. Blood 1997; 89:4531–4536.
14. McSweeney PA, Niederwieser D, Shizuru JA, Sandmaier BM, Molina AJ, Maloney DG, Chauncey TR, Gooley TA, Hegenbart U, Nash RA, Radich J, Wagner JL, Minor S, Appelbaum FR, Bensinger WI, Bryant E, Flowers ME, Georges GE, Grumet FC, Kiem HP, Torok-Storb B, Yu C, Blume KG, Storb RF. Hematopoietic cell transplantation in older patients with hematologic malignancies: replacing high-dose cytotoxic therapy with graft-versus-tumor effects. Blood 2001; 97(11):3390–3400.
15. Johnson BD, Drobyski WR, Truitt RL. Delayed infusion of normal donor cells after MHC-matched bone marrow transplantation provides an antileukemia reaction without graft-versus-host disease. Bone Marrow Transplant 1993; 11:329–336.
16. Kolb HJ, Mittermueller J, Holler E, Clemm C, Ledderose G, Brehm G, Wilmanns W. Treatment of recurrent chronic myelogenous leukemia posttransplant with interferone alpha (INFa) and donor leukocyte transfusions. Blut 61, 122–122. 1990. Ref Type: Abstract
17. Bar BMAM, Schattenberg A, Mensink EJBM, Van Kessel AG, Smetsers TFCM, Knops GHJN, Linders EHP, De Witte T. Donor leukocyte infusions for chronic myeloid leukemia relapsed after allogeneic bone marrow transplantation. J Clin Oncol 1993; 11:513–519.

18. van Rhee F, Lin F, Cullis JO, Spencer A, Cross NCP, Chase A, Garicochea B, Bungey J, Barrett AJ, Goldman JM. Relapse of chronic myeloid leukemia after allogeneic bone marrow transplant: The case for giving donor leukocyte transfusions before the onset of hematological relapse. Blood 1994; 83:3377–3383.
19. Porter DL, Roth MS, McGarigle C, Ferrara JLM, Antin JH. Induction of graft-versus-host disease as immunotherapy for relapsed chronic myeloid leukemia. New Engl J Med 1994; 330:100–106.
20. Giralt S, Hester J, Huh Y, Hirsch-Ginsberg C, Rondon G, Seong D, Lee M, Gajewski J, Van Besien K, Khouri I, Mehra R, Przepiorka D, Körbling M, Talpaz M, Kantarjian H, Fischer H, Deisseroth A, Champlin R. CD8-depleted donor lymphocyte infusion as treatment for relapsed chronic myelogenous leukemia after allogeneic bone marrow transplantation. Blood 1995; 86:4337–4343.
21. Mackinnon S, Papadopoulos EB, Carabasi MH, Reich L, Collins NH, Boulad F, Castro-Malaspina H, Childs BH, Gillio AP, Kernan NA, Small TM, Young JW, OReilly RJ. Adoptive immunotherapy evaluating escalating doses of donor leukocytes for relapse of chronic myeloid leukemia after bone marrow transplantation: separation of graft-versus-leukemia responses from graft-versus-host disease. Blood 1995; 86:1261–1268.
22. Slavin S, Naparstek E, Nagler A, Ackerstein A, Samuel S, Kapelushnik J, Brautbar C, Or R. Allogeneic cell therapy with donor peripheral blood cells and recombinant human interleukin-2 to treat leukemia relapse after allogeneic bone marrow transplantation. Blood 1996; 87:2195–2204.
23. Collins RH, Shpilberg O, Drobyski WR, Porter DL, Giralt S, Champlin R, Goodman SA, Wolff SN, Hu W, Verfaillie C, List A, Dalton W, Ognoskie N, Chetrit A, Antin JH, Nemunaitis J. Donor leukocyte infusions in 140 patients with relapsed malignancy after allogeneic bone marrow transplantation. J Clin Oncol 1997; 15:433–444.
24. Alyea EP, Soiffer RJ, Canning C, et al. Toxicity and efficacy of defined doses of CD4+ donor lymphocytes for treatment of relapse after allogeneic bone marrow transplantation. Blood 91, 3671–3677. 1998.
25. Mutis T, Verdijk R, Schrama E, Esendam B, Brand A, Goulmy E. Feasability of immunotherapy of relapsed leukemia with ex vivo generated cytotoxic T lymphocytes specific for hematopoietic system-restricted minor histocompatibility antigens. Blood 1999; 93(7):2336–2341.
26. Childs R, Chernoff A, Contentin N, Bahceci E, Schrump D, Leitman S, Read EJ, Tisdale J, Dunbar C, Linehan WM, Young NS, Barrett AJ. Regression of metastatic renal-cell carcinoma after nonmyeloablative allogeneic peripheral-blood stem-cell transplantation. N Engl J Med 2000; 343(11):750–758.
27. Papadopoulos EB, Ladanyi M, Emanuel D, Mackinnon S, Boulad F, Carabasi MH, Castro-Malaspina H, Childs BH, Gillio AP, Small TN, Young JW, Kernan NA, OReilly RJ. Infusions of donor leukocytes to treat Epstein-Bar virus- associated lymphoproliferative disorders after allogeneic bone marrow transplantation. N Engl J Med 1994; 330:1185–1191.
28. Rooney CM, Smith CA, Heslop HE. Control of virus-induced lymphoproliferation: Epstein-Barr virus- induced lymphoproliferation and host immunity. Mol Med Today 1997; 3(1):24–30.
29. Walter EA, Greenberg PD, Gilbert MJ, Finch RJ, Watanabe KS, Thomas ED, Riddell SR. Reconstitution of cellular immunity against cytomegalovirus in recipients of allogeneic bone marrow by transfer of T-cell clones from the donor. N Engl J Med 1995; 333:1038–1044.
30. Weber M, Lange C, Kolb HJ, Kolb HJ. CFU-suppression by T-Cells primed with DLA-identical dendritic cells. Bone Marrow Transplant 2000; 25(Suppl 1):S23–abstract.
31. Weiden PL, Storb R, Tsoi M-S, Graham TC, Lerner KG, Thomas ED. Infusion of donor lymphocytes into stable canine radiation chimeras: Implications for mechanism of transplantation tolerance. J Immunol 1976; 116:1212–1219.
32. Bonini C, Ferrari G, Verzelletti S, Servida P, Zappone E, Ruggieri L, Ponzoni M, Rossini S, Mavilio F, Traversari C, Bordignon C. HSV-TK gene transfer into donor lymphocytes for control of allogeneic graft-versus-leukemia. Science 1997; 276:1719–1724.
33. Weissinger EM, Franz M, Voss C, Kremmer E, Kolb H-J. Expression of HSV-TK suicide gene in primary T-lymphocytes: The dog as a preclinical model. Cytokines, Cellular & Molecular Therapy 2000; 6(1):25–33.

The Roles of the Chemokine SDF-1 and its Receptor CXCR4 in Human Stem Cell Migration and Repopulation of NOD/SCID and B2mnull NOD/SCID mice

T. Lapidot

The Weizmann Institute of Science, Rehovot 76100, Israel

Abstract

The mechanism of hematopoieitc stem cell migration and repopulation involve a complex interplay between stromal cells, chemokines, cytokines and adhesion molecules, however details of this regulatory process are not fully understood. During development hematopoietic stem cells migrate from the fetal liver into the blood circulation, home to the bone marrow and repopulate it wkth immature and maturing blood cells which in turn are released into the circulation. Murine fetuses which lack the chemokine Stromal Derived Factor One (SDF-1null) or its receptor CXCR4 (CXCR4null) have multiple defects which are lethal, including impaired bone marrow hematopoiesis. These results suggest a major role for SDF-1/CXCR4 interactions in murine fetal liver stem cell homing into the bone marrow and its repopulation. Human and murine SDF-1 are cross reactive and differ in one amino acid. Recently, we reported that SDF-1 and CXCR4 interactions are essential for homing and repopulation of immune deficient NOD/SCID and B2mnull NOD/SCID mice by human stem cells. In the present manuscript we review the central roles of this chemokine and its receptor in human stem cell migration and repopulation of transplanted immune deficient mice.

Introduction

The establishemnt of functional in vivo transplantation assays for human stem cells, using immune deficient SCID, NOD/SCID and B2mnull NOD/SCID mice as recipients

During development, blood forming stem cells migrate from the fetal liver into the blood, home to the bone marrow and repopulate it with immautre and maturing myeloid and lymphoid cells [2]. Similarly, in clinical bone marrow transplantation and in experimental stem cell transplantation assays, using animal models, transplanted stem and progenitor cells migrate in the circulation, home to the bone marrow and repopulate it with high levels of immature and maturing myeloid and lymphoid cells which in turn are released into the blood circulation [3]. Since blood forming stem cells are identified based on their functional ability to home in transplantation assays to the host bone marrow and to repopulate it with high levels of immature and maturing myeloid and lymphoid cells, functional in vivo models for the characterization of human stem cells were in need. Homing and repopulation assays for human stem cells which are based on intravenous transplantation into sublethally irradiated immune deficient SCID, NOD/SCID and more recently B2mnull NOD/SCID mice have been developed by us, and by other laboratories [4–7]. In these assays, transplanted human stem and progenitor cells gave rise to high levels multilineage hematopoiesis in the murine bone marrow. These assays were further used to identify a rare population of primitive human $CD34^{+}/CD38^{-}$ SCID repopulating cells (SRC), with the potential to repopulate the bone marrow of transplanted immune deficient NOD/SCID mice with high levels of both myeloid and lymphoid cells [8]. B2mnull NOD/SCID mice lack natural killer cell activity due the absence of class one B2 microglobulin [9]. The reduced innate immunity of these mice makes them superior recipients for preclinical human stem cell assays, which better resemble auotologous stem cell transplantation. The increased immune deficiency of these mice led to increased frequencies of transplanted SRC by up to 11 fold, higher levels of multilineage repopulation in serially transplanted mice and significantly faster homing of primitive human $CD34^{+}/CD38^{-/low}/CXCR4^{+}$ stem and progenitor cells into the murine bone marrow [7, 10, 11].

The chemokine stromal derived factor one (SDF-1)

Stromal cells regulate the continuous production of maturing blood cells and their release into the blood circulation while maintaining a small pool of primitive, undifferentiated stem cells throughout life, by the secretion of chemokines, cytokines and activation of adhesion molecules, however details of stem cell regulation by stromal cells are poorly understood [1]. The most primitive stem and progenitor cells reside within the bone marrow microenvironment in direct contact with immature bone forming osteoblast cells along the endosteum region and to a lesser degree also in periarterial regions (ref). Van Dyke et al reported in 1969 that endosteal trauma induces reactions in the surrounding bone that provide a growth stimulus for hematopoietic cells within the bone marrow. One possible explanation for this result is that chemokines produced by the immature osteoblasts are released due to the endosteal trauma and provide a growth stimulus for the hematopoietic progenitor cells in the bone marrow.

Chemokines are small signaling molecules which are part of the cytokine superfamily and are best known for their ability to selectively attract subsets of leukocytes to sites of inflammation by chemotaxis [12]. The chemokine stromal derived factor one (SDF-1) is produced by bone marrow stromal cells and also by epithelial cells in many other organs [13]. Human and murine SDF-1 are cross reactive and differ in one amino acid [14]. The SDF-1 receptor, CXCR4 is expressed by a wide variety of cells including endothelial, neuronal, and a wide range of hematopoietic cells which include myeloid, lymphoid and immature $CD34^{+}$ cells. In contrast to most chemokines, SDF-1 is produced by bone marrow stromal cells also in the absence of external stimuli generated by viral or bacterial infections, suggesting a major role for this chemokine in steady-state homeostatic processes such as leukocyte trafficking. In the developing murine embryo, lack of SDF-1 or CXCR4 led to severe defects which are lethal. These include defective formation of the ventricular septum of the heart [15], gastrointestinal blood vessel formation [16], defective formation of neuronal networks in the cerebellum [17], reduced B cell development in the liver and impaired myeloid and lymphoid bone marrow hematopoiesis [14]. These results suggest a major role for SDF-1 and CXCR4 interactions in murine fetus development processes which require cell migration, including homing of fetal liver stem cells into the bone marrow and its repopulation. SDF-1 synergizes with VEGF to form blood vessels in adult mice by stimulating endothelial cells which express CXCR4 [18]. SDF-1 is a survival factor for both human and murine colony forming progenitor cells [19], In vivo administration of high doses of SDF-1 once a day for two consecutive days prevented primitive human repopulating cells from cycling in transplanted NOD/SCID mice which lead to higher levels of engraftment by these cells in serially transplanted recipients compared to mice which were serially transplanted with human cells without SDF-1 treatment [20]. Low doses of this chemokine together with other cytokines increase proliferation of immature human and murine colony forming progenitor cells [21, 22]. SDF-1/CXCR4 interactions are involved in stem cell differentiation into the B lymphocyte [15], and Megakaryocyte lineage's [23] while suppressing development into the erythroid lineage by activation of FAS ligand [24]. Within the immature $CD34^+$ cell population, the more primitive and rare $CD38^{-/low}$ cells express higher levels of surface CXCR4 while the more differentiated $CD38^+$ cells also secrete low levels of SDF-1 [25, 26]. This chemokine is a powerful chemoattractant for immature and mature hematopoietic cells of several lineages including immature human $CD34^+$ cells [27–29]. Transgenic mice expressing human CXCR4 and CD4 on their $CD4^+$ T cells had increased levels of these cells in their bone marrow and only very low levels in the circulation [30]. In addition to stimulating of a wide array of normal cells, there are also CXCR4+ malignant cells which also respond to stimulation with SDF-1. These include many types of leukemic cells, including multiple myeloma as well as some breast and prostate cancer cells. In a recent report the group of Zlotnik et al demonstrated that metastatic breast cancer cells functionally express CXCR4 and that their spread into the lungs of SCID mice can be inhibited by in vivo treatment with neutralizing anti CXCR4 antibodies . This study shows involvement of chemokines such as SDF-1 in metastasis of cancer cells into secondary organs [31]. Taken together the above results suggest a major role for SDF-1/CXCR4 interactions in stem cell homing and repopulation, however the role that chemokines and their receptors play in human stem cell migration and development is not fully understood.

Stem cell homing and repopulation

Stem cell homing and engraftment is presumably a multi step process, sharing some common features with migration of leukocytes to inflammatory sites and homing of lymphocytes into lymph nodes [32, 33]. Transplanted human stem cells, which migrate through the blood circulation, must interact with the bone marrow vascular endothelial cells. This results in rolling on P and E selectins followed by firm shear resistant adhesion to the vessel wall. These interactions are mediated by the coordinated action of activated adhesive molecules. Adhesive activation processes are triggered specifically by chemokines, such as SDF-1, and vascular ligands such as VCAM-1 and ICAM-1 [32–36]. Following immobilization on the bone marrow microvasculature, stem cells extravasate through the endothelium and into the hematopoietic compartment. One protein involved in the extravasation process is the β2 integrin, lymphocyte function associated-1 (LFA-1). This molecule is involved in the spontaneous transendothelial migration of immature human $CD34^+$ cells in vitro [36]. Furthermore, activation of LFA-1 present on human $CXCR4^+$ T lymphocytes by SDF-1, led to firm shear resistant adhesion to endothelial ICAM-1 [37]. Other proteins involved are the major b1 integrins, very late antigen–4 (VLA-4) and VLA-5, which have been implicated in the adhesive interactions of human, primate and mouse stem cells with the bone marrow extracellular matrix (ECM) and stromal cells [38–40]. SDF-1 was also found to mediate the migration of immature human $CD34^+$ cells across bone marrow blood vessels subendothelial basement membranes by regulating production of matrix degrading metalloproteinases (MMPs) MMP2 and MMP9. These enzymes which are produced by hematopoietic, endothelial and epithelial cells participate in homing and release of hematopoietic cells which require penetration across the blood endothelium and bone marrow stroma by degrading all the components of the extracellular matrix (ECM) [41].

Release and mobilization from the bone marrow

Release of maturing cells from the bone marrow into the circulation as well as mobilization of immature and maturing hematopoietic cells in response to multiple cytokine stimulations such as G-CSF, both involve a complex interplay between stromal cells, cytokines, chemokines and adhesion molecules, though details of this regulatory process are poorly understood. The cytokine SCF has a membrane bound form which is also expressed on some stromal cells. Blocking interactions between hematopoietic stem and progenitor cells via their integrin VLA-4 and also their SCF receptor c-kit with neutralizing antibodies lead to mobilization of the immature cells from the bone marrow into the circulation, suggesting a major role for SCF and VLA-4 in the mobilization process [20, 42–43]. Recent results demonstrate that G-CSF or Cyclophosphamide mediated mobilization induces disruption of VLA-4/VCAM-1 adhesion interactions by reduction of VCAM expression on bone marrow stromal cells followed by increase of soluble VCAM-1 in the circulation during mobilization [44]. A single dose of human G-CSF decreased by ten fold the levels of human SDF-1 in the bone marrow of treated patients within 24 hours [45]. Furthermore, immune deficient SCID mice infected with a SDF-1 expressing virus had increased plasma levels of SDF-1 which induced stem and progenitor cell mobilization from the bone marrow into the circulation [46]. Sulfated polysaccharides also rapidly induce stem cell mobilization by preventing interacions with P and E selectins [35] and by causing the secretion of SDF-1 from the bone marrow into the circulation most probably by competing for binding of SDF-1 to the bone marrow endothelium and stromal cells via the c-terminus [47]. Lastly, preliminary experiments to test the toxicity of in vivo administration of the CXCR4 blocker AMD3100 to healthy volunteers as a possible treatment for HIV patients led to rapid and significant increase in their white blood cell counts suggesting hematopoietic cell mobilization from the bone marrow by preventing SDF-1/CXCR4 interactions [48].

In summery, the mechanism of human stem cells development and function are tightly linked to their motility and migration patterns. Therefor a better understanding of human stem cells development and regulation requires deciphering the mechanisms governing their homing, repopulation, release, and/or mobilization.

Results and Discussion

Dependence of human stem cell repopulation of NOD/SCID and B2mnull NOD/SCID mice on CXCR4

We discovered that concomitant expression of the chemokine SDF-1 and its receptor CXCR4 by the host bone marrow cells and by the transplanted donor cells respectively, is essential for NOD/SCID and B2mnull NOD/SCID bone marrow engraftment by human SRC. Pretreatment of donor human $CD34^+$ enriched cells from cord blood, bone marrow or mobilized PBL with neutralizing anti CXCR4 antibodies blocked engraftment. Moreover, we found that SRC are true stem cells capable of high level multilineage repopulation of serially transplanted primary NOD/SCID and secondary B2mnull NOD/SCID mice in a CXCR4 dependent mannar. Our data characterizes human SRC further as $CD38^{-/low}CXCR4^+$ cells with major stem cell properties. The activity of SDF-1 on immature human $CD34^+$ enriched cells was regulated by cytokines such as SCF and IL-6, which induced the expression of CXCR4 on immature human $CD34^+/CXCR4^{-/low}$ and primitive $CD34^+/CD38^{-/low}/CXCR4^{-/low}$ cells during short term in vitro stimulation (16–48hr.) prior to transplantation, which increased in vitro migration to a gradient of SDF-1 in transwells and converted non repopulating cells into SRC in both primary and serially transplanted NOD/SCID and B2mnull NOD/SCID mice [10]. This approach of CXCR4 upergulation between primary and serially transplanted NOD/SCID mice by short term in vitro stimulation with SCF and IL-6 in order to increase the levels of repopulation in serially transplanted mice was successfully repeated by the group of Dick et al in a recent report describing the fate of marked SRC clones by gene transfer [49]. Rosu-Myles and Bhatia et al transplanted sorted $CD34^+/CD38^-/Lin^-/CXCR4^-$ and $CXCR4^+$ cells from cord and fetal blood into NOD/SCID mice [50]. This work is based on an earlier study by Bhatia and Dick et al which determined the frequency of SRC in sorted human cord blood $CD34^+/CD38^-/Lin^-$ cells [51]. Transplantation of 1,000-5,000 sorted $CD34^+/CD38^-/Lin^-$ cord blood cells per mouse into 22 mice by Bhatia and Dick et al led to 5/22 mice with no engraftment,13/22 mice with low levels of engraftment (0.1%–1%), 3/22 mice with medium levels of engraftment (1%–10%), and also one mouse with high levels of engraftment. In sharp contrast, transplantation of 1,000–5,000 or 5,000–10,000 sorted $CD34^+/CD38^-/Lin^-/CXCR4^-$ cord and fetal blood cells per mouse by Rosu-Myles and Bhatia et al into 5 and 4 mice respectively, led to no engraftment in 3/5 and 1/4 mice respectively and only very low levels of human engraftment in 2/5 and 3/4 mice (0.2% and 0.23% respectively). These results suggest very low repopulation potential and/or proliferation pressure on the engrafting cells. Moreover, transplantation of a broad cell dose ranging between 330-300000 sorted $CD34^+/CD38^-/Lin^-/CXCR4^-$ cells (up to 60 fold increase in the transplanted cell dose compared to the work of Bhatia and Dick) by Rosu-Myles and Bhatia et al gave rise to no engraftment in 9/20 mice, low levels of engraftment (0.1%-1%) in 8/20 mice, no mice with medium range engraftment (1%-10%) and only 3/20 mice were highly engrafted! Similarly $CXCR4^+$ sorted $CD34^+/CD38^-/Lin^-$ cells also gave rise to low levels of engraftment, however the anti CXCR4 antibody (12G5) used for cell sorting binds the same sites as SDF-1 and thus inhibits its function i.e the CXCR4+ cells were partially inhibited by neutralising anti CXCR4 ab used for their enrichment. Comparing the two studies reveals a 10-60 fold decrease in the repopulation potential of sorted $CXCR4^-$ and partially inhibited $CXCR4^+$ $CD34^+/CD38^-/Lin^-$ cord and fetal blood cells compared to sorting of the entire $CD34^+/CD38^-/Lin^-$ cord blood cell population. In addition, we have shown that transplantation of $3x10^4$ sorted $CD34^+/CD38^{-/low}$ cord blood cells which also migrated to a gradient of SDF-1 in vitro gave rise to high levels of engraftment in transplanted NOD/SCID mice (>40%) while transplantation of $3x10^4$ non migrating $CD34^+/CD38^{-/low}$ cells led to very low levels of engraftment (<1%). More important, short term 48hr. in vitro stimulation of non migrating, sorted $CD34^+/CD38^{-/low}$ cells with SCF has increased CXCR4 expression, migration towards a gradient of SDF-1 and converted the repopulation potential of these cells to that of SRC, i.e. with high level multi lineage engraftment (in one case from 0.3% human engraftment before treatment with SCF, to 50% after 48hr. SCF stimulation and on average from <1% for non migrating $CD34^+/CD38^{-/low}$ cells to >35% after short term stimulation with SCF [10]. Lastly, preliminary results from our studies reveal that non migrating, non repopulating human cord blood $CD34^+$ enriched cells and sorted $CD34^+/CXCR4^-$ cells contain high levels of internal CXCR4 which can be re-expressed either by short term in vitro stimulation with cytokines such as SCF and IL-6 or to a lesser degree also in vivo in transplanted NOD/SCID and B2mnull NOD/SCID mice during the first 24–48hr. post transplantation which can convert some of these cells into functional SRC. However, this in vivo CXCR4 upregulation is not very efficient and therefor requires transplantation of extremely high cell doses (up to 60 fold increase). Similarly, Rosu-Myles and Bhatia et al also demonstrate that sorted $CD34^+/CD38^-/Lin^-/CXCR4^-$ cord and fetal blood cells can express surface CXCR4 expression after short term, 24hr. stimulation with a cytokine cocktail which contains SCF and IL-6 and is known to maintain the repopulation potential of SRC in serum free media. This surface CXCR4 expression by sorted $CD34^+/CD38^-/Lin^-/CXCR4^-$ cord and fetal blood cells is sensitive to SDF-1, since in the presence of SDF-1, lower levels of CXCR4 expression were documented. Moreover, preliminary results from our experiments show that co-transplantation of sorted cord blood $CD34^+/CXCR4^-$ cells together with neutralizing anti CXCR4 antibodies prevented CXCR4 re-expression and blocked their repopulation potential in transplanted NOD/SCID and B2mnull NOD/SCID mice! Based on all the above, we suggest that the high levels of engraftment documented by Rosu-Myles and Bhatia et al in 3 out of 20 mice transplanted with up to 300,000 sorted $CD34^+/CD38^-/Lin^-/CXCR4^-$ cord and fetal blood cells are also due to in vivo surface CXCR4 expression. In support of our hypothesis, a recent report demonstrated that immature human $CD34^+$ enriched PBL cells from patients treated with chemotherapy and G-CSF induced mobilization, which better migrated in vitro (both spontaneously and to a gradient of SDF-1) initiated significantly faster hematological recovery in autologous transplantation compared to patients transplanted with $CD34^+$ cells which had reduced motility. This study demonstrates for the first time a direct link between the motility of enriched human $CD34^+$ cells in vitro and their homing and repopulation potential in vivo, in clinical autologous stem cell transplantation [52].

Rapid and efficient homing of human $CD34^+CD38^{-/low}CXCR4^+$ stem and progenitor cells to the bone marrow and spleen of NOD/SCID and B2mnull NOD/SCID mice

Stem cell homing into the bone microenvironment is the first step in the initiation of marrow derived blood cells. In a recent study we have found that human SRC home and accumulate rapidly, within a few hours, in the bone marrow and spleen of B2mnull NOD/SCID mice and at a significantly slower rate in the BM and spleen of NOD/SCID mice, both previously conditioned with total body irradiation. Primitive human $CD34^+CD38^{-/low}CXCR4^+$ from freshly isolated cord blood $CD34^+$ cells capable of engrafting primary NOD/SCID and secondary B2mnull NOD/SCID recipient mice homed to the bone marrow and spleen while $CD34^-CD38^{-/low}$ cord blood cells which also contain a minority of $CXCR4^+$ cells (about 20%) were not detected. Moreover, $CD34^-CD38^{-/low}$ cord blood cells had superior in vitro random migration but inferior migration to a gradient of SDF-1 in transwells compared to $CD34^+CD38^{-/low}$ cord blood cells from the same donors. These results suggest that directional migration towards a gradient of SDF-1 in vitro is the dominant factor and not random migration for in vivo SRC repopulation potential in transplanted NOD/SCID and B2mnull NOD/SCID mice. A recent report demonstrated that mobilized human $CD34^+$ enriched cells from patients treated with chemotherapy and G-CSF, which better migrated across fibronectin coated transwell filters both spontaneously and to a gradient of SDF-1 in vitro, initiated significantly faster hematological recovery in autologous transplanted patients, compared to patients transplanted with $CD34^+$ cells with reduced in vitro migratory capacities. This study demonstrates for the first time a direct link between the motility of enriched human $CD34^+$ cells in vitro and their homing and repopulation potential in vivo, in clinical autologous stem cell transplantation (ref blood). Sorting of primitive $CD34^+CD38^{-/low}$ cells (about 20% of the total $CD34^+$ cord blood cell population) and the more differentiated, $CD34^+CD38^{+/high}$ cells (about 80% of the total $CD34^+$ cord blood cell population) revealed that only the more primitive cells could home to the bone marrow and spleen of B2mnull NOD/SCID and NOD/SCID mice. While freshly isolated cord blood $CD34^+CD38^{+/high}$ cells did not home to the murine bone marrow and spleen, in vivo stimulation with human G-CSF as part of the mobilization process, or in vitro stimulation with SCF for 2-4 days, potentiated the homing capabilities of cytokine stimulated $CD34^+CD38^+$ cells from cord blood or G-CSF mobilized PBL cells into the bone marrow and spleen of NOD/SCID mice. These cytokine induced $CD34^+/CD38^+$ cells engrafted NOD/SCID mice transiently for 1-2 weeks and were not detected one month post transplantation. More important, cytokine induced $CD34^+/CD38^+$ cord blood cells were mostly cycling G1 cells which could increase the migration levels of quiescent Go $CD34^+/CD38^{-/low}$ cells to low gradients of SDF-1 in vitro and also increase their levels of repopulation in transplanted NOD/SCID and B2mnull NOD/SCID mice [53].

Interestingly, Auiti et al have demonstrated that while both primitive $CD34^+CD38^{-/low}$ cells and the more differentiated $CD34^+CD38^+$ cells express surface CXCR4, only the more differentiated $CD34^+CD38^+$ cells also secrete low levels of SDF-1, which may explain their reduced repopulation potential in transplanted immune deficient mice [25]. Homing of enriched human cord blood $CD34^+$ cells to the bone marrow and spleen of NOD/SCID and B2mnull NOD/SCID mice was inhibited by pretreatment with anti CXCR4 antibodies. Moreover, primitive human $CD34^+CD38^{-/low}CXCR4^+$ cord blood cells also homed in response to a gradient of human SDF-1, directly injected into the bone marrow or spleen of non-irradiated NOD/SCID mice in a CXCR4 dependent manner. Homing to the bone marrow and spleen of B2mnull NOD/SCID mice was significantly reduced by pretreatment of $CD34^+$ cells with antibodies for the major integrins VLA-4, VLA-5, or LFA-1. Pertussis-toxin (PTX), an inhibitor of signals mediated by Ga_i proteins, inhibited SDF-1 mediated in vitro migration but not adhesion or in vivo homing of $CD34^+/CXCR4^+$ cells. Homing of immature human cord blood $CD34^+$ cells and murine $Sca\text{-}1^+/Lin^-$ cells was blocked by pretreatment with chelerythrine chloride, a broad range PKC inhibitor. This study reveals rapid and efficient homing to the murine bone marrow by primitive human $CD34^+CD38^{-/low}CXCR4^+$ cells which is integrin mediated and depends on activation of the PKC signal transduction pathway by SDF-1 [11, 52–53].

The chemokine SDF-1 stimulates integrin-mediated arrest of immature CD34+ cells on vascular endothelium under shear flow

To extravasate into the bone marrow, a stem cell must first firmly arrest on vascular endothelium under physiological blood flow. Enriched human $CD34^+$ progenitor cells were found to efficiently roll on human endothelial P and E selectins under physiological shear flow, and rapidly developed firm LFA-1 mediated adhesion to ICAM-1 in the presence of surface-bound human SDF-1. SDF-1 also promoted VLA-4 mediated firm adhesion to VCAM-1 and spreading. Interestingly, we found that in vivo SDF-1 is highly expressed on the surface of human bone marrow endothelial cells. In support of our work, Imai et al reported in vivo expression of SD-1 on murine bone marrow endothelium and the secretion of SDF-1 by immortalized endothelial cell lines, derived from murine bone marrow endothelial cells Thus, SDF-1 displayed on vascular human and murine endothelium is crucial for translating rolling adhesions of human progenitor cells into firm adhesion, this occurs through the activation of VLA-4 and LFA-1-adhesiveness to the respective endothelial ligands, VCAM-1 and ICAM-1. Our studies suggest that SDF-1 expressed by bone marrow endothelial cells is critically involved in the homing of immature human stem and progenitor cells to the bone marrow [54].

The chemokine SDF-1 activates the integrins LFA-1, VLA-4 and VLA-5 on immature human CD34+ cells: role in transendothelial/stromal migration and engraftment of NOD/SCID mice

Stem cell engraftment is a multi step process utilizing activation of specific adhesion molecules. We found that engraftment of NOD/SCID mice by human SRC/stem cells is dependent on the major integrins VLA-4, VLA-5 and to a lesser degree on LFA-1. Treatment of enriched human cord blood $CD34^+$ cells with antibodies to either VLA-4 or VLA-5 prevented engraftment and treatment with anti LFA-1 antibodies significantly reduced the levels of engraftment. Activation by SDF-1 of enriched immature $CD34^+$ cells, bearing the chemokine receptor CXCR4, led to firm shear resistant LFA-1/ICAM-1 and VLA-4/VCAM-1 dependent adhesion and to transendothelial migration across both human and murine endothelial cells. Furthermore, SDF-1-induced polarization and extravasation of $CD34^+$/$CXCR4^+$ cells through the extracellular matrix underlining the endothelium was shown to be dependent on both VLA-4 and VLA-5. Thus, SDF-1 activates all the major adhesion molecules which are crucial for the multi step process of SRC/stem cell homing and engraftment [55].

Increased expression of the chemokine SDF-1 following DNA damage: relevance for human stem cell function in transplanted NOD/SCID mice

The expression patterns of SDF-1 by different bone marrow stromal cells is currently unknown. We found that within the human bone marrow, SDF-1 is mainly produced by immature bone forming osteoblasts in the endosteum region along the bones as well as by bone marrow endothelial cells. Previous reports demonstrated that the most primitive undifferentiated progenitor cells largely localize to the endosteum region along the bone, and to a lesser degree to periarterial regions [56]. Our results suggest that SDF-1 secreted by immature osteoblasts along the endosteum region and by endothelial cells in periarterial regions is crucial for stem cell retention and development. Consistent with our concept, Van Dyke et al reported that endosteal trauma induces reactions in the surrounding bone that provide a growth stimulus for hematopoietic cells within the bone marrow [57]. Pretransplantation conditioning of the recipient by DNA damaging agents is essential for successful stem cell engraftment. Unexpectedly, we found increased expression of SDF-1 following conditioning of mice with DNA damaging agents, such as ionizing irradiation or treatment with cytotoxic drugs. The elevated production of SDF-1 correlated with an increase in CXCR4 dependent homing and repopulation by human SRC/stem cells transplanted into NOD/SCID mice. Thus, SDF-1 appears to play a role both in stem cell homing, retention and repopulation as well as in host defense responses to protect stem cells from DNA damage [58].

Activation of PKC-zeta by SDF-1 is essential for migration of human $CD34^+$ cells towards SDF-1 in vitro and for SRC engraftment of NOD/SCID mice

Signaling following binding of SDF-1 to its receptor CXCR4 on immature human $CD34^+$ cells and the role of PKC activation in stem cell migration is poorly understood. Preliminary results indicate that while the Ca^{++} and DAG dependent PKC inhibitors staurosporine and GF had no effect on migration of immature human $CD34^+$ cells and leukemic Pre B ALL cells, SDF-1 chemotaxis was blocked by chelerythrine chloride (CC), a broad range PKC inhibitor known to also block Ca^{++} and DAG-independent PKC isoforms, suggesting a role for an atypical PKC in migration of hematopoietic cells. Inhibiton of atypical PKC-z by pseudosubstrate (PS) peptides, prevented Pre B ALL and $CD34^+$ cell migration towards SDF-1. SDF-1 induced translocation of PKC-z to the plasma membrane of these cells was wortmanin- sensitive, suggesting that activation of PI3-Kinase is upstream of PKC-z. In addition, SDF-1-induced actin polymerization was also blocked by CC and PKC-z PS peptides. Moreover, pretreatment of human $CD34^+$ cells and murine Sca-1+Lin- stem and progenitor cells with chelerythrine chloride blocked in vivo homing to the bone marrow of transplanted NOD/SCID mice. Inhibition of PKC-z by PS peptides significantly reduced engraftment by human SRC. Surprisingly, PKCab PS peptides which do not inhibit migration of $CD34^+$ cells to SDF-1, could also efficiently block SRC engraftment, suggesting an additional role for PKCab in homing and repopulation of the bone marrow. Our data suggest that activation of PKC-z is essential for SDF-1 mediated migration of human CD34+ cells, in vivo homing and repopulation by SRC/stem cells [53].

SDF-1 induces survival, adhesion, and migration in 3D ECM like gels of murine CXCR4null fetal liver cells via another receptor

During development hematopoietic stem cells migrate from the fetal liver into the blood circulation and home to the bone marrow. Murine fetuses which lack the chemokine SDF-1 (SDF-1null) or its receptor CXCR4 (CXCR4null) have multiple defects including impaired bone marrow hematopoiesis [15–17]. Unexpectedly, recent reports demonstrated that CXCR4null fetal liver cells from murine embryos can engraft the bone marrow of sublethaly irradiated wild type (WT) syngeneic mice [59–60]. Since we have demonstrated that total body irradiation increases the levels of SDF-1 production within the murine bone marrow and spleen [58], we tested whether CXCR4null fetal liver cells can respond to SDF-1 stimulation via another receptor. While CXCR4null cells did not migrate in vitro to a gradient of SDF-1 in transwells, they developed as efficient VLA-4 dependent chemokine-stimulated adhesion to VCAM-1/SDF-1 co-substrates as WT fetal liver cells. Denatured SDF-1 or a non-signaling SDF-1 mutant (PTG) did not induce adhesion. Pretreatment with the CXCR4 blocker AMD3100 reduced the adhesion of WT cells while the adherence of CXCR4null cells was not affected. In addition, both cell types migrated in a 3D ECM-like gel towards a gradient of SDF-1 while in the absence of SDF-1 no migration could be observed. In vitro stimulation with low levels (0.5 ng/ml) of SDF-1 significantly increased the viability of both CXCR4null and WT cells while high doses of this chemokine (50-100ng/ml) significantly reduced the levels of viable cells in both WT and CXCR4null fetal liver cultures. These results suggest that CXCR4null cells express an alternative SDF-1 receptor which partially compensates for the absence of CXCR4. Alternative mechanisms for homing and engraftment by hematopoietic stem cells may exist, however, they are secondary to the SDF-1 pathway since both SDF-1null and CXCR4null embryos have impaired bone marrow hematopoieis and transplanted CXCR4null fetal liver cells can interact with SDF-1 via another receptor [61].

In conclusion, our results delineate key events in the multi step process of stem cell migration and repopulation and suggest upregulation of SDF-1 and CXCR4 expression in order to increase their interactions as a novel approach to improve clinical stem cell transplantation.

References

1. Weissman IL. Translating stem and progenitor cell biology to the clinic: barriers and opportunities. Science. 2000;287:1442–1446.
2. McGrath KE, Koniski AD, Maltby KM, McGann JK, Palis J. Embryonic expression and function of the chemokine SDF-1 and its receptor, CXCR4. Dev Biol. 1999;213:442-456.
3. Moore MA. „Turning brain into blood“-clinical applications of stem-cell research in neurobiology and hematology. N Engl J Med. 1999;341:605-607.
4. McCune JM, Namikawa R, Kaneshima R, Schultz LD, Leiberman K, Weissman IL. The SCID-hu mouse: murine model for the analysis of human hematolymphoid differentiation and function. Science. 1988;241:1632.
5. Lapidot T, Pflumio F, Doedens M, Murdoch B, Williams DE, Dick JE. Cytokine stimulation of multilineage hematopoiesis from immature human cells engrafted in SCID mice. Science. 1992;255:1137.
6. Cashman JD, Lapidot T, Wang JC, et al. Kinetic evidence of the regeneration of multilineage hematopoiesis from primitive cells in normal human bone marrow transplanted into immunodeficient mice. Blood. 1997;89:4307–4316.
7. Kollet O, Peled A, Byk T, et al. beta2 microglobulin-deficient (B2m(null)) NOD/SCID mice are excellent recipients for studying human stem cell function. Blood. 2000;95:3102–3105.
8. Larochelle A, Vormoor J, Hanenberg H, et al. Identification of primitive human hematopoietic cells capable of repopulating NOD/SCID mice using retroviral gene marking and cell purification: implications for gene therapy. Nat Med. 1996;2:1329–1337.
9. Christianson SW, Greiner DL, Hesselton RA, et al. Enhanced human CD4+ T cell engraftment in beta2-microglobulin-deficient NOD-scid mice. J Immunol. 1997;158:3578–3586.
10. Peled A, Petit I, Kollet O, et al. Dependence of human stem cell engraftment and repopulation of NOD/SCID mice on CXCR4. Science. 1999;283:845–848.
11. Kollet O, Spiegel A, Peled A, et al. Rapid and efficient homing of human CD34+CD38-/low-CXCR4+ stem and progenitor cells to the bone marrow and spleen of NOD/SCID and NOD/SCID/B2m*null* mice. Blood. 2001;In Press.
12. Kim CH, Broxmeyer HE. SLC/exodus2/6Ckine/TCA4 induces chemotaxis of hematopoietic progenitor cells: differential activity of ligands of CCR7, CXCR3, or CXCR4 in chemotaxis vs. suppression of progenitor proliferation. J Leukoc Biol. 1999;66:455–461.
13. Maekawa T, Ishii T. Chemokine/receptor dynamics in the regulation of hematopoiesis. Intern Med. 2000;39:90–100.
14. Nagasawa T, Tachibana K, Kishimoto T. A novel CXC chemokine PBSF/SDF-1 and its receptor CXCR4: their functions in development, hematopoiesis and HIV infection. Semin Immunol. 1998;10:179–185.

15. Nagasawa T, Hirota S, Tachibana K, et al. Defects of B-cell lymphopoiesis and bone-marrow myelopoiesis in mice lacking the CXC chemokine PBSF/SDF-1. Nature. 1996;382:635–638.
16. Tachibana K, Hirota S, Iizasa H, et al. The chemokine receptor CXCR4 is essential for vascularization of the gastrointestinal tract [see comments]. Nature. 1998;393:591–594.
17. Zou YR, Kottmann AH, Kuroda M, Taniuchi I, Littman DR. Function of the chemokine receptor CXCR4 in haematopoiesis and in cerebellar development. Nature. 1998;393:595–599.
18. Salcedo R, Wasserman K, Young HA, et al. Vascular endothelial growth factor and basic fibroblast growth factor induce expression of CXCR4 on human endothelial cells: In vivo neovascularization induced by stromal-derived factor-1alpha. Am J Pathol. 1999;154:1125–1135.
19. Lataillade JJ, Clay D, Dupuy C, et al. Chemokine SDF-1 enhances circulating CD34(+) cell proliferation in synergy with cytokines: possible role in progenitor survival. Blood. 2000;95:756–768.
20. Cashman J, Clark-Lewis I, Eaves C. SDF-1 and TGF-b enhance the detection of transplantable human stem cells regenerating in NOD/SCID mice. Exp. Hematol. 2000;28:85 [abstr].
21. Grafte-Faure S, Leveque C, Ketata E, et al. Recruitment of primitive peripheral blood cells: synergism of interleukin 12 with interleukin 6 and stromal cell-derived FACTOR-1. Cytokine. 2000;12:1–7.
22. Broxmeyer HE, Hangoc G, Cooper S, Kim CH. Enhanced myelopoiesis in SDF-1 transgenic mice: SDF-1 modulates myelopoeisis by regulat-ing progenitor cell survival and inhibitory effects of myelosuppresive chemokines. Blood. 1999;94:650a [abstr].
23. Hodohara K, Fujii N, Yamamoto N, Kaushansky K. Stromal cell-derived factor-1 (SDF-1) acts together with thrombopoietin to enhance the development of megakaryocytic progenitor cells (CFU-MK). Blood. 2000;95:769–775.
24. Gibellini D, Bassini A, Re MC, et al. Stroma-derived factor 1alpha induces a selective inhibition of human erythroid development via the functional upregulation of Fas/CD95 ligand [In Process Citation]. Br J Haematol. 2000;111:432–440.
25. Aiuti A, Turchetto L, Cota M, et al. Human CD34(+) cells express CXCR4 and its ligand stromal cell-derived factor-1. Implications for infection by T-cell tropic human immunodeficiency virus. Blood. 1999;94:62–73.
26. Viardot A, Kronenwett R, Deichmann M, Haas R. The human immunodeficiency virus (HIV)-type 1 coreceptor CXCR-4 (fusin) is preferentially expressed on the more immature CD34+ hematopoietic stem cells. Ann Hematol. 1998;77:193–197.
27. Bleul CC, Farzan M, Choe H, et al. The lymphocyte chemoattractant SDF-1 is a ligand for LESTR/fusin and blocks HIV-1 entry. Nature. 1996;382:829–833.
28. Aiuti A, Webb IJ, Bleul C, Springer T, Gutierrez-Ramos JC. The chemokine SDF-1 is a chemoattractant for human CD34+ hematopoietic progenitor cells and provides a new mechanism to explain the mobilization of CD34+ progenitors to peripheral blood. J Exp Med. 1997;185:111–120.
29. Jo DY, Rafii S, Hamada T, Moore MA. Chemotaxis of primitive hematopoietic cells in response to stromal cell-derived factor-1. J Clin Invest. 2000;105:101–111.
30. Sawada S, Gowrishankar K, Kitamura R, et al. Disturbed CD4+ T cell homeostasis and in vitro HIV-1 susceptibility in transgenic mice expressing T cell line-tropic HIV-1 receptors. J Exp Med. 1998;187:1439–1449.
31. MuÈ ller A., Homey B, Soto H, et al. Involvement of chemokine receptors in breast cancer metastasis. Nature. 2001, 410: 50
32. Springer TA. Traffic signals for lymphocyte recirculation and leukocyte emigration: the multistep paradigm. Cell. 1994;76:301–314.
33. Butcher EC, Picker LJ. Lymphocyte homing and homeostasis. Science. 1996;272:60–66.
34. Quesenberry PJ, Becker PS. Stem cell homing: rolling, crawling, and nesting. Proc Natl Acad Sci USA. 1998;95:15155–15157.
35. Frenette PS, Subbarao S, Mazo IB, von Andrian UH, Wagner DD. Endothelial selectins and vascular cell adhesion molecule-1 promote hematopoietic progenitor homing to bone marrow. Proc Natl Acad Sci U S A. 1998;95:14423–14428.
36. Mohle R, Moore MA, Nachman RL, Rafii S. Transendothelial migration of CD34+ and mature hematopoietic cells: an in vitro study using a human bone marrow endothelial cell line. Blood. 1997;89:72–80.

37. Campbell JJ, Hedrick J, Zlotnik A, Siani MA, Thompson DA, Butcher EC. Chemokines and the arrest of lymphocytes rolling under flow conditions. Science. 1998;279:381–384.
38. Verfaillie CM. Adhesion receptors as regulators of the hematopoietic process. Blood. 1998;92:2609–2612.
39. Hirsch E, Iglesias A, Potocnik AJ, Hartmann U, Fassler R. Impaired migration but not differentiation of haematopoietic stem cells in the absence of beta1 integrins. Nature. 1996;380:171–175.
40. van der Loo JC, Xiao X, McMillin D, Hashino K, Kato I, Williams DA. VLA-5 is expressed by mouse and human long-term repopulating hematopoietic cells and mediates adhesion to extracellular matrix protein fibronectin. J Clin Invest. 1998;102:1051–1061.
41. Janowska-Wieczorek A, Marquez LA, Dobrowsky A, Ratajczak MZ, Cabuhat ML. Differential MMP and TIMP production by human marrow and peripheral blood CD34(+) cells in response to chemokines. Exp Hematol. 2000;28:1274–1285.
42. Sanchez X, Cousins-Hodges B, Aguilar T, Gosselink P, Lu Z, Navarro J. Activation of HIV-1 coreceptor (CXCR4) mediates myelosuppression. J Biol Chem. 1997;272:27529–27531.
43. Coulomb-L'Hermin A, Amara A, Schiff C, et al. Stromal cell-derived factor 1 (SDF-1) and antenatal human B cell lymphopoiesis: expression of SDF-1 by mesothelial cells and biliary ductal plate epithelial cells. Proc Natl Acad Sci U S A. 1999;96:8585–8590.
44. Levesque JP, Takamatsu Y, Nilsson SK, Haylock DN, Simmons PJ. Mobilization of hemopoietic progenitor cells into peripheral blood is associated with VCAM-1 proteolytic cleavage in the bone marrow. Blood. 96:221a [abstr].
45. Lapidot T, Szyper-Kravitz M, Peled A, et al. A single dose of human G-CSF inhibited production of sdf-1 in the bone marrow and upregulated cxcr4 expression on immature and mature hematopoietic cells prior to their mobilization. Blood. 1999;94:606a [abstr].
46. Hattori K, Heissig B, Tashiro M, et al. Overexpression of SDF-1 by adenoviral vectors induced mobilization of myeloid and megakaryocytic progenitors and precoursor cells. Blood. 1999;94:605a [abstr].
47. Sweeney EA, Priestley G, Nakamoto B, Papayannopoulou T. Sulfated polysaccharides increase plasma levels of sdf-1 in monkeys and mice: involvement in mobilization of stem/progenitor cells. Blood. 2000;96:540a [abstr].
48. Hendrix C, Flexner C, Cfarland T, et al. Pharmacokinetics and Safety of AMD-3100, a Novel Antagonist of the CXCR-4 Chemokine Receptor, in Human Volunteers. Antimicrobial agents and chemotherapy, 2000, p. 1667–1673.
49. Guenechea G, Gan O, Dorrell C, Dick JE. Distinct classes of human stem cells that differ in proliferative and self-renewal potential. Nat Immunol. 2001;2:75–82.
50. Rosu-Myles M, Gallacher L, Murdoch B, et al. The human hematopoietic stem cell compartment is heterogeneous for CXCR4 expression. Proc Natl Acad Sci U S A. 2000;97:14626–14631.
51. Bhatia M, Wang JCY, Kapp U, Bonnet D, Dick JE. Purification of primitive human hematopoietic cells capable of repopulating immune-deficient mice. Proc Natl Acad Sci U S A. 1997;94:5320–5325.
52. Byk T, Kahn J, Kollet O, et al. G1 CD34+/CD38+ cells potentiate the motility and engraftment of quiescent Go CD34+/CD38-/low SCID repopulating cells. Blood. 2000;[abst].
53. Petit I, Spiegel A, Kollet O, et al. Activation of PKC zeta by SDF-1 is essential for migration of human CD34+ cells towards SDF-1 in vitro and for SRC engraftment of NOD/SCID mice. Blood. 2000;[abst].
54. Peled A, Grabovsky V, Habler L, et al. The chemokine SDF-1 stimulates integrin-mediated arrest of CD34(+) cells on vascular endothelium under shear flow. J Clin Invest. 1999;104:1199–1211.
55. Peled A, Kollet O, Ponomaryov T, et al. The chemokine SDF-1 activates the integrins LFA-1, VLA-4, and VLA-5 on immature human CD34(+) cells: role in transendothelial/stromal migration and engraftment of NOD/SCID mice. Blood. 2000;95:3289–3296.
56. Lambertsen RH, Weiss L. A model of intramedullary hematopoietic microenvironments based on stereologic study of the distribution of endocloned marrow colonies. Blood. 1984;63:287–297.
57. Van Dyke D, Harris N. Bone marrow reactions to trauma: Stimulation of erythropoietic marrow by mechanical disruption, fracture or endosteal curettage. Blood. 1969;34:257--275.

58. Ponomaryov T, Peled A, Petit I, et al. Induction of the chemokine stromal-derived factor-1 following DNA damage improves human stem cell function. JCI. 2000;106:1331–1339.
59. Ma Q, Jones D, Springer TA. The chemokine receptor CXCR4 is required for the retention of B lineage and granulocytic precursors within the bone marrow microenvironment. Immunity. 1999;10:463–471.
60. Kawabata K, Ujikawa M, Egawa T, et al. A cell-autonomous requirement for CXCR4 in long-term lymphoid and myeloid reconstitution. Proc Natl Acad Sci U S A. 1999;96:5663–5667.
61. Kollet O, Grabovsky V, Franitza S, Lider O, Alon R, Lapidot T. SDF-1 induces survival, adhesion, and migration in 3D-ECM like gels of murine CXCR4 null fetal liver cells. Blood. 2000;96:65a [abstr]

Towards Adoptive Immunotherapy Using High Affinity T Cell Receptors

M. Theobald

Johannes Gutenberg-University, Department of Hematology & Oncology, Langenbeckstr. 1, D-55101 Mainz, Germany

Results and Discussion

The hdm2 oncoprotein is frequently overexpressed in a variety of human malignancies, including acute myeloid and lymphoblastic leukemia. Synthetic peptides representative of hdm2 sequences were tested for their binding to A2.1. HLA-A2.1 ($/K^b$)-Tg mice were immunized with A2.1-binding hdm2 peptides in order to induce A2.1-restricted and hdm2-specific CTL. A2.1-restricted CTL lines obtained from both A2.1 and HuCD8 x A2.1/K^b-Tg mice were able to recognize a synthetic 8-mer peptide representative of a N-terminal hdm2 sequence. These CTL were capable of recognizing and lysing Saos-2 cells transfected with the hdm2 gene as opposed to the parental cell line that lacks any detectable hdm2 expression, thereby indicating that the 8-mer peptide is being naturally processed and presented by A2.1. The identity of the naturally presented hdm2 CTL epitope and the synthetic hdm2 8-mer peptide was confirmed by extracting peptides from class I MHC molecules of hdm2-transfectants. Subsequent HPLC-purification allowed the reconstitution of CTL lysis by those natural and synthetic HPLC-fractions which had an identical retention time. CTL specific for the hdm2 8-mer epitope were of sufficiently high avidity to specifically kill $A2.1^+$ human leukemia and myeloma targets provided that these cells displayed high level hdm2 protein expression as ascertained by Western blotting. In contrast, a variety of non-transformed human cells, such as PBMC, resting T and B cells, and antigen-activated T lymphocytes, all of them which did not express detectable amounts of hdm2, were not susceptible to lysis by these CTL. The full length a and b chains of high affinity T cell receptors (TCRs) derived from A2.1-restricted and hdm2-specific murine CTL clones have been cloned and sequenced. Hu A2.1-positive dendritic cells pulsed with the leukemia-associated hdm2 self-epitope were able to induce peptide-specific autologous human CTL. These autologous CTL, however, appeared to be of low avidity, thereby indicating that the hdm2 epitope does represent a self-tolerogen for high avidity CTL *in vivo*.

It has been recently shown in a Mu system that T cell tolerance to widely expressed proteins was also circumvented by raising CTL from MHC-mismatched donors (Sadovnikova and Stauss 1996). In a collaborative effort with Hans J. Stauss (London), peripheral blood mononuclear cells from A2.1-negative and -positive donors were stimulated with ($A2.1^+$) T2 cells pulsed with the synthetic hdm2 8-mer peptide. Cloning of bulk cultures revealed that CTL clones derived from A2.1-mismatched as opposed to A2.1-matched donors were peptide-specific. $A2.1^+$ and hdm2 overexpressing leukemia and lymphoma cells, in contrast to nontransformed peripheral blood cells, were killed by an allo-A2.1-restricted CTL clone specific for the hdm2 8-mer peptide and derived from an A2.1-negative allogeneic donor.

The CD19 signal transduction molecule is expressed by more than 95% of Hu B-lymphoid malignancies and is therefore likely to serve as an attractive B-cell associated target for class I MHC-restricted CTL. Targeting of peptides representative of single sequence differences between Mu and Hu in HLA-A2.1(/K^b) and HuCD8 x A2.1/K^b-Tg mice allowed the circumvention of CTL-based self-tolerance to HuCD19. A selection of HuCD19 peptides with potential A2.1-binding motifs was synthesized and tested for their actual A2.1-binding affinity. The immunogenicity of peptides with sufficiently high binding affinity to A2.1 was determined by testing their ability to induce A2.1-restricted CTL in Tg mice. Polyclonal CTL lines specific for 7 different HuCD19 peptides were generated after peptide challenge of both A2.1 and HuCD8 x A2.1/K^b-Tg mice. Mu EL4 transfectants that expressed the Hu A2.1 gene (EA2) were co-transfected with HuCD19 cDNA (EA2/19) and used as targets for the HuCD19-specific CTL lines in order to analyse as to whether immunogenic CD19 peptides were endogenously processed and presented. Two CTL lines specific for either a 9-mer and a 10-mer peptide, both of which were derived from the extracellular domain of the CD19 molecule, demonstrated specific recognition and lysis of EA2/19 as opposed to the parental EA2 transfectants, thereby indicating that these peptides serve as natural A2.1-bound CTL epitopes. Consistent with this finding, A2.1$^+$ EBV-transformed B-lymphoblastoid cell lines as well as B-cell derived lymphoma and leukemia lines were efficiently killed by A2.1-restricted and HuCD19 peptide-specific CTL.

In situations in which the host immune system is devoid of such high avidity, leukemia-reactive CTL, the Mu genes for A2.1-restricted, hdm2 or HuCD19 epitope-specific TCRs could be transfered into patient T cells. High affinity tumor- and leukemia-specific TCR genes could also be isolated from allo-A2.1-restricted Hu CTL clones. High-affinity TCRs derived from tumor- and leukemia-specific A2.1-restricted Tg and Hu CTL could be modified and used to transfer antigen specificity (Chung et al. 1994, Cole et al. 1995). The most attractive approach is to attach to the TCR an intracellular domain that enables direct signal transduction (Chung et al. 1994). This would override the necessity of relying upon appropriate interaction with the endogenous TCR-CD3 complex in order to transduce a stimulatory signal. Hooking up the TCR molecules with the intracellular domains of $CD3_{\varepsilon}, _{\zeta}$ (Chung et al. 1994), or FcR_{γ}, or with cytoplasmic tyrosine kinases (Syk, ZAP 70) (Eshhar et al. 1996) is supposed to be an attractive approach. The extracellular domains could consist of either a single (sc) or double chain (dc) TCR molecule. In order to prevent competition with endogenous TCR Va and Vb chains and to increase the expression efficiency of the desired TCR specificity, sc TCRs are likely to be of advantage (Chung et al. 1994). The designed TCR molecules could be equipped with an Ig or CD8 hinge (in order to allow the extension of the TCR from the transmembrane region) and short spacers (in order to enhance the three-dimensional flexibility of the TCR molecule) (Eshhar et al. 1996). Retroviral gene transfer allows efficient transduction of Hu T lymphocytes with both high affinity tumor- and leukemia-specific sc and dc TCRs as well as suitable suicide genes. Crosslinking of transduced Hu T cells by anti-CD3 and anti-CD28 monoclonal antibodies results in short term clonal expansion required for adpotive transfer into leukemia patients. Constant TCR regions of human origin could be enployed to humanize designer sc and dc TCRs obtained from A2.1-Tg mice, thereby preventing a potential immune reponse directed against sc or dc TCR transduced human T lymphocytes during therapeutic intervention *in vivo*.

As another therapeutic option, allo-restricted Hu CTL raised against peptides that are preferentially expressed in transformed cells would be particularly useful for adoptive immunotherapy of leukemia patients (Sadovnikova et al. 1998). As these patients may receive bone marrow transplants from partially MHC-mismatched donors, it is likely that they would accept injections of MHC-mismatched, donor-derived CTL clones specific for leukemia-associated proteins.

As an alternative, T cells with low avidity for hdm2 and CD19-derived peptide epitopes that have escaped negative selection could be expanded by a variety of different vaccination strategies. Under certain circumstances, such as low tumor burden and high density antigen expression, even the amplification of a low avidity T cell repertoire could be of some therapeutic value (Sherman et al. 1998).

Provided that the peripheral T cell repertoire is not devoid of high avidity CTL specific for tumor- or leukemia-associated peptide antigens not being expressed intrathymically, TCR technology could be used to express selected high affinity TCRs in hemopoetic stem cells. Depending on the efficiency of hemopoetic stem cell transduction, this would, in theory, give rise to a high frequency of tumor- or leukemia-reactive CTL in the peripheral T cell repertoire.

The identification of hdm2 and HuCD19-derived peptides representing broad-spectrum, leukemia-associated CTL epitopes provides the molecular background for a hdm2- and CD19-directed and TCR-based immunotherapy of hematologic malignancies.

Acknowledgementes. This work was supported by grants to Matthias Theobald from the Deutsche Forschungsge-meinschaft (DFG) (SFB 432 A3), the „Stiftung Rheinland-Pfalz für Innovation", and the „Mainzer Forschungsförderungs-programm des Fachbereichs Medizin (MAIFOR)". We fully appreciate the expert contributions by Edite Antunes Ferreira and Ulrike Liewer.

Summary

Peptides presented by class I major histocompatibility complex (MHC) molecules and derived from normal self-proteins that are expressed at elevated levels by cells from a variety of human (Hu) malignancies provide, in theory, potential target antigens for a broad-spectrum, cytotoxic T lymphocyte (CTL)-based immunotherapy of hematologic malignancies and cancer. However, as leukemia-associated self-proteins are also expressed at low level in some types of normal tissues, such as thymus, spleen, and lymphohemopoetic cells, these self-MHC-self-peptide complexes may also represent thymic and/or peripheral tolerogens, thereby preventing immune responses. This is particularly true for class I MHC-peptide complexes expressed by bone marrow derived cells in the thymus, as such expression would cause negative selection of immature thymic T cells with high avidity for self-MHC-self-peptide complexes. This intrathymic deletion of potentially self-reactive T cells could result in a peripheral T cell repertoire purged of CTL precursors with sufficient avidity to recognize natural tumor associated self-epitopes presented by class I MHC molecules on tumor cells. HLA-transgenic (Tg) mice provide the basis of an experimental strategy that exploits species differences between Hu and murine (Mu) protein sequences in order to circumvent self-tolerance and obtain HLA-restricted CTL specific for epitopes derived from tumor- and leukemia-associated Hu self proteins, such as p53, Her-2/neu, hdm2, and CD19 (Theobald et al. 1995, Lustgarten et al. 1997, Theobald et al. 1997, Lindauer et al. 1997, Sherman et al. 1997, Theobald et al. 1998).

References

Chung S, Wucherpfennig KW, Friedman SM, Hafler DA, Strominger JL (1994) Functional three-domain single-chain T-cell receptors. Proc Natl Acad Sci USA 91:12654-12658

Cole DJ, Weil DP, Shilyansky J, Custer M, Kawakami Y, Rosenberg SA, Nishimura MI (1995) Characterization of the functional specificity of a cloned T-cell receptor heterodimer recognizing the MART-1 melanoma antigen. Cancer Res 55:748-752

Eshhar Z, Bach N, Fitzer-Attas CJ, Gross G, Lustgarten J, Waks T, Schindler DG (1996) The T-body approach: Potential for cancer immunotherapy. Springer Semin. Immunopathol. 18:199-209

Lindauer M, Stanislawski T, Häußler A, Antunes E, Cellary A, Huber C, Theobald M (1998) The molecular basis of cancer immunotherapy by cytotoxic T lymphocytes. J Mol Med 76:32-47

Lustgarten J, Theobald M, Labadie C, LaFace D, Peterson P, Disis ML, Cheever MA, Sherman LA (1997) Identification of Her-2/neu CTL epitopes using double transgenic mice expressing HLA-A2.1 and human CD8. Human Immunol 52:109-118

Sadovnikova E, Stauss HJ (1996) Peptide-specific cytotoxic T lymphocytes restricted by nonself major histocompatibility complex class I molecules: Reagents for tumor immunotherapy. Proc Natl Acad Sci USA 93:13114-13118

Sadovnikova E, Jopling LA, Soo KS, Stauss HJ (1998) Generation of human tumor-reactive cytotoxic T cells against peptides presented by non-self HLA class I molecules. Eur J Immunol 28:193-200

Sherman LA, Theobald M, Morgan D, Hernandez J, Bacik I, Yewdell J, Bennink J, Biggs J (1998) Strategies for tumor elimination by cytotoxic T lymphocytes. Crit Rev Immunol 18:47-54

Theobald M, Biggs J, Dittmer D, Levine AJ, Sherman LA (1995) Targeting p53 as a general tumor antigen. Proc Natl Acad Sci USA 92:11993-11997

Theobald M, Biggs J, Hernandez J, Lustgarten J, Labadie C, Sherman LA (1997) Tolerance to p53 by A2.1-restricted cytotoxic T lymphocytes. J Exp Med 185:833-841

Theobald M, Ruppert T, Kuckelkorn U, Hernandez J, Häussler A, Antunes Ferreira E, Liewer U, Biggs J, Levine AJ, Huber C, Koszinowski UH, Kloetzel P-M, Sherman LA (1998) The sequence alteration associated with a mutational hotspot in p53 protects cells from lysis by cytotoxic T lymphocytes specific for a flanking peptide epitope. J Exp Med 188:1017-1028

New Antigens and Avenues to Immunotherapy of Cancer

J. L Schultze

Department of Adult Oncology, Dana-Farber Cancer Institute, Department of Medicine, Brigham and Women's Hospital, Department of Medicine, Harvard Medical School, Boston, Massachusetts 02115

Abstract

Tumor immunology has seen many exciting developments in the last few years. In addition to tumor antigens that are defined by anti-tumor T and B cell responses in patients the human telomerase reverse transcriptase has been identified by „reverse immunology" as the most widely expressed tumor antigen. Molecular remission has been associated with a cancer vaccine targeting the clonal idiotype of B cell malignancies and sophisticated cellular vaccines including fusions of tumor cells and antigen presenting cells have demonstrated promising results. Moreover, our capabilities to measure immunity have been significantly enhanced by novel technology such as ELISPOT and MHC/peptide tetramer analysis. With these techniques, antigen-specific T cells are tracked on the single cell level.

Introduction

Based on the fact that the majority of spontaneous tumors in animal models were non-immunogenic and disappointing results in clinical trials for many decades cancer immunotherapy was judged as an impossible task (Hewitt et al., 1976). With rapidly increasing knowledge about basic immunological mechanisms, the prospects of cancer immunotherapy, including cell-based approaches to induce strong cellular immune responses has dramatically changed over the last decade and this field of research has now emerged as a viable therapeutic strategy. This important change started with the seminal work of Boon et al demonstrating that the reason for an insufficient anti-tumor immune response is not due to the lack of tumor antigens but rather due to an inappropriate activation of the immune system by tumor cells (Boon et al., 1994). Since then multiple tumor antigens have been identified both for murine and human tumors and these findings have fueled recent efforts to develop molecularly defined immunization strategies.

Several important questions are currently addressed as the field of tumor immunotherapy moves forward. Most of the tumor antigens identified to date have not been demonstrated to be powerful tumor rejection antigens (Gilboa, 1999; Rosenberg, 1999). Tumor regression antigens are not only associated with malignant cells but if targeted by T cells will lead to clinically significant tumor regression. Furthermore, there is no consensus about the most effective treatment modality in cancer immunotherapy. Vaccination strategies include cellular as well as non-cellular approaches, antigen-specific and tumor-specific approaches. Moreover, the role of antigen-specific T cell therapy is still not defined.

New cellular treatment modalities

Over the last decade there has been an exponential growth of new and exciting strategies to induce immunity against cancer. Clearly, the major focus is the development of cancer vaccines, however, a small group of highly sophisticated laboratories is still attempting to develop adoptive transfer strategies of antigen-specific T cells (Yee et al., 1997). Adoptive T cell transfer has been demonstrated to successfully eradicate tumor cells, however, the technical obstacles are still very high. This is clearly the major reason why the majority of investigators have turned to therapeutic vaccination although most pre-clinical models and the experience from viral diseases do not support „post-exposure" vaccination. Vaccination is likely to be more effective in a prophylactic setting, as has been clearly demonstrated for infectious diseases. Since only a few cancer types have been associated with viruses such as hepatocellular carcinoma (Wild and Hall, 2000) or cervical carcinoma (Cain and Howett, 2000), it is unlikely that we will be able to develop prophylactic vaccine strategies for the majority of cancer patients in the near future.

Nevertheless, several important and promising results from therapeutic vaccination have been reported recently. Bendandi et al reported an association of vaccination against the idiotype protein in patients with lymphoma with molecular remission in a large number of patients treated on this study at a stage of minimal residual disease induced by chemotherapy (Bendandi et al., 1999). In context with other vaccine trials these findings strongly suggest that vaccination is likely to be successful in minimal residual disease. Moreover, this study also addressed the need for potent adjuvants – in this case KLH and GM-CSF.

An incredible amount of work has been the development of cellular vaccines, particularly dendritic cell based immunotherapy. Dendritic cells have been shown to be potent inducers of anti-tumor immune responses in numerous pre-clinical models (Ashley et al., 1997; Fields et al., 1998; Mayordomo et al., 1995; Paglia et al., 1996; Shimizu et al., 1999) and clinical trials (Hsu et al., 1996; Nestle et al., 1998). One of the most prominent studies in this field was conducted by Nestle et al, demonstrating tumor regression in melanoma patients vaccinated directly into lymph nodes with autologous dendritic cells loaded with peptides derived from melanoma tumor antigen and KLH (Nestle et al., 1998). The fusion of allogeneic dendritic cells with autologous tumor cells is a similarly sophisticated approach to cancer vaccination (Gong et al., 2000; Gong et al., 1997; Gong et al., 1998). Pioneered here at the Dana-Farber Cancer Institute by D. Kufe in murine models, this approach has been recently translated into clinical trials (Kugler et al., 1998; Kugler et al., 2000). Kugler et al demonstrated the clinical feasibility of fusing autologous B cells, allogeneic B cells or allogeneic dendritic cells. The direct comparison of autologous and allogeneic B cells as fusion partners addressed the role of the APC in this approach (Kugler et al., 1998). While there was no clinical response using autologous B cells, the response observed after vaccination using allogeneic B cells as fusion partners was comparable to that seen with allogeneic dendritic cells. These results clearly point to an allogeneic adjuvant effect of the APC used in this cellular vaccine approach. Taking the potential risks of applying allogeneic APC from multiple donors into account additional studies have to carefully address whether the cellular component to induce enough „danger“ could be supplemented by simpler and safer technology.

Postulating that the APC is not only delivering a „danger“ signal and taking into account Zinkernagel's suggestion about the need to dose-intensify therapeutic vaccination (Ochsenbein et al., 1999), we have started to exploit alternative sources of APC that can be expanded to large quantities for multiple vaccinations. One such source are CD40-activated B cells generated from small amounts of peripheral blood (Schultze et al., 1997). CD40-activated B cells expand 3-4 fold of magnitude in less than a month of continuous culture and are are very efficient antigen presenting cells. We have established a clinically applicable culture system and are planning to test these cells in clinical trials in the near future.

New tumor antigens

Tumor antigens have been identified by analyzing patients $CD4^+$ T cell responses (Wang et al., 1999), $CD8^+$ T cell responses (Boon et al., 1994) or by antibody based techniques (see reviews (Boon et al., 1994; Gilboa, 1999; Pardoll, 1994; Rosenberg, 1999; Sahin et al., 1997; Van den Eynde and van der Bruggen, 1997)). These classical approaches have revealed neo-antigens based on mutations (e.g. a CDK4 mutant (Wolfel et al., 1995) or the bcr-abl fusion protein (Mannering et al., 1997)) and developmental tumor antigens (e.g. the MAGE genes (Van den Eynde and van der Bruggen, 1997)). Most of these tumor antigens are restricted to a small subset of tumors and cannot be targeted for widely applicable cancer immunotherapy. In an attempt to identify genes that are widely expressed in cancer we have recently identified the human telomerase reverse transcriptase (hTERT) by „reverse immunology“ (Vonderheide et al., 1999). hTERT is expressed in >85% of all human cancers, yet it is not expressed in the vast majority of normal tissue (Kim et al., 1994; Kolquist et al., 1998) Its expression in telomerase-positive tumors has been linked to tumor growth and development; (Hahn et al., 1999) (Greenberg et al., 1999). Co-transfection of oncogenes in human fibroblasts is only tumorogenic in the presence of hTERT expression (Hahn et al., 1999). Moreover, the blockade of hTERT function in tumor cells leads to growth arrest (Hahn et al., 1999). hTERT contains immunogenic epitopes that are expressed and presented by tumor cells and that elicit CTL responses *ex vivo* in cancer patients and healthy individuals (Vonderheide et al., 1999; Vonderheide et al., 2000). This strategy has thus far revealed several immunogenic HLA-A2-binding peptides (Vonderheide et al., 1999) and one HLA-A3 binding peptide (Vonderheide et al., 2000). Our findings for the HLA-A2 peptide were recently confirmed by another group using the identical approach (Minev et al., 2000). Using tetramer and ELISPOT analysis we have not been able to detect hTERT-specific T cells in peripheral blood or in tumor infiltrating T cell populations. However, such T cells have been expanded from peripheral blood of multiple donors *ex vivo*, demonstrating that hTERT-specific CTL exist in the T cell repertoire. It is too early to know whether hTERT is a tumor rejection antigen. However, if efficient immunity can be successfully delivered to cancer patients without the induction of severe autoimmunity – and current evidence points away from the latter – it can be speculated that hTERT is clearly a prime candidate to become the most widely expressed tumor rejection antigen. This is the prime goal of currently ongoing clinical efforts targeting hTERT by immunotherapy.

Assessment of T-cell immunity on the single cell level

The inability to track T cell responses on the single cell level was one of the major drawbacks of tumor immunotherapy for a long time. Quantification of antigen-specific T cells was based on indirect measurements linked to functional readouts such as cytokine release, proliferation (limiting dilution analysis) or cytotoxicity. With the development of single cell analysis including cytokine ELISPOT and MHC/peptide tetramer analysis (Altman et al., 1996) it is now possible to directly monitor immunotherapy *ex vivo*. The sensitivity of these assays is currently only between 1/1000 and 1/5000 T cells in peripheral blood, tumor-infiltrating T lymphocytes or *ex vivo* cultured T cell lines. However, short-term *ex vivo* expansion can increase the sensitivity of these assays by up to 100-fold, making it possible to detect antigen-specific T cells at extremely low frequencies. Tetramers have been used to detect T cells against a variety of tumor antigens including Melan-A/Mart-1 (Anichini et al., 1999; Gervois et al., 2000; Ogg et al., 1998; Pittet et al., 1999; Romero et al., 1998; Valmori et al., 2000; Valmori et al., 1999; Yee et al., 1999), tyrosinase (Valmori et al., 1999), proteinase-3 (Molldrem et al., 1999) and p53 (Hernandez et al., 2000). These studies revealed several important facts that were not appreciated before. It was convincingly demonstrated that the frequency of Melan-A-specific T cells is closely correlated with the induction of vitiligo, an autoimmune condition characterized by loss of epidermal melanocytes (Ogg et al., 1998) while there was an inverse correlation between frequency of antigen-specific T cells and tumor burden suggesting that the frequency of Melan-A/Mart-1-specific T cells is not a surrogate marker for tumor regression (Anichini et al., 1999). Furthermore, a surprisingly high frequency of Melan-A/Mart-1 specific T cells was found in lymph node metastasis (Romero et al., 1998), but also in peripheral blood of healthy individuals (Pittet et al., 1999). Moreover, Melan-A/Mart-1 specific T cells were mostly of a naïve phenotype and no clonal expansion was observed in both, healthy donors and patients (Valmori et al., 2000).

Combining MHC/peptide tetramer analysis with functional readouts such as ELISPOT analysis or extracellular cytokine staining further facilitates the characterization of antigen-specific T cells. Striking findings were recently reported for cancer patients. Lee et al demonstrated a state of *in vivo* anergy in tumor antigen-specific T cells by using multi-color flow analysis, cytotoxicity assays and mitogenic stimulation to measure cytokine production while EBV-specific T cells in the same patient were functioning normally (Lee et al., 1999). There was also an almost complete loss of tumor antigen-specific T cells in a patient with melanoma after treatment with chemotherapy while there was no change in frequency of EBV-specific CTL. These data strongly suggest that it is critical to carefully monitor the immune response to cancer-associated antigens during any therapeutic intervention if immunotherapy is considered as additional modality of therapy.

Summary

The last 10 years have seen an enormous increase in knowledge in the field of tumor immunology. Many exciting tumor antigens have been discovered, multiple new ways to induce immunity against such antigens have been developed and the methods to analyze immunity on the single-cell level are now in place. If we keep in mind that it took almost 20 years from the first treatment with a monoclonal antibody to the commercialization of monoclonal antibodies for the treatment of cancer, we should see cancer vaccines to become a reality in the near future.

References

Altman, J. D., Moss, P. A. H., Goulder, P. J. R., Barouch, D. H., McHeyzer-Williams, M. G., Bell, J. I., McMichael, A. J., and Davis, M. M. (1996). Phenotypic analysis of antigen-specific T lymphocytes. Science *274*, 94–6.

Anichini, A., Molla, A., Mortarini, R., Tragni, G., Bersani, I., Di Nicola, M., Gianni, A. M., Pilotti, S., Dunbar, R., Cerundolo, V., and Parmiani, G. (1999). An expanded peripheral T cell population to a cytotoxic T lymphocyte (CTL)-defined, melanocyte-specific antigen in metastatic melanoma patients impacts on generation of peptide-specific CTLs but does not overcome tumor escape from immune surveillance in metastatic lesions. J Exp Med *190*, 651–67.

Ashley, D. M., Faiola, B., Nair, S., Hale, L. P., Bigner, D. D., and Gilboa, E. (1997). Bone marrow-generated dendritic cells pulsed with tumor extracts or tumor RNA induce antitumor immunity against central nervous system tumors. J Exp Med *186*, 1177–82.

Bendandi, M., Gocke, C. D., Kobrin, C. B., Benko, F. A., Sternas, L. A., Pennington, R., Watson, T. M., Reynolds, C. W., Gause, B. L., Duffey, P. L., Jaffe, E. S., Creekmore, S. P., Longo, D. L., and Kwak, L. W. (1999). Complete molecular remissions induced by patient-specific vaccination plus granulocyte-monocyte colony-stimulating factor against lymphoma. Nat Med *5*, 1171–7.

Boon, T., Cerottini, J. C., Van den Eynde, B., van der Bruggen, P., and Van Pel, A. (1994). Tumor antigens recognized by T lymphocytes. Annual Review of Immunology *12*, 337–365.

Cain, J. M., and Howett, M. K. (2000). Preventing cervical cancer. Science *288*, 1753–1755.

Fields, R. C., Shimizu, K., and Mule, J. J. (1998). Murine dendritic cells pulsed with whole tumor lysates mediate potent antitumor immune responses in vitro and in vivo. Proc Natl Acad Sci U S A *95*, 9482–7.

Gervois, N., Labarriere, N., Le Guiner, S., Pandolfino, M. C., Fonteneau, J. F., Guilloux, Y., Diez, E., Dreno, B., and Jotereau, F. (2000). High avidity melanoma-reactive cytotoxic T lymphocytes are efficiently induced from peripheral blood lymphocytes on stimulation by peptide- pulsed melanoma cells. Clin Cancer Res *6*, 1459–67.

Gilboa, E. (1999). The makings of a tumor rejection antigen. Immunity *11*, 263–70.

Gong, J., Avigan, D., Chen, D., Wu, Z., Koido, S., Kashiwaba, M., and Kufe, D. (2000). Activation of antitumor cytotoxic T lymphocytes by fusions of human dendritic cells and breast carcinoma

cells [published erratum appears in Proc Natl Acad Sci U S A 2000 Apr 25;97(9):5011]. Proc Natl Acad Sci U S A *97*, 2715–8.
Gong, J., Chen, D., Kashiwaba, M., and Kufe, D. (1997). Induction of antitumor activity by immunization with fusions of dendritic and carcinoma cells. Nat Med *3*, 558–61.
Gong, J., Chen, D., Kashiwaba, M., Li, Y., Chen, L., Takeuchi, H., Qu, H., Rowse, G. J., Gendler, S. J., and Kufe, D. (1998). Reversal of tolerance to human MUC1 antigen in MUC1 transgenic mice immunized with fusions of dendritic and carcinoma cells. Proc Natl Acad Sci U S A *95*, 6279–83.
Greenberg, R. A., Chin, L., Femino, A., Lee, K. H., Gottlieb, G. J., Singer, R. H., Greider, C. W., and DePinho, R. A. (1999). Short dysfunctional telomeres impair tumorigenesis in the INK4a-(delta2/3) cancer-prone mouse. Cell *97*, 515–25.
Hahn, W. C., Counter, C. M., Lundberg, A. S., Beijersbergen, R. L., Brooks, M. W., and Weinberg, R. A. (1999). Creation of human tumour cells with defined genetic elements. Nature *400*, 464–8.
Hahn, W. C., Stewart, S. A., Brooks, M. W., York, S. G., Eaton, E., Kurachi, A., Beijersbergen, R. L., Knoll, J. H., Meyerson, M., and Weinberg, R. A. (1999). Inhibition of telomerase limits the growth of human cancer cells. Nat Med *5*, 1164–70.
Hernandez, J., Lee, P. P., Davis, M. M., and Sherman, L. A. (2000). The use of HLA A2.1/p53 peptide tetramers to visualize the impact of self tolerance on the TCR repertoire. J Immunol *164*, 596–602.
Hewitt, H. B., Blake, E. R., and Walder, A. S. (1976). A critique of the evidence for active host defence against cancer, based on personal studies of 27 murine tumours of spontaneous origin. Br J Cancer *33*, 241–59.
Hsu, F. J., Benike, C., Fagnoni, F., Liles, T. M., Czerwinski, D., Taidi, B., Engleman, E. G., and Levy, R. (1996). Vaccination of patients with B-cell lymphoma using autologous antigen-pulsed dendritic cells. Nature Medicine *2*, 52–58.
Kim, N. W., Piatyszek, M. A., Prowse, K. R., Harley, C. B., West, M. D., Ho, P. L., Coviello, G. M., Wright, W. E., Weinrich, S. L., and Shay, J. W. (1994). Specific association of human telomerase activity with immortal cells and cancer. Science *266*, 2011–5.
Kolquist, K. A., Ellisen, L. W., Counter, C. M., Meyerson, M., Tan, L. K., Weinberg, R. A., Haber, D. A., and Gerald, W. L. (1998). Expression of TERT in early premalignant lesions and a subset of cells in normal tissues. Nat Genet *19*, 182–6.
Kugler, A., Seseke, F., Thelen, P., Kallerhoff, M., Muller, G. A., Stuhler, G., Muller, C., and Ringert, R. H. (1998). Autologous and allogenic hybrid cell vaccine in patients with metastatic renal cell carcinoma. Br J Urol *82*, 487–93.
Kugler, A., Stuhler, G., Walden, P., Zoller, G., Zobywalski, A., Brossart, P., Trefzer, U., Ullrich, S., Muller, C. A., Becker, V., Gross, A. J., Hemmerlein, B., Kanz, L., Muller, G. A., and Ringert, R. H. (2000). Regression of human metastatic renal cell carcinoma after vaccination with tumor cell-dendritic cell hybrids. Nat Med *6*, 332–6.
Lee, P. P., Yee, C., Savage, P. A., Fong, L., Brockstedt, D., Weber, J. S., Johnson, D., Swetter, S., Thompson, J., Greenberg, P. D., Roederer, M., and Davis, M. M. (1999). Characterization of circulating T cells specific for tumor-associated antigens in melanoma patients. Nat Med *5*, 677–85.
Mannering, S. I., McKenzie, J. L., Fearnley, D. B., and Hart, D. N. (1997). HLA-DR1-restricted bcr-abl (b3a2)-specific CD4+ T lymphocytes respond to dendritic cells pulsed with b3a2 peptide and antigen-presenting cells exposed to b3a2 containing cell lysates. Blood *90*, 290–7.
Mayordomo, J. I., Zorina, T., Storkus, W. J., Zitvogel, L., Celluzzi, C., Falo, L. D., Melief, C. J., Ildstad, S. T., Kast, W. M., DeLeo, A. B., and a, e. (1995). Bone marrow-derived dendritic cells pulsed with synthetic tumour peptides elicit protective and therapeutic antitumour immunity. Nature Medicine *1*, 1297–1302.
Minev, B., Hipp, J., Firat, H., Schmidt, J. D., Langlade-Demoyen, P., and Zanetti, M. (2000). Cytotoxic T cell immunity against telomerase reverse transcriptase in humans. Proc Natl Acad Sci U S A *97*, 4796–801.
Molldrem, J. J., Lee, P. P., Wang, C., Champlin, R. E., and Davis, M. M. (1999). A PR1-human leukocyte antigen-A2 tetramer can be used to isolate low- frequency cytotoxic T lymphocytes from healthy donors that selectively lyse chronic myelogenous leukemia. Cancer Res *59*, 2675–81.
Nestle, F. O., Alijagic, S., Gilliet, M., Sun, Y., Grabbe, S., Dummer, R., Burg, G., and Schadendorf, D. (1998). Vaccination of melanoma patients with peptide- or tumor lysate-pulsed dendritic cells. Nat Med *4*, 328–32.

Ochsenbein, A. F., Klenerman, P., Karrer, U., Ludewig, B., Pericin, M., Hengartner, H., and Zinkernagel, R. M. (1999). Immune surveillance against a solid tumor fails because of immunological ignorance. Proc Natl Acad Sci U S A *96*, 2233–8.

Ogg, G. S., Rod Dunbar, P., Romero, P., Chen, J. L., and Cerundolo, V. (1998). High frequency of skin-homing melanocyte-specific cytotoxic T lymphocytes in autoimmune vitiligo. J Exp Med *188*, 1203–8.

Paglia, P., Chiodoni, C., Rodolfo, M., and Colombo, M. P. (1996). Murine Dendritic Cells Loaded In Vitro with Soluble Protein Prime Cytotoxic T Lymphocytes against Tumor Antigen In Vivo. Journal of Experimental Medicine *183*, 317–322.

Pardoll, D. M. (1994). A new look for the 1990s. Nature *369*, 357–358.

Pittet, M. J., Valmori, D., Dunbar, P. R., Speiser, D. E., Lienard, D., Lejeune, F., Fleischhauer, K., Cerundolo, V., Cerottini, J. C., and Romero, P. (1999). High frequencies of naive Melan-A/MART-1-specific CD8(+) T cells in a large proportion of human histocompatibility leukocyte antigen (HLA)-A2 individuals. J Exp Med *190*, 705–15.

Romero, P., Dunbar, P. R., Valmori, D., Pittet, M., Ogg, G. S., Rimoldi, D., Chen, J. L., Lienard, D., Cerottini, J. C., and Cerundolo, V. (1998). Ex vivo staining of metastatic lymph nodes by class I major histocompatibility complex tetramers reveals high numbers of antigen- experienced tumor-specific cytolytic T lymphocytes. J Exp Med *188*, 1641–50.

Rosenberg, S. A. (1999). A new era for cancer immunotherapy based on the genes that encode cancer antigens. Immunity *10*, 281–7.

Sahin, U., Tureci, O., and Pfreundschuh, M. (1997). Serological identification of human tumor antigens. Curr Opin Immunol 9, 709–16.

Schultze, J. L., Michalak, S., Seamon, M. J., Dranoff, G., Jung, K., Daley, J., Delgado, J. C., Gribben, J. G., and Nadler, L. M. (1997). CD40 activated human B cells: an alternative source of highly efficient antigen presenting cells to generate autologous antigen-specific T cells for adoptive immunotherapy. Journal of Clinical Investigation *100*, 2757–2765.

Shimizu, K., Fields, R. C., Giedlin, M., and Mule, J. J. (1999). Systemic administration of interleukin 2 enhances the therapeutic efficacy of dendritic cell-based tumor vaccines. Proc Natl Acad Sci U S A *96*, 2268–73.

Valmori, D., Dutoit, V., Lienard, D., Lejeune, F., Speiser, D., Rimoldi, D., Cerundolo, V., Dietrich, P. Y., Cerottini, J. C., and Romero, P. (2000). Tetramer-guided analysis of TCR beta-chain usage reveals a large repertoire of melan-A-specific CD8+ T cells in melanoma patients. J Immunol *165*, 533–8.

Valmori, D., Pittet, M. J., Rimoldi, D., Lienard, D., Dunbar, R., Cerundolo, V., Lejeune, F., Cerottini, J. C., and Romero, P. (1999). An antigen-targeted approach to adoptive transfer therapy of cancer. Cancer Res *59*, 2167–73.

Valmori, D., Pittet, M. J., Vonarbourg, C., Rimoldi, D., Lienard, D., Speiser, D., Dunbar, R., Cerundolo, V., Cerottini, J. C., and Romero, P. (1999). Analysis of the cytolytic T lymphocyte response of melanoma patients to the naturally HLA-A*0201-associated tyrosinase peptide 368–376. Cancer Res *59*, 4050–5.

Van den Eynde, B. J., and van der Bruggen, P. (1997). T cell defined tumor antigens. Curr Opin Immunol 9, 684–93.

Vonderheide, R. H., Hahn, W. C., Schultze, J. L., and Nadler, L. M. (1999). The telomerase catalytic subunit is a widely expressed tumor-associated antigen recognized by cytotoxic T lymphocytes. Immunity *10*, 673–679.

Vonderheide, R. H., Schultze, J. L., Anderson, K. S., Maecker, B., Butler, M. O., Kuroda, M. J., von Bergwelt-Baildon, M. S., Bedor, M. M., Hoar, K. M., Schnipper, D. R., Brooks, M. W., Letvin, N. L., Stephans, K. F., Wucherpfennig, K. W., Hahn, W. C., and Nadler, L. M. (2000). Telomerase-specific cytotoxic T lymphocytes from tumor-bearing patients are spared functional inactivation due to immunological ignorance. submitted.

Wang, R. F., Wang, X., Atwood, A. C., Topalian, S. L., and Rosenberg, S. A. (1999). Cloning genes encoding MHC class II-restricted antigens: mutated CDC27 as a tumor antigen. Science *284*, 1351–4.

Wild, C. P., and Hall, A. J. (2000). Primary prevention of hepatocellular carcinoma in developing countries. Mutat Res *462*, 381–93.

Wolfel, T., Hauer, M., Schneider, J., Serrano, M., Wolfel, C., Klehmann-Hieb, E., De Plaen, E., Hankeln, T., Meyer zum Buschenfelde, K. H., and Beach, D. (1995). A p16INK4a-insensitive CDK4 mutant targeted by cytolytic T lymphocytes in a human melanoma. Science *269*, 1281–4.

Yee, C., Riddell, S. R., and Greenberg, P. D. (1997). Prospects for adoptive T cell therapy. Curr Opin Immunol *9*, 702–8.
Yee, C., Savage, P. A., Lee, P. P., Davis, M. M., and Greenberg, P. D. (1999). Isolation of high avidity melanoma-reactive CTL from heterogeneous populations using peptide-MHC tetramers. J Immunol *162*, 2227–34.

Allogeneic Cell Therapy with Antigen-Specific Cytotoxic T Lymphocytes (CTL) for Malignant Melanoma

A. Nolte, J. Slotty, C. Beike, W. E. Berdel, and J. Kienast

Dept. of Internal Medicine – Hematology/Oncology, University of Muenster, Germany

Background

Melanoma cells express numerous melanoma-associated antigens (MAA) which are recognized by cytotoxic T lymphocytes (CTL) in an HLA-restricted manner [1-7]. However, in most patients a tumor-specific immune response seems to be hampered by tolerance induction. In principal, tumor tolerance should be overcome by transplantation of an HLA-identical immune system followed by transfer of melanoma-specific CTL of the donor. We therefore evaluated strategies for adoptive immunotherapy with allogeneic, major histocompatibility complex (MHC) matched CTL specific for MAA. Several peptide epitopes derived from MAA with known HLA-A*0201-restriction were investigated for their ability to reproducibly induce a melanoma-specific CTL response.

Methods

Peripheral blood lymphocytes (PBL) from HLA-A*0201+ healthy donors were serially stimulated under GMP-like conditions with irradiated autologous dendritic cells (DC) or mononuclear cells (MNC) pulsed with 40 µg/ml of the following HLA-A*0201-associated melanoma peptides: AAGIGILTV ($MT_{27\text{-}35}$ from Melan-A/MART-1), IMDQVPFSV ($G_{209\text{-}2M}$ from gp100, modified in position 2), or FLWGPRALV (271-279 from MAGE-3). Alternatively, tumor lysate of MAA+ melanoma cell lines D10 or HBL was used. Interleukin-2 (IL-2) was added after the first restimulation (50 U/ml). After three rounds of stimulation, cytolytic activity and cytokine secretion were measured in standard chromium release assays and IFN-γ or IL-4 ELISAs.

Results

Melanoma-reactive recognition could be detected in CTL stimulated with AAGIGILTV ($MT_{27\text{-}35}$) and IMDQVPFSV ($G_{209\text{-}2M}$) with lysis of peptide pulsed target cells as well as HLA-A2+/Ag+ melanoma cells (Fig. 1). The peptide FLWGPRALV ($MAGE3_{271\text{-}279}$) appeared to induce a peptide-specific recognition of target cells only. In contrast, tumor lysate of MAA+ melanoma cell lines did not effectively induce melanoma-specific CTL; several CTL lines stimulated with dif-

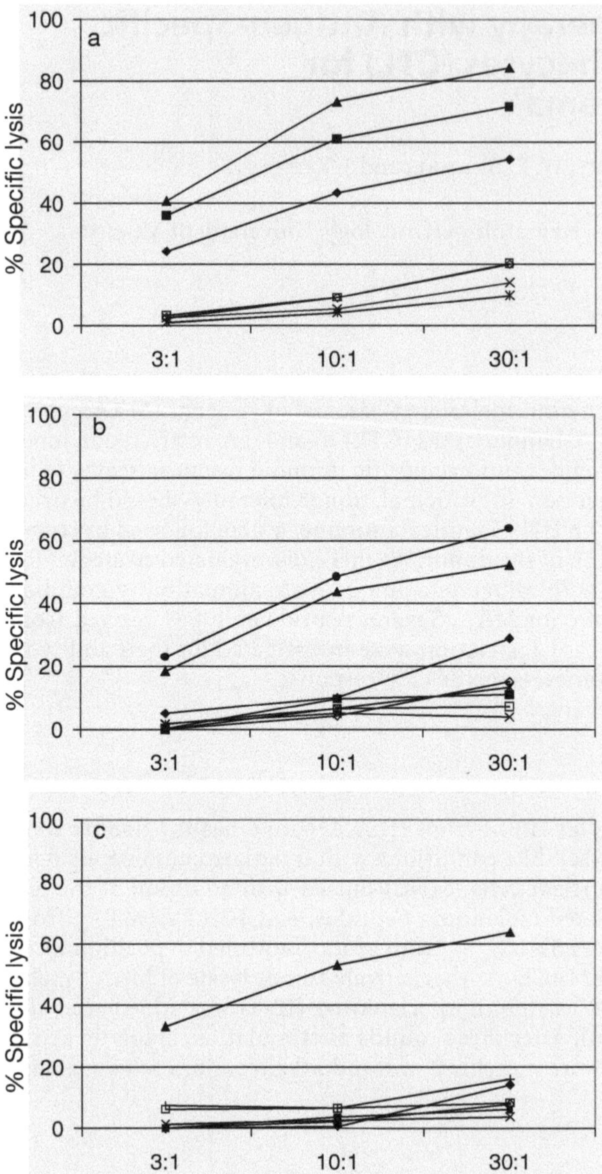

Fig. 1a–c. After three rounds of stimulation with different melanoma-associated peptides, CTL were tested for cytolytic activity against different target cells, including TAP-deficient and HLA-A2+ T2 cells (◊), T2 cells loaded with the stimulator peptide (▲) or an irrelevant peptide (□), the HLA-A2+ and MAA+ melanoma cell lines D10 (◆) and HBL (■), the HLA-A2+ and MAA- melanoma line Na8-mel (*), and the K562 line (×). For $G_{209\text{-}2M}$-stimulated CTL, T2 cells loaded with the native peptide G_{209} were also included (•). Data for representative stimulator peptides are shown. Stimulator peptides during the three week CTL culture were: (A) AAGIGILTV ($MT_{27\text{-}35}$), (B) IMDQVPFSV ($G_{209\text{-}2M}$), (C) FLWGPRALV (MAGE-$3_{271\text{-}279}$).

ferent concentrations of the two tumor lysates (50 or 100 µg/ml) showed no recognition of lysate-pulsed target cells or intact melanoma cells (data not shown). Peptide- and melanoma-specific cytolytic activity was paralleled by IFN-γ secretion of CTL lines (Fig. 2). IL-4 could not be detected in the supernatant of cocultures, indicating that a T1 response was induced by the culture conditions (data not shown).

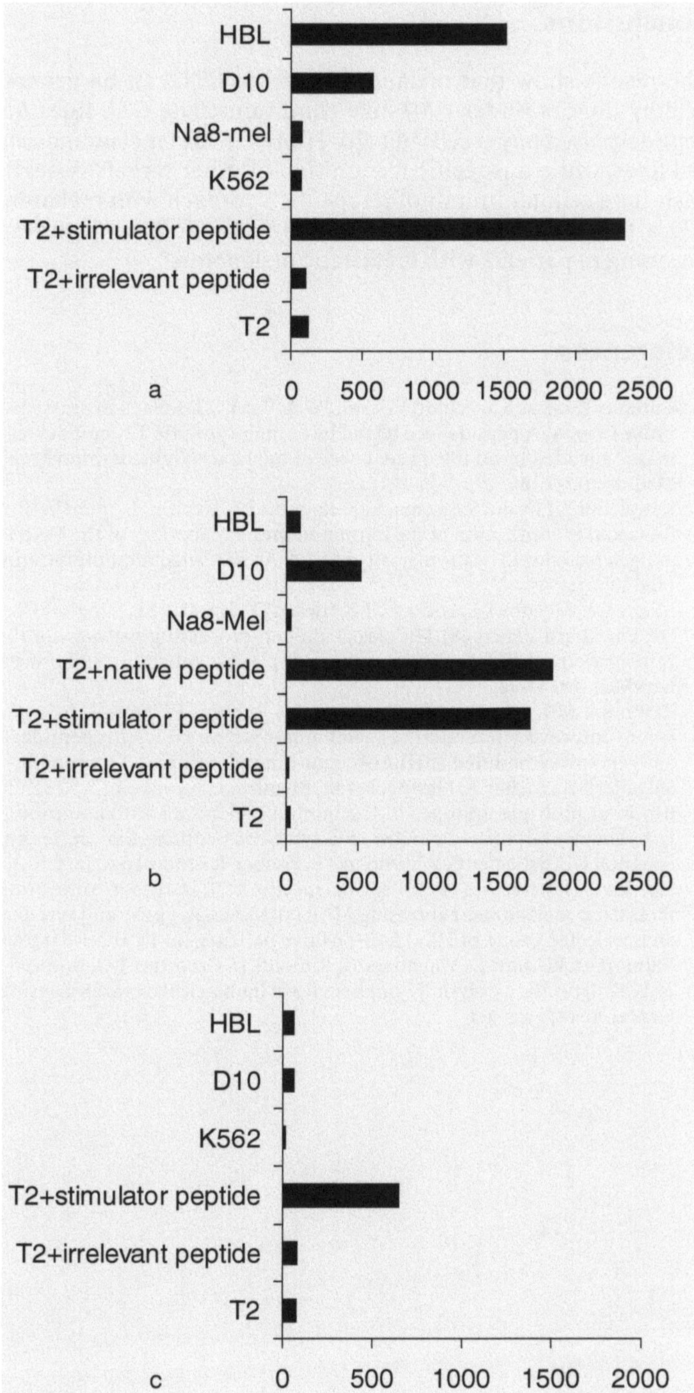

Fig. 2a–c. IFN-γ secretion of peptide-induced CTL-lines (representative data of at least 3 independent assays, mean of duplicate samples). CTL-lines were stimulated with (a) AAGIGILTV from Melan-A/MART-1, (b) IMDQVPFSV from gp100, (c) FLWGPRALV from MAGE-3. On the y-axes, different stimulator cells used for coincubation with the CTL lines are indicated.

Conclusions

The results show that melanoma-specific CTL can be generated from PBL of healthy donors under GMP-like conditions. The CTL lines not only recognize peptide-pulsed target cells but also HLA-A2+ and melanoma-antigen+ melanoma cell lines, while unspecific recognition of other targets is negligible. This is the basis for a cellular immunotherapeutic approach with melanoma-specific donor CTL after allogeneic stem cell transplantation following non-myeloablative conditioning in patients with metastatic melanoma.

References

1. Guilloux Y, Lucas S, Brichard VG, Van Pel A, Viret C, De Plaen E, Brasseur F, Lethé B, Jotereau F, Boon T (1996) A peptide recognized by human cytolytic T lymphocytes on HLA-A2 melanomas is encoded by an intron sequence of the N-acetylglucosaminyltransferase V gene. J Exp Med 183: 1173-1183
2. Kawakami Y, Eliyahu S, Sakaguchi K, Robbins PF, Rivoltini L, Yannelli JB, Appella E, Rosenberg SA (1994) Identification of the immunodominant peptides of the MART-1 human melanoma antigen recognized by the majority of HLA-A2 restricted tumor infiltrating lymphocates. J Exp Med 180: 347-352
3. Mosse CA, Meadows L, Luckey CJ, Kittlesen DJ, Huczko EL, Slingluff CL, Shabanowitz J, Hunt DF, Engelhard VH (1998) The class I antigen-processing pathway for the membrane protein tyrosinase involves translation in the endoplasmic reticulum and processing in the cytosol. J Exp Med 187: 37-48
4. Parkhurst MR, Salgaller ML, Southwood S, Robbins PF, Sette A, Rosenberg SA, Kawakami Y (1996) Improved induction of melanoma-reactive CTL with peptides from the melanoma antigen gp100 modified at HLA-A*0201-binding residues. J Immunol 157: 2539-2548
5. Salgaller ML, Afshar A, Marincola FM, Rivoltini L, Kawakami Y, Rosenberg SA (1995) Recognition of multiple epitopes in the human melanoma antigen gp100 by peripheral blood lymphocytes stimulated in vitro with synthetic peptides. Cancer Res 55: 4972-4979
6. Spagnoli GC, Schaefer C, Willimann TE, Kocher T, Amoroso A, Juretic A, Zuber M, Luscher U, Harder F, Heberer M (1995) Peptide-specific CTL in tumor-infiltrating lymphocytes from metastatic melanomas expressing MART-1/Melan-A, gp100 and tyrosinase genes: A study in an unselected group of HLA-A2.1-positive patients. Int J Cancer 64: 309-315
7. Valmori D, Liénard D, Waanders G, Rimoldi D, Cerottini J-C, Romero P (1997) Analysis of MAGE-3-specific cytolytic T lymphocytes in human leukocyte antigen-A2 melanoma patients. Cancer Res 57: 735-741

New Conditioning Strategies in Allogeneic Stem Cell Transplantation

Intensification of the Conditioning Regimen for Patients with high-risk AML and MDS: 3 year Experience of using an ^{188} Re – Labelled anti – CD 66 Monoclonal Antibody

D. Bunjes[1], I. Buchmann[2], Ch. Duncker[1], U. Seitz[2], J. Kotzerke[2], M. Wiesneth[3], D. Dohr[4], M. Stefanic[1], A. Buck[2], St. v. Harsdorf[1], G. Glatting[2], W. Grimminger[1], R. Schlenk[1], G. Munzert[1], H. Döhner[1], L. Bergmann[1], and S. N. Reske[2] *

Department of Haematology/Oncology[1], Department of Nuclear Medicine[2], Department of Transfusion Medicine[3] and Department of Radiotherapy[4]

Abstract

We have intensified the conditioning regimen prior to stem cell transplantation in 42 patients with high-risk AML and MDS by treating patients with a ^{188} Re – labeled anti – CD 66 monoclonal antibody. Dosimetry was performed prior to therapy and a favourable dosimetry was observed in all cases. Radioimmunotherapy with the labeled antibody provided a mean of 15.3 Gy of additional radiation to the marrow, the kidney was the normal organ receiving the highest dose of supplemental radiation (mean 7.3 Gy): Radioimmunotherapy was followed by standard full-dose conditioning with total body irradiation (12 Gy) or busulfan and high – dose cyclophosphamide ± thiotepa. Patients subsequently received a T cell depleted allogeneic graft from a HLA – identical family donor (n = 16) or an alternative donor (n = 22). In 4 patients without an allogeneic donor an unmanipulated autologous graft was used. Infusion – related toxicity due to the labeled antibody was minimal and no increase in treatment – related mortality due to the radioimmunoconjugate was observed. Day +30 and day +100 mortalities were 2% and 5% respectively and after a median follow-up of 22 months treatment-related mortality was 24%. Late renal toxicity was observed in 14% of patients. The relapse rate of 19 patients transplanted in 1.CR or 2.CR was 16%, in 23 patients not in remission at the time of transplant we observed a 36% relapse rate.

Introduction

Patients with high – risk AML in first complete remission (CR), with disease refractory to induction chemotherapy, with relapsed AML or high-risk MDS (RAEB; RAEB – T) are essentially incurable by currently available chemotherapy and have a poor outcome after allogeneic stem cell transplantation with conventional conditioning (Greenberg et al. 1997; Mrozek et al. 1997; Wheatley et al. 1999;

---

* The study was supported by Deutsche Krebshilfe (grant 70 – 2388 – Bu 1).

Thomas et al. 1977; Clift et al. 1987; Biggs et al. 1992; Anderson et al. 1993; Gale et al. 1995; Appelbaum 1997; Ferrant et al. 1997; Horowitz 1999). This poor outcome is the result of both a significantly higher relapse rate and a higher transplant – related mortality.

In view of the high radiation sensitivity of leukemic cells it is not surprising that several investigators have attempted to reduce the relapse rate after BMT by increasing the dose of total body irradiation (TBI) (Clift et al. 1990; Clift et al. 1991). Increasing the TBI dose from 12 to 15,75 Gy significantly reduced the relapse rate in patients with both AML in 1.CR and CML in chronic phase with cyclosporine/methotrexate as GvHD-prophylaxis. This did not translate into an improved survival because patients treated with the higher dose of external beam radiation had a higher incidence of GvHD and more hepatotoxicty which resulted in a higher transplant-related mortality (Clift et al. 1990; Clift et al. 1991).

A different experience was reported by Papadopoulos et al who treated patients with AML in 1.CR with 15.75 Gy plus chemotherapy and transplanted T-cell depleted grafts. They reported a relapse rate of 3% and a low rate of transplant-related mortality resulting in a DFS of 80%. (Papadopoulos et al. 1998) No data on the feasibility of this approach have been reported in patients with advanced acute leukaemia because of concerns about the importance of the GvHD-associated GVL effect in curing advanced leukaemias (Horowitz et al. 1990; Marmont et al. 1991).

An alternative approach would be to target the radiation to the marrow using radiolabeled antibodies and thus avoiding excessive organ toxicity. This approach has been pioneered in both animal models and patients by investigators from Seattle and New York using antibodies with specificity for CD33 or CD45 labeled with Iodine – 131 (^{131} I) (Matthews et al. 1991; Appelbaum et al. 1992; Jurcic et al. 1995; Matthews et al. 1996).

For the study reported here we chose an anti – CD66 (a, b, c, e) monoclonal antibody labeled with Rhenium – 188 (^{188} Re). The anti-CD 66 antibody (anti – Granulocyte, anti-NCA 95, BW 250/183) is well characterized with respect to biokinetic data and clinical application in bone marrow scintigraphy and localization of infections (Reske et al. 1989; Reske 1991; Becker et al. 1994) . The CD66 antigen is expressed at a high densitiy (2 x 10^5 molecules/cell) on normal myelopoetic cells from the promyelocyte onwards but not on AML blasts. (Noworolska et al. 1985; Noworolska et al. 1989; Bordessoule et al. 1993; Boccuni et al. 1998). The high affinity of the antibody for its target epitope and the abundant expression of the epitope in the marrow results in the accumulation of approximately 50% of the antibody in the marrow within 2 hours (Reske et al. 1989; Schubinger et al. 1989; Reske 1991). ^{188} Re is an almost pure β-emitter with just enough γ-radiation to permit imaging and a physical half-life of 17 h (Press et al. 1995). These properties substantially reduce the radioprotection requirements compared with ^{131} I. We report our initial experience of combining the strategies of radioimmunotherapy with ^{188} Re – labeled anti CD - 66 antibody and T cell depletion of the graft in 42 patients at high risk of both relapse and transplant-related death.

Patients and Methods

Patients

The aim of the study was to include patients with a relapse risk of ≥ 40–50% after a conventional stem cell transplant. Thus we included patients with AML beyond 1.CR, with AML in 1.CR if high-risk cytogenetic features were present or there was a poor response to primary induction chemotherapy and patients with high-risk MDS (RAEB, RAEB – T). Patients were required to be in remission or good partial remission defined as no blasts in the periperal and ≤ 25% blasts in the marrow. The age limits were 16 to 65 years. We accepted HLA – identical and mismatched family members or a haploidentical sibling or parent as well as matched unrelated volunteers as donors. If no allogeneic donor was available autologous peripheral blood progenitor cells (PBPC) were acceptable as an alternative stem cell source. Patients were also required to be free of medical conditions excluding them from high – dose chemoradiotherapy and to have a favourable dosimetry. Favourable dosimetry was defined as a marrow or spleen dose higher than that of any other normal organ.

Over a period of 3 years a total of 42 patients were recruited. The patient population consisted of 18 males and 24 females, the median age was 45 years (range 17–63 years). The diagnosis was AML in 38 patients and MDS in 4 pts (see table 1). Of the 38 patients with AML 27 were beyond 1.CR (19 in PR, 8 in 2.CR), 11 patients with high – risk cytogenetic features and/or poor response to primary induction chemotherapy were transplanted in 1. CR . Primary study endpoints were feasibility and toxicity of the procedure, secondary endpoints the incidence of acute and chronic GvHD and the frequency of relapses. The protocol for the study was approved by the Ethics Committee of Ulm University and all patients and donors gave their written, informed consent.

Antibody labeling

The antibody used for radioimmunotherapy was the anti – CD 66 (a, b, c, e) monoclonal antibody (anti – Granulocyte, Scintec Diagnostics, Zug, Switzerland). This is a mouse IgG1 antibody with a high affinity for the CD 66 antigen (2 x 10^9 mol/l) (Schubinger et al. 1989). ^{188}Re was obtained from a ^{188}W/^{188}Re radionuclide generator as a solution of sodium perrhenate in saline. The generator was supplied by the Oak Ridge National Laboratory (Oak Ridge, Tenn. USA). Full details of generator performance have been published elsewhere (Knapp and Mirzadeh 1994). The labeling procedure for the antibody has been previously described (Seitz et al. 1999). ^{188}Re incorporation was > 95% in the final product with < 3% unbound ^{188}Re perrhenate and < 2% colloid. Immunoreactivity of the antibody after labeling was evaluated by FACS analysis and was determined to be 99.3%.

Dosimetry

The methodology used for dosimetry in our study has been published recently (Kotzerke et al. 2000). In all patients, individual dosimetry was performed after i.v. infusion of 1–2 mg of anti – CD66 antibody labeled with 1.2 ± 0.6 GBq. Biodistribution of radioimmunoconjugates was measured with whole body imaging by means of a γ-camera (Whole Body Imager, Siemens, Erlangen, FRG) in anterior and posterior projections at 1.5, 3, 20, 26 and 44 hrs p.i. Radioactivity excretion in the urine was quantitatively determined until 48 hrs p.i. Since the radioimmunoconjugates used are not excreted with the faeces, no sampling of stool was performed. Percent injected dose in organs was determined by the geometric mean of count rates sampled from anterior and posterior regions of interest by γ-camera images of respective tissue or organs. After calibration and subtraction of radioactivity excreted with urine, whole body radioactivity measured by γ-camera was normalized to the injected dose. Radioactivity in the remainder of the body was calculated by subtracting the sum of organ radioactivity from whole body radioactivity. Decay corrected radioactivity of organs with significant radioactivity retention (bone marrow, liver, spleen, kidneys) and remainder of body were fitted with up to 3 coupled exponential functions with up to four parameters. Organ residence times were determined and radioactive exposure calculated using MIRDOSE 3 software (Stabin 1996).

Radioimmunotherapy

Patients with a favourable biodistribution as defined above were treated. The intention of the study was to give each patient the highest tolerable dose. No dose escalation study was performed. The dose injected was determined by the results of the biodistribution studies, the activity of the generator and the type of conditioning. For patients receiving additional TBI with 12 Gy the limiting organ doses for the bone marrow and liver were derived from the studies of Matthews et al and set at 25 Gy and 7–10 Gy respectively (Matthews et al. 1996; Matthews, Appelbaum et al. 1999). The upper limit for the kidney was defined as 12 Gy based on published studies on the radiation tolerance of the kidneys (Luxton and Kunkler 1964; Emami et al. 1991). For patients not receiving TBI the dose limits were 35 Gy for the marrow, 19–24 Gy for the liver and 20 Gy for the kidney (Emami et al. 1991). The therapeutic antibody was given i.v. over a period of 10 minutes in 1 to 2 fractions of 1–2 mg of labeled antibody 24 to 48 h after the completion of dosimetry and on day – 14 relative to the transplant to ensure elimination of the nuclide. To prevent ^{188}Re uptake into the thyroid gland and gastric mucosa all patients were treated with 3 x 480mg perchlorate (Irenat, Bayer, Leverkusen, FRG) beginning 24h before dosimetry and continued for 1 week after the last antibody infusion. Radioimmunotherapy (RIT) was performed in radiation isolation rooms and patients usually remained there for 48 hrs as required by German radioprotection regulations.

Conditioning

All patients were given additional conditioning therapy after RIT. Three protocols were used. Patients with matched family donors , matched unrelated donors and receiving autologous PBPC were treated with either TBI 12 Gy plus cyclophosphamide 120mg/kg (n = 24) or i.v. Busulfan 12,8 mg/kg plus cyclophosphamide 120mg/kg (n = 12). Patients with haploidentical family donors (n = 6) were conditioned with TBI 12 Gy plus Thiotepa 10mg/kg plus cyclophosphamide 120mg/kg. In all patients receiving TBI renal shielding was used to reduce the radiation exposure of the kidneys from TBI to 6 Gy. In patients with mismatched family donors or receiving a graft from a matched unrelated donor conditioning was intensified by adding ATG 5 mg/kg d – 4 to d - 1 (Fresenius, Bad Homburg, FRG) to prevent graft rejection.

Donors and grafts

Thirty - six patients received G – CSF mobilized peripheral blood progenitor cell (PBPC) grafts, bone marrow was the source of stem cells in 6 cases. PBPC were obtained by treating donors with G – CSF 2 x 6µg/kg/d for 4–6 days. Between days 4 and 6 of G – CSF treatment, one to three leukaphereses were performed using the COBE Spectra (COBE, Lakewood, CO) cell separator. Bone marrow was harvested by multiple aspirations under general anaesthesia. Thirty - seven patients received an allogeneic PBPC or bone marrow graft, 1 patient syngeneic PBPC and 4 patients were given unmanipulated autologous PBPC. The donors for the 38 patients receiving an allogeneic transplant were HLA – identical siblings in 16 cases, matched unrelated donors in 13 cases, a mismatched family donor in 2 cases, a haploidentical family member in 6 cases and a twin in 1 case.

GvHD – Prophylaxis

Thirty - six of the 38 allogeneic stem cell grafts were T – cell depleted. Two methods of T cell depletion were employed depending on the risk of GvHD. In patients with HLA – compatible family donors 16/18 grafts (14 PBPC, 2 BM) were T – cell depleted by adding the humanized anti – CD 52 monoclonal antibody Campath 1H to the leukaphereses (Hale et al. 2000). Depending on the nucleated cell count 10mg, 20mg or 30mg of Campath 1H were added to each PBPC or BM graft and the antibody and cell suspension were gently mixed for 30 minutes at room temperature. In patients receiving a PBPC graft from a matched unrelated donor or a haploidenical family donor T – cell depletion was performed by CD 34+ – selection using the immunomagnetic CliniMACS device (Miltenyi Biotec GmbH, Bergisch Gladbach FRG) (Handgretinger et al. 1999). The target T cell doses were $< 1 \times 10^5$/kg and $< 5 \times 10^4$ CD3 + cells/kg respectively. Bone marrow from matched unrelated donors was T – cell depleted using the Campath 1H in the bag approach in 3 cases (Jacobs et al. 1994). T cell depletion was the sole GvHD

– prophylaxis in 26 patients. In 1 patient given a matched unrelated bone marrow graft we gave cyclosporine, mycophenolate mofetil and steroids as GvHD – prophylaxis and 9 patients were given additional cyclosporine.

Supportive care

Patients were treated in single rooms. Irradiated erythrocytes and platelets were transfused if the haemoglobin dropped below 8g/dl or the platelet count below 20000/µl. CMV – seronegative blood donors were used if both stem cell donor and recipient were CMV – seronegative. All patients were given prophylactic ofloxacin, fluconazole, acyclovir and cotrimoxazol. CMV seropositive patients (n = 18) received prophylactic gancyclovirâ (5mg/kg/d i.v.) from d+7 to d+21. Preemptive therapy with gancyclovir 2 x 5mg/kg i.v. or foscavir 3 x 60 mg/kg was instituted if patients became positive in the CMV – antigenemia test (Hertenstein et al. 1995). Ten patients (24%) were treated with amphotericin for definite or very probable aspergillus pneumonia during induction chemotherapy and required amphotericin prophylaxis (0.5 mg/kg) during the transplant period. Prophylaxis with acyclovir, fluconazole and cotrimoxazol was maintained until patients had achieved > 200 CD4+ T cells/µl. 31 patients were treated with G – CSF 5 µg/kg from d + 7 until a stable neutrophil count of > 1000/µl was reached.

Diagnosis of GvHD

Patients were evaluable for acute GvHD if they engrafted and survived at least 21 days and for chronic GvHD if they survived more than 90 days posttransplant. The diagnosis of acute and chronic GvHD was established by using standard clinical and/or histopathological criteria (Glucksberg et al. 1974).

Evaluation of regimen – related toxicity (RRT)

Evaluation of RRT was performed using the Bearman Scale which was specifically designed to evaluate organ toxicity after high-dose chemoradiotherapy and which excludes the effects of infections, GvHD and bleeding (Bearman et al. 1988).

Results

Dosimetry

The results of dosimetry for some of these patients have been previously published (Kotzerke et al. 2000). The tracer dose consisted of 1–2 mg of anti – CD 66 antibody labeled with 1.2 ± 0.6 GBq of ^{188}Re. The application of the tracer dose

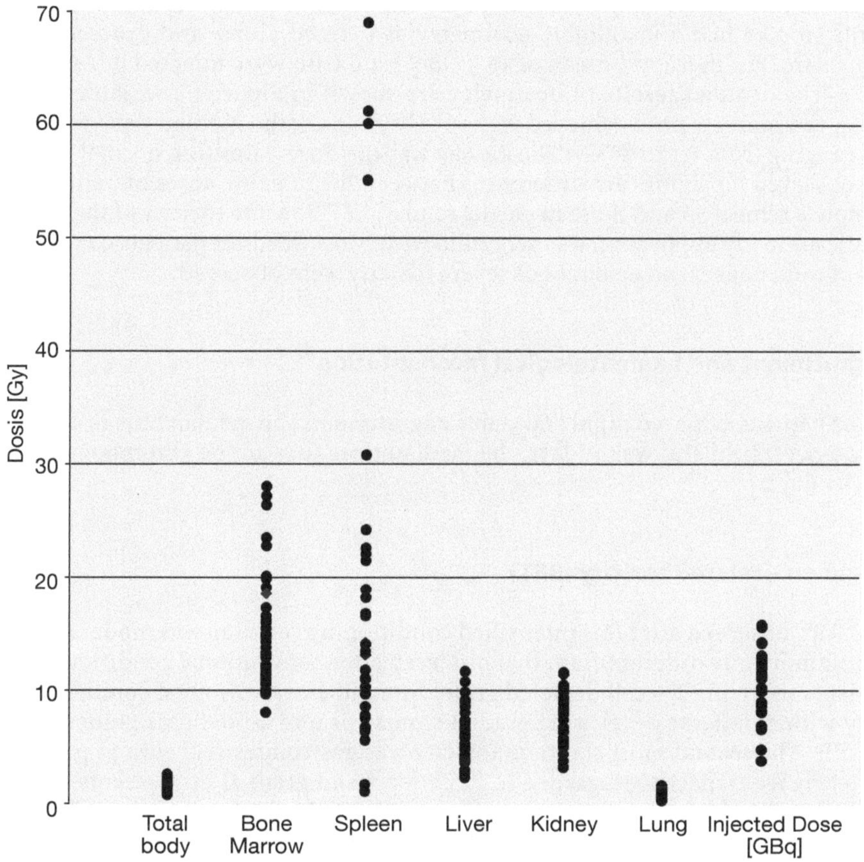

Fig. 1. Biodistribution of ^{188} Re – labelled anti – CD 66 antibody. Dose distribution of ^{188} Re – labeled anti – CD 66 antibody in all 36 patients in GyOrgan. The injected dose of ^{188} Re is given in GBq.

Table 1. Results of dosimetry

Organ	Rad. abs.dose Gy/G Bq	Total dose in Gy Mean ± SD	Total dose in Gy Median (Range)
Bone Marrow	1.5 ± 0.6	15.3 ± 5.1	14.5 (8.1 – 28)
Spleen	1.7 ± 1.3	14.1 ± 5,1	14.0 (1.1 – 69)
Liver	0.5 ± 0.2	5.7 ± 2.2	5.3 (2.3 – 11.7)
Kidney	0.7 ± 0.2	7.3 ± 2.9	6.7 (3.3 – 11.6)
Lung	0.1 ± 0.1	0.7 ± 0.8	0.7 (0.3 – 1.6)
Total body	0.1 ± 0.04	1.5 ± 0.4	1.5 (0.8 – 2.6)

Rad. abs. dose: Radatiation absorbed Dose

was tolerated without any significant reaction by all 42 patients. All of these patients (100%) had a favourable dosimetry as defined above and proceeded to transplant. For therapy a mean of 10.5 GBq ± 2.6 GBq were injected in 1–2 fractions. The detailed results of dosimetry are shown in Figure 1 and Table 1. The mean red marrow dose achieved was 15.3 Gy ± 5,1 Gy, the median dose was 14.5 Gy, ranging from 8.1 to 28 Gy. The kidney was the dose – limiting normal organ. We observed no significant differences between the marrow doses of patients in complete remission and those in partial remission. The acute toxicity of the therapeutic antibody application was very mild with two – thirds of patients complaining of mild nausea, no episodes of severe toxicity were observed.

Engraftment and haematological reconstitution

All 42 patients achieved rapid and stable engraftment. The median time to achieve > 500 neutrophils/µl was 11 days, the median time to > 20000 thrombocytes/µl was 12 days.

Regimen – related toxicity (RRT)

The RRT observed after this intensified conditioning regimen was moderate and not significantly different from that observed after conventional conditioning in patients receiving T – cell depleted grafts. Stomatitis was the most common toxicity with 2 patients developing grade I stomatitis and 40 patients grade II stomatitis. The second most common toxicity was gastrointestinal with 19 patients suffering from diarrhoea, grade I in 22 patients and grade II in 3 patients. Grade I renal toxicity was observed in 11 patients, grade II in 2 patients and grade III in 1 patient. The more severe renal toxicity developed > 6 months after transplant. Renal biopsies are available for the patient requiring dialysis and for one of the patients with grade II toxicity. In the case of the patient with end–stage renal disease the renal pathologist suggested a viral aetiology (CMV, BK virus), in the second case a radiation nephropathy was diagnosed. Overall 5 patients showed the clinical syndrome of bone marrow radiation nephropathy with hypertension, raised serum creatinine, anaemia and urinary abnormalities (Cohen et al. 1995). Grade I hepatic toxicity was seen in 7 patients and 1 patient developed VOD (grade III). Finally 1 case of grade II cardiac toxicity was observed.

Graft – versus – host disease

No patient developed severe acute GvHD. Grade I–II acute GvHD developed in 40% of patients, 17% grade II disease. Extensive mild to moderate chronic GvHD was documented in 36%.

Table 2

Subgruppe	Relapse	TRM	DFS
Patients in Remission (N = 19)	16%	5%	79%
Patients not in remission (N = 23)	36%	38%	26%
Allogeneic (N = 38)	22%	26%	52%
HLA - compatible Fam. Donor (N = 19)	26%	16%	58%
MUD (N = 13)	31%	23%	46%

TRM : Transplant - related mortality; DFS : Disease - free survival; MUD : Matched unrelated donor; Fam .: Family

Relapse

After a median follow-up period of 22 months (range 5–37 months) 11 of 41 (27%) evaluable patients have relapsed, 2 out of 4 autologous cases (50%) and 9 of 37 (24%) allogeneic cases. The relapse rate for patients transplanted in remission was 16% and that for patients not in remission at the time of transplant 36% (Table 2). Three of the 11 relapses occurred primarily in extramedullary sites (skin, lymphnode, muscle).

Transplant – related mortality (TRM)

Overall 10 out of 42 (24%) patients have died of transplant-related toxicity. In the subgroup of patients receiving an allogeneic transplant (n = 38) TRM was 26%. One patient died within the first 30 days (2%) and a total of 2 patients (5%) within the first 100 days. The risk of dying of transplant-related toxicity was dependent on the type of graft. None of the patients with an autologous graft died of toxicity, whereas TRM was 16% with a compatible family donor, 23% with a matched unrelated donor and 67% after a haploidentical transplant (Table 2).

Causes of death

9 of the 12 patients who relapsed have died, one patient. For the 10 patients who died of transplant-related toxicity the causes of death were : cerebral haemorrhage (n = 1), sepsis (n = 2), pneumonia (1 influenza, 1 CMV, 1 Aspergillus, 1 unknown pathogen), EBV -LPD (n = 1), viral encephalitis (n = 1), cerebral toxoplasmosis (n = 1)

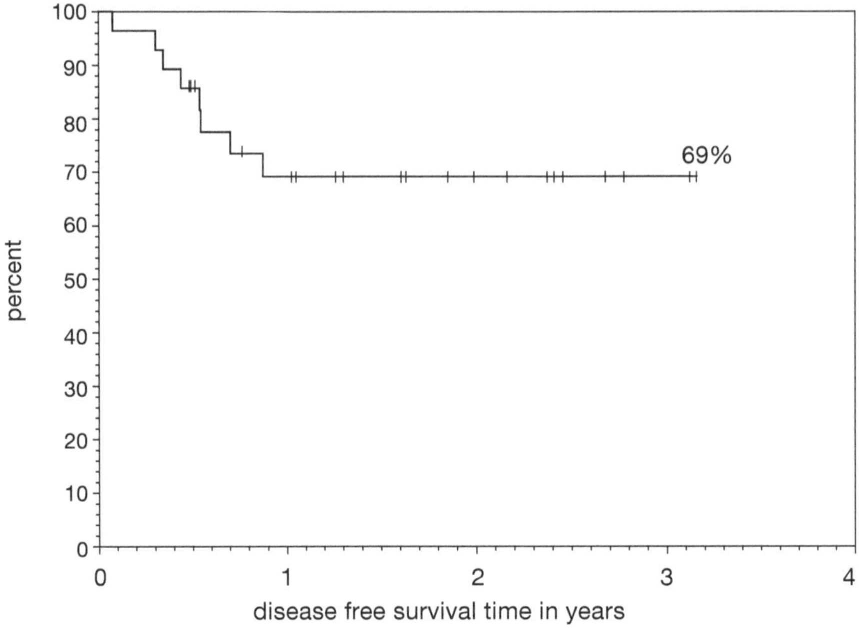

Fig. 2. Kaplan – Meier estimate of disease – free survival of 28 patients with = 15% at the time of transplant

Survival and disease – free survival

After a median follow – up of 22 months 24 patients are alive, 2 with recurrent disease . DFS for the whole group is 52%. 79% of patients transplanted in remission are currently surving free of disease, whereas the figure is only 26% for those transplanted with up to 25% blasts in the marrow at the time of transplant. These results clearly indicate that the antileukaenic efficacy of this approach is dependent on the tumor burden The cut–off point in terms of the degree of leukaemic marrow infiltration is approximately 15%. The probability of disease–free survival of patients with less than 15% blasts in the marrow is 68% (Fig. 2).

Discussion

The primary aim of this study was to evaluate the feasibility and safety of intensifying the conditioning regimen for patients with high–risk myeloid malignancies prior to stem cell transplantation by adding a ^{188} Re – labeled anti–CD 66 (a, b, c, e) monoclonal antibody. We have attempted to improve the feasibility of radioimmunotherapy in the context of stem cell transplantation by replacing ^{131} I with ^{188} Re as the therapeutic nuclide and by using the anti – Granulocyte (anti – CD 66) monoclonal antibody. ^{188} Re was chosen as therapeutic nuclide because it is an almost pure β-emitter (85%), the high energy of its β-emissions (2,1 MeV) and the short half-life of 17 hrs (Press et al. 1995). These favourable properties should make it possible to limit the radioprotective measures required. The anti - CD 66 antibody (Anti - Granulocyte) was chosen for a number of reasons and feasibility was a major consideration. The antibody has been extensively used in immunoscintigraphy over the past 10 years and is commercially available as a kit. In these diagnostic studies no relevant binding to normal tissues other than bone marrow has been observed (Reske et al. 1989; Reske 1991). Thanks to the large number of target sites and its high affinity the antibody rapidly and quantitatively accumulates in the marrow thus ensuring a potent crossfire effect (Reske et al. 1989; Schubinger et al. 1989; Nourigat et al. 1990) (Matthews et al. 1999; Reske et al. 2000) . We felt that these advantageous properties outweighed potential disadvantages such as a lack of binding to myeloid leukaemic blasts. (Noworolska et al. 1985; Noworolska et al. 1989; Bordessoule et al. 1993; Carrasco et al. 2000). This reliance on the crossfire effect clearly imposes certain limitations on the kinds of patients which can be treated with this approach. Thus we restricted ourselves to treating patients in remission or partial remission.

The results presented in this paper clearly confirm our hypothesis with respect to the feasibility of our approach. A favourable dosimetry was observed in all patients tested, and we were able to recruit 42 patients over a period of 3 years.

The acute toxicity of the application of both the tracer and the therapeutic antibody dose compares favourably with that reported by Matthews et al. In contrast to the Seattle experience no cytokine release reaction was observed in our cohort after infusion of the anti - CD 66 antibody. This difference is probably due to the very much lower amount of foreign protein infused into our patients. The total dose of anti - CD 66 injected ranged from 2–4mg compared with 50–74 mg of ^{131} I - labeled anti - CD 45 antibody in the Seattle study (Matthews et al. 1996; Matthews et al. 1999).

The biodistribution studies showed that it was possible to deliver on average an additional 15.3 Gy to the marrow while exposing liver, kidney and lung to mean of 5.7 Gy, 7.3 Gy and 0.8 Gy respectively. Taken at face value these data suggest that we have more than doubled the therapeutic radiation dose to the marrow compared with standard TBI - based conditioning regimens.. This statement has to be qualified, however, in view of the limitations of the dosimetric techniques available for estimating the red marrow dose, and the uncertainty concerning the biological efficacy of low–dose rate radiation (Sgouros 1993; Plaizier et al. 1994; Buchsbaum and Roberson 1996; Sgouros et al. 1996).

The mean therapeutic ratio of radiation delivered to the marrow as compared to the liver of 3.0 was very similar to that reported by the Seattle team, whereas the therapeutic ratios for the lung (15. 0) and for the kidney (2.1) were substiantially different, favouring the anti - CD 66 antibody in the case of the lungs and the anti - CD 45 antibody in the case of the kidneys (Matthews et al. 1996; Matthews et al. 1999). These differences in biodistribution are probably the result of choosing ^{188} Re as therapeutic nuclide. Radiometals such as ^{188} Re tend to accumulate in the kidney by the tubular reabsorption of labeled peptides (Behr et al. 1997).

Acute regimen–related organ toxicity was low and no higher than anticipated for this group of high–risk patients. Only one patient experienced grade III liver toxicity and the day +30 (2%) and day + 100 (5%) mortalities observed are considerably lower than expected from data reported by the IBMTR for similar patients (Rowlings et al. 1998). This is also true for early renal toxicity. No patient experienced more than grade I toxicity and the incidence of 10% is at the lower end of what is reported in the literature (Zager 1994). More worrying is the fact that a rise in serum creatinine was observed in 6 patients (14%) 6–12 months after transplant. This late renal toxicity was mild (grade I) in 2 patients, moderate (grade II) in 3 patients and severe (grade III) in one patient. Chronic radiation nephritis was identified as the cause by renal biopsy in only one patient, however four of the 5 patients fulfill the diagnostic criteria for BMT nephropathy as defined by Cohen et al i.e. a rise in creatinine occurring more than 100 days after BMT with concurrent hypertension and anaemia in the absence of an identifiable nephrotoxin (Cohen et al. 1995). In the most severely affected patient who went to develop end-stage renal disease no evidence for the typical histological features of radiation nephritis could be found in two sequential renal biopsies, and the chronic renal failure was ascribed to drug toxicity (gancyclovir) and infection of the kidney with polyoma virus and cytomegalovirus.

BMT nephropathy is a fairly common complication after both autologous and allogeneic stem cell transplantation with an incidence ranging from 5–50% (Guinan et al. 1988; Lawton et al. 1991; Rabinowe et al. 1991; Cohen et al. 1995; Miralbell et al. 1996). Several studies in recent years have identified TBI as the main cause of this complication (Paller 1994; Zager 1994; Cohen et al. 1995). The most convincing evidence for this hypothesis is the fact that BMT nephropathy is practically never observed after conditioning regimens excluding TBI, that there is a clear dose – response relationship and finally that the risk of BMT nephropathy can be reduced by renal shielding (Lucarelli et al. 1990; Miralbell et al. 1996; Lawton et al. 1997).

We had anticipated some renal toxicity and renal shielding was used in all patients receiving TBI. This reduced the radiation exposure of the kidney due to TBI to 6 Gy. The mean kidney dose due to the radiolabeled antibody was 7.0 Gy resulting in a mean total dose to the kidney of 13.0 Gy in those patients receiving TBI. The mean kidney dose of the 5 patients with the diagnosis of BMT nephropathy was 14.7 Gy. The incidence of BMT nephropathy in patients with a kidney dose of > 12 Gy was 29% compared with 5% in those with a kidney dose of < 12 Gy. The incidence of BMT nephropathy we have observed so far is thus similar to that in patients being conditioned with TBI doses of > 12 Gy reported in other studies (Miralbell et al. 1996; Lawton et al. 1997). So far no case of BMT nephropathy has been observed in patients conditioned with Bu/Cy.

Engraftment was rapid and durable in all 42 patients, and we therefore have no evidence of any stromal damage due to the radioimmunoconjugates although marrow doses of up to 40 Gy were observed.

The intensified conditioning regimen has had no negative impact on other important variables of outcome after allogeneic stem cell transplantation such as the incidence of GvHD and transplant-related mortality. In our study only 17% of patients developed clinically relevant acute GvHD, no cases of severe acute GvHD were observed. Slightly more than one third of the patients developed mild to moderate chronic GvHD.Since > 50% of patients received allogeneic stem cell grafts from alternative donors the incidence of acute and chronic GvHD is low

(Szydlo et al. 1997; Hansen et al. 1998). This low incidence of clinically relevant GvHD is due to the use of in-vivo/ex-vivo T-cell depletion which effectively reduces the risk of acute and chronic GvHD while ensuring stable engraftment (Bunjes et al. 1995; Hale et al. 1998; Papadopoulos et al. 1998).

The age of the patient, the stage of disease, the type of donor and the intensity of the conditioning regimen are the main factors determining transplant-related mortality (Bearman et al. 1988; Rowlings et al. 1998; Horowitz 1999). If one takes these variables into account one would anticipate a transplant-related death rate of 30–40% for our cohort of high-risk patients. We therefore consider the overall incidence of transplant-related deaths of 24% to be encouraging. The risk of transplant-related death in our study was mainly determined by the stem cell donor ranging from 16% for a HLA-compatible sibling donor to 67% for a haploidentical family donor. Overall our results provide no evidence that intensification of the conditioning regimen with ^{188}Re – labeled anti – CD 66 monoclonal antibody has increased the risk of treatment – related death although the potential long - term impact of the late renal toxicity remains to be determined.

Although antileukaemic efficacy was not the primary endpoint of this phase I–II study the impact of using T-cell depletion as GvHD-prophylaxis in this cohort of patients at high risk of relapse should be considered. In patients given standard conditioning regimens T-cell depletion has been associated with an increased risk of early relapse in both early and advanced AML (Marmont et al. 1991). In our cohort of patients we have observed a relapse rate of 16% in patients transplanted in first or second remission and of 36% for those transplanted while not in remission. Since the IBMTR reports relapse rates of 40% and 60% - 70% respectively at 1 year for these two subgroups of patients after T-cell depleted HLA-identical sibling transplants, we are confident that our T cell depletion strategy has not had a major negative impact on relapse rates. We also believe that after median follw-up of almost two years some tentative conclusions concerning the antileukaemic efficacy of this approach are permissible. We have observed a statistically significant difference in disease-free survival between those patients transplanted in first and second remission (79%) and those transplanted in partial remission (26%). A more detailed analysis of the impact of tumor burden at the time of transplantation on outcome shows that the cutoff-point is a leukaemic marrow infiltration of 15%. Patients with < 15% have a highly encouraging outcome (DFS 68%) compared with the very poor outcome of patients with > 15% blasts (17%). These results are entirely compatible with the radiobiology of our approach which relies entirely on the crossfire effect and is therefore dependent on the presence of a significant amount of normal granulopoiesis in the marrow.

In summary, we report a feasible approach to the intensification of conditioning for patients with high-risk myeloid malignancies using a ^{188}Re – labeled anti - CD 66 antibody.

Acknowledgements. We would like to thank Dr. G. Hale and Prof. H. Waldmann (Oxford University) for providing Campath 1H. We would also like to acknowledge the efforts of the technical staff of the Red Cross Bloodbank in Ulm as well as the technical staff in the Department of Nuclear Medicine. Above all we would like to thank the nursing staff of the Adult BMT Unit for their outstanding patient care.

References

Anderson J, Appelbaum F, Fisher L et al. (1993). Allogeneic bone marrow transplantation for 93 patients with myelodysplastic syndrome. Blood 82: 677 - 681

Appelbaum F. (1997). Allogeneic hematopoietic stem cell transplantation for acute leukemia. Sem. Oncol 24: 114 -123

Appelbaum F, Matthews D, Eary J et al. (1992). The use of radiolabelled anti - CD33 antibody to augment marrow irradiation prior to marrow transplantation for acute myelogenous leukemia. Transplantation 54: 629 - 633

Bearman S, Appelbaum F, Buckner C et al. (1988). Regimen - related toxicity in patients undergoing bone marrow transplantation. J Clin Oncol 6: 1562 - 1568

Becker W, Goldenberg D, Wolf F et al. (1994). The use of monoclonal antibodies and antibody fragments in the imaging of infectious lesions. Sem Nucl Med 25: 1 - 13

Behr T, Sharkey R, Sgouros G et al. (1997). Overcoming the nephrotoxicity of radiometal - labeled immunoconjugates. Cancer 80 (suppl): 2591 - 2610

Biggs J, Horowitz M, Gale R et al. (1992). Bone Marrow transplants may cure patients with acute leukemia never achieving remission. Blood 80: 1090 - 1093

Boccuni P, Di Noto R, Lo Pardo C et al. (1998). CD66c antigen expression is myeloid restricted in normal bone marrow but is a common feature of of CD10+ early B - cell malignancies. Tissue Antigens 52: 1 - 8

Bordessoule D, Jones M, Gatter K et al. (1993). Immunohistological patterns of myeloid antigens: tissue distribution of CD13, CD14, CD16, CD31, CD36, CD65, CD66 and CD67. Br J Haematol 83: 370 - 383

Buchsbaum D, Roberson P (1996). Experimental Radioimmunotherapy : biological effectiveness and comparison with external beam radiation. In : Sautter - Bihl M -L, Bihl H, Wannenmacher M (eds) Systemic Radiotherapy with Monoclonal Antibodies. Springer. Berlin, 141: 9 -18

Bunjes D, Hertenstein B, Wiesneth M et al. (1995). In vivo/ ex vivo T cell depletion reduces the morbidity of allogeneic transplantation in patients with acute leukaemias in first remission without increasing the risk of treatment failure: comparison with cyclosporin/methotrexate. Bone Marrow Transplant 15: 563 - 568

Carrasco M, Munoz L, Bellido M et al. (2000). CD66 expression in acute leukaemia. Ann Haematol 79: 299 - 303

Clift R, Buckner C, Thomas E et al. (1987). The treatment of acute nonlymphocytic leukemia by allogeneic bone marrow transplantation. Bone Marrow Transplant 2: 243 - 258

Clift R, Buckner C, Appelbaum F et al. (1990). Allogeneic marrow transplantation in patients with acute myeloid leukemia in first remission: a randomized trial of two irradiation regimens. Blood 76: 1867-1871

Clift R, Buckner C, Appelbaum F et al. (1991). Allogeneic marrow transplantation in patients with chronic myeloid leukemia in the chronic phase . A randomized trial of two irradiation regimens. Blood 77: 1660 - 1665

Cohen E, Lawton C, Moulder J. (1995). Bone marrow transplant nephropathy : radiation nephritis revisited. Nephron 70: 217 - 222

Emami B, Lyman J, Brown A et al. (1991). Tolerance of normal tissue to therapeutic irradiation. Int J Radiation Oncology Biol Phys 21: 109 - 122

Ferrant A, Labopin M, Frassoni F et al. (1997). Karyotype in acute myeloblastic leukemia: prognostic significance for bone marrow transplantation in first remission: a European Group for Blood and Marrow Transplantation study. Blood 90: 2931 - 2938

Gale R, Horowitz M, Weiner R et al. (1995). Impact of cytogenetic abnormalities on outcome of bone marrow transplantats in acute myelogenous leukemia in first remission. Bone Marrow Transplant 16: 203 - 208

Glucksberg H, Storb R, Fefer A et al. (1974). Clinical manifestations of graft-versus-host disease in human recipients of marrow from HLA-matched sibling donors. Transplantation 18: 295-304

Greenberg P, Cox C, LeBeau M et al. (1997). International scoring system for eveluating prognosis in myelodysplastic syndromes. Blood 89: 2079 - 2088

Guinan E, Tarbell N, Niemeyer C et al. (1988). Intravascular hemolysis and renal insufficiency after bone marrow transplantation. Blood 72: 451 - 455

Hale G, Zhang M - J, Bunjes D et al. (1998). Improving the outcome of bone marrow transplantation by using CD52 monoclonal antibodies to prevent graft - versus - host disease and graft rejection. Blood 92: 4581 - 4590

Hale G, Jacobs P, Wood L et al. (2000). CD52 antibodies for prevention of graft - versus - host disease and graft rejection following transplantation of allogeneic peripheral blood stem cells. Bone Marrow Transplant 26: 69 - 76

Handgretinger R, Schumm M, Lang P et al. (1999). Transplantation of megadoses of purified haploidentical stem cells. Ann NY Acad Sci 872: 351 - 360

Hansen J, Gooley T, Martin P et al. (1998). Bone marrow transplants from unrelated donors for patients with chronic myeloid leukemia. N Engl J Med 338: 962- 968

Hertenstein B, Hampl W, Bunjes D et al. (1995). In vivo/ex-vivo T cell depletion for GVHD prophylaxis influences onset and course of active cytomegalovirus infection and disease after BMT. Bone Marrow Transplant 15: 387 - 397

Horowitz, M. (1999). Results of allogeneic stem cell transplantation for malignant disorders. In Hoffman R, Benz E, Shattil S et al (eds) Hematology, Basic Priciples and Practice. Churchill Livingstone, Philadelphia 1: 1573 - 1587

Horowitz M, Gale R, Sondel P et al. (1990). Graft-versus-leukemia reactions after bone marrow transplantation. Blood 75: 555-562

Jacobs P, Wood L, Fullard L et al. (1994). T-cell depletion by exposure to Campath-1G in vitro prevents graft-versus-host disease. Bone Marrow Transplant 13: 763 - 769

Jurcic J, Caron P, Nikula T et al. (1995). Radiolabeled anti - CD33 monoclonal antibody M195 or myeloid leukemias. Cancer Res (Suppl) 55: 5908a - 5910a

Knapp, F. and S. Mirzadeh (1994). The continuing important role of radionuclide generator systems for nuclear medicine. Eur J Nucl Med 20: 1151 - 1165

Kotzerke J, Glatting G, Seitz et al. (2000). Radioimmunotherapy for the intensification of conditioning prior to stem cell transplantation: differences in dosimetry and biokinetics of Re 188 and Tc - 99m - labeled monoclonal anti NCA - 95 antibodies. J Nucl Med 41: 531 - 537

Lawton C, Cohen E, Barber - Derus S et al. (1991). Late renal dysfunction in adult survivors of bone marrow transplantation. Cancer 67: 2795 - 2800

Lawton C, Cohen E, Murray K et al. (1997). Long - term results of selective renal shielding in patients undergoing total body irradiation in preparation for bone marrow transplantation. Bone Marrow Transplant 20: 1069 - 1074

Lucarelli G, Galimberti M, Polchi P et al. (1990). Bone marrow transplantation in patients with thalassaemia. N Engl J Med 336: 850 - 854

Luxton R. and P. Kunkler (1964). Radiation nephritis. Acta Radiol Ther Phys Biol 2: 169 - 178.

Marmont A, Horowitz M, Gale R et al. (1991). T-cell depletion of HLA-identical transplants in leukemia. Blood 78: 2120-2130

Matthews D, Appelbaum F, Eary J et al. (1996). Development of a marrow transplant regimen for acute leukemia using targeted hematopoietic irradiation delivered by 131 - I labelled anti CD45 antibody combined with cyclophosphamide and total body irradiation. Blood 85: 1122 - 1131

Matthews D, Appelbaum F, Eary J et al. (1999). Phase I study of 131 I - anti CD45 antibody plus cyclophosphamide and total body irradiation for advanced acute leukemia and myelodysplastic syndrome. Blood 94: 1237 - 1247

Matthews D, Appelbaum F, Eary et al. (1991). Radiolabeled ant - CD45 monoclonal antibodies target lymphohematopoetic tissue in the macaque. Blood 78: 1864 - 1874

Miralbell R, Bieri S, Mermillod B et al. (1996). Renal toxicity after allogeneic bone marrow transplantation: the combined effects of total body irradiation and graft - versus - host disease. J Clin Oncol 14: 579 - 585

Mrozek K, Heimonen K, De la Chapelle A et al. (1997). Clinical significance of cytogenetics in acute myeloid leukemia. Sem Oncol 24: 17 - 31
Nourigat C, Badger C, Bernstein I et al. (1990). Treatment of lymphoma with radiolabeled antibody.: elimination of tumor cells lacking target antigen. J Natl Cancer Inst 82: 47 - 50
Noworolska A, Hardoszinska A, Richter R et al. (1985). Non - specific cross - reacting antigen (NCA) in the individual maturation stages of myeloid cell series. Br J Cancer 51: 371 - 377
Noworolska A, Hardozinska A, Buchegger F et al. (1989). Expression of non - specific cross - reacting antigen species in myeloid leukemic patients and healthy subjects. Blut 58: 69 - 73
Paller M. (1994). Bone marrow transplantation nephropathy. J Lab Clin Med 124: 315 - 317
Papadopoulos E, Carabasi M, Castro - Malespina C et al. (1998). T - cell - depleted allogeneic bone marrow transplantation as postremission therapy for acute myelogenous leukemia: freedom from relapse in the absence of graft - versus - host disease. Blood 91: 1083 - 1090
Plaizier M, Roos J, Teule G et al. (1994). Comparison of non - invasive approaches to red marrow dosimetry for radiolabelled monoclonal antibodies. Eur J Nucl Med 21: 216 - 222
Press O, Appelbaum F, Eary J et al. (1995). Radiolabeled antibody therapy of lymphomas. In : De Vita VT, Hellmann S, Rosenberg S (eds) Important advances in oncology 1995. Lippincott, Philadelphia : 157 - 171
Rabinowe S, Soiffer R, Tarbell N et al. (1991). Hemolytic , uremic syndome following bone marrow transplantation in adults for hematologic malignancies. Blood 77: 1837 - 1844
Reske S. (1991). Recent advances in bone marrow scanning. Eur J Nucl Med 18: 203 -221.
Reske S, Bunjes D, Buchmann I et al. (2000). Tumor cell kill by friendly fire: radioimmunotherapy with a bone marrow selective Rhenium - 188 CD66a, b, c, e antibody in the conditioning of high risk leukaemia patients prior to stem cell transplantation. (submitted)
Reske S, Karstens J, Gloeckner W et al. (1989). Radioimmunoimaging for diagnosis of bone marrow involvement in breast cancer and malignant lymphoma. Lancet i: 299 - 301
Rowlings P, Sobocinsky K, Zhang M - J et al. (1998). Multicentre observational databases in bone marrow transplantation. In : Barrett J, Treleaven J (eds) The Clinical Practice of Stem - Cell Transplantation. Isis, Oxford : 896 - 911
Schubinger P, Hasler P, Novak - Hofer I et al. (1989). Assessment of the binding properties of Granuloszint. Eur J Nucl Med 15: 605 - 608
Seitz U, Neumaier B, Glatting G et al. (1999). Preparation and evaluation of the rhenium - 188 - labelled anti - NCA antigen monoclonal antibody BW 250/183 for radioimmunotherapy of leukaemia. Eur J Nucl Med 26: 1265 - 1273
Sgouros G. (1993). Bone marrow dosimetry for radioimmunotherapy : theoretical considerations. J Nucl Med. 34: 689 - 694
Sgouros G, Jureidini I, Scott A et al. (1996). Bone marrow dosimetry : regional variability of marrow - localizing antibody. J Nucl Med. 37: 695 - 698
Stabin M. (1996). MIRDOSE: the personal computer software for use in internal dose assessment in nuclear medicine. J Nucl Med 37: 538 - 546
Szydlo R, Goldman G, Klein J et al. (1997). Results of bone marrow transplants for leukemia using donors other than HLA - identical siblngs. J Clin Oncol 15: 1767 - 1777
Thomas E, Buckner C, Banaji M et al. (1977). One hundred patients with acute leukemia treated by chemotherapy, total body irradiation, and allogeneic bone marrow transplantation. Blood 49: 511-533
Wheatley K, Burnett A, Goldstone A et al. (1999). A simple, robust, validated and highly predictive index for the determination of risk - directed therapy in acute myeloid leukaemia derived from the MRC AML 10 trial. Br J Haematol 107: 69 - 79
Zager R. (1994). Acute renal failure in the setting of bone marrow transplantation. Kidney International 46: 1443 - 1458

Dose Reduced Conditioning for Allogeneic Blood Stem Cell Transplantation from Sibling and Unrelated Donors in 51 Patients

M. Bornhäuser, C. Thiede, F. Kroschinsky, A. Neubauer*, and G. Ehninger

Med. Klinik und Poliklinik I, Universitätsklinikum Carl Gustav Carus, Dresden
*Medizinische Klinik, Phillips Universität, Marburg, Germany

Abstract

Between February 1998 and July 1999 fifty-one patients with progressed or refractory leukemia, lymphoma and solid tumors of whom most had a reduced performance status received either bone marrow (BM) or peripheral blood stem cells (PBSC) from sibling (n=18) and unrelated (n=33) donors after dose reduced conditioning therapy. Conditioning therapy consisted out of 3.3 mg/kg intravenous busulfan x 2 days, 30 mg/m^2 fludarabine x 5 days. In unrelated or mismatched transplants 2.5 mg/kg ATG x 4 days were added. GvHD prophylaxis was performed with cyclosporine A (CsA) and short course methotrexate or mycophenolate mofetil in patients receiving unmanipulated grafts. Low dose CsA was given after transplantation with CD34 positive selected grafts. The regimen was tolerable for all patients with only mild toxicity. The day 100 survival was 92% for the whole group. Primary engraftment was reached in 50 patients after 14 days (range, 9–24) and 18 days (range, 7–38) for neutrophils and platelets, respectively. The median time with a neutrophil count of $< 0.5 \times 10^9$/L was 8 days (range, 2 to 20). Secondary graft-failure was observed in 8 patients, all with unrelated donors and no prior intensive chemotherapy. In 6 patients autologous blood stem cells were reinfused as a rescue. Relapse of disease and toxicity associated with retreatment or second transplantation were the main causes of death. Symptoms of acute GvHD were observed in 17 patients. CMV antigenemia was detected in 9 patients. The actuarial 12 month overall/event-free survival is 57/23% for related transplants and 32/27% for unrelated transplants, respectively. Graft-versus-tumor responses were observed in patients with metastatic renal cell carcinoma and melanoma. Reduced-intensity conditioning is feasible without ATG in related transplants and leads to a reduction of transplant-related mortality.

Introduction

Allogeneic hematopoietic stem cell transplantation after conditioning regimen with reduced doses of cytostatic drugs has been shown to combine the known antitumor effects of allogeneic immunotherapy with less toxicity. Especially older patients with reduced performance status and prior infectious complications might benefit from this treatment modality.

Significant graft-versus-leukemia effects have been demonstrated in patients with recurrent leukemia after allogeneic bone marrow transplantation (BMT). Prolonged remission can be achieved by donor leukocyte infusions in 70 to 80% of patients with relapsing chronic myeloid leukemia [1, 2]. Therefore the success of allogeneic BMT seems to depend mostly on graft-versus-tumor effects which can also be obtained after less intensive preparative regimens when a persistent hematopoietic chimerism is achieved.

There are several reports in the literature on the establishment of mixed lymphohematopoietic chimerism after nonmyeloablative radio-/chemotherapy in animal models [3, 4]. Encouraging clinical results have been achieved by using reduced doses of alkylating agents together with purine analogues for conditioning therapy [5, 6]. Only recently, stable engraftment was achieved in patients after 200 rad total body irradiation (TBI) combined with immunosuppressive drugs [7]. Most of these studies have used blood stem cell grafts from HLA-identical sibling donors. Since there is evidence for graft-versus tumor reactions in solid tumors [8-10] we felt that allogeneic cell therapy with less toxic conditioning therapy might be one way to explore these effects in a greater proportion of patients with non-hematological malignancies in the near future.

In this study we observed successful engraftment in recipients of blood stem cell grafts from HLA identical siblings without ATG and from unrelated donors in most cases. Prolonged remissions were achieved in patients with limited tumor burden at the time of transplant. Graft-versus tumor effects were observed in patients with renal cell carcinoma and malignant melanoma.

Patients and Methods

Fifty one patients were included after having given informed consent from February 1998 to July 1999. The study had been approved by the local ethical board. Only patients not eligible for standard allogeneic BMT were included. Table 1 gives an overview on the whole patient population. The disease characteristics of the patients receiving grafts from unrelated donors (n=33) are summarized in Table 2, those of the related group (n=18) in Table 3. In brief, most patients belonged to a high-risk category with either a reduced performance status or extensive pretreatment including autologous PBSCT. Invasive aspergillosis or other severe infec-

Table 1. Patient characteristics (n=51)

• Age	46 (r= 16–63)
• Sex:	36 M/15F
• Months from diagnosis:	18 (r=4–95)
• Sibling/UD.:	18/33
• After autologous Tx:	7
• Prior aspergillosis:	10
• Septic complications:	4
• HLA-match unrelated:	21 A, B, C + DRB1 ident 2 B + Cw Mismatch 10 Cw + DRB1 Micromismatch

Table 2. Related Transplants (n=18)

• AML:	7	2 1st CR, 4 Ref
• CML:	2	1 BC, 1st CP
• MDS:	2	1 CMMol, 1 s-MDS
• Hodgkin's D:	2	2 relapsing after HDT
• SCLC	1	PR after ACO
• CLL	1	
• Melanoma	1	
• Renal-Cell Ca	2	One patient with a 2 AG-mism

Table 3. Unrelated transplants (n=22)

• AML:	13	2 s-AML, 10 PR/Refr, 1 CR (2.)
• CML:	7	1 1st CP, 4 AP, 1 BC, 1 2nd CP
• ALL:	3	2 Ref, 1 PR
• MDS:	5	1 RAEB, 4 RAEB-t
• NHL:	3	1 Richter's Transformation 1 Relapse after auto PBSCT
• Multiple Myeloma	1	1 Relapse after auto PBSZT

tious complications had occurred during pretreatment in 12 out of 51 patients. 4 patients with solid tumors were included (2 renal cell carcinoma, 1 small cell lung cancer and 1 melanoma).

HLA matching

All patients and donors were tested serologically for HLA-A and B and with high-resolution PCR-SSP typing for HLA-C, DRB1 and DQB1 according to standard procedures [11]. In the unrelated transplants complete matching was possible in 22 patients. DRB1/DQB1 micromismatches were detected in 9 transplants with an additional HLA-C mismatch in 5 patients. In three patient-donor pairs an one antigen mismatch in the HLA-A or B locus was accepted.

Stem cell collection

The sources of blood stem cells used are summarized in Table 4. Bone marrow was harvested after informed consent of the donors in general anesthesia. Mobilization of PBSC was performed using 7.5 µg/ml lenograstim or 10 µg/kg filgrastim for 5 days and two subsequent aphereses on days 5 and 6 of the stimulation period. The product was cryopreserved when indicated. CD34 positive selection of PBSC from 9 unrelated donors was performed using an immunomagnetic device (CliniMACS, Milteny Biotec, Bergisch Gladbach, Germany) according to the manufacturers instructions. Briefly, PBSC were washed once to reduce platelet

Table 4. Sources of stem cells

Related		Unrelated	
• BM:	0	• BM:	8
• PBSC:	17	• PBSC:	16
• $CD34^+$ PBSC:	1	• $CD34^+$ PBSC:	9

BM = bone marrow, PBSC = peripheral blood stem cells, $CD34^+$ PBSC = CD34 positive selected PBSC

contamination. The washed cells were incubated with QBEND-10 antibody (mouse antihuman CD34) for 30 minutes at room temperature. Two centrifugation steps followed to reduce unbound antibody. The labeled cells were loaded onto the CliniMACS column and a semiautomated separation process was started. Marked cells were bound in the column and flushed out with buffer after removing the column out of the magnetic field. The negative fraction was recovered and stored as was the CD34 positive fraction. Purity and content of CD3 positive T cells of each graft were measured by flow cytometric analysis using a FACSCAN (Becton Dickinson, San Jose). All patients who had received CD34 selected PBSC were infused with 1×10^5/kg CD3 positive donor T cells on day 14 and 1×10^6/kg on day 21 when no signs of GvHD were detectable. Those T cells had been collected and frozen before G-CSF stimulation. When $< 4 \times 10^6$ CD34 positive cells/kg were obtained with the first apheresis, unmanipulated PBSC were infused. Bone marrow was infused without prior manipulation.

Chemotherapy

Conditioning therapy started with 3.3 mg/kg busulfan (Sigma-Aldrich, Deisenhofen, Germany) dissolved in 10 ml of dimethyl sulphoxide and further diluted by 1000 ml saline. The daily dose was infused over 3 hours on day -6 and -5. Prior studies had shown 3.3 mg/kg iv to be equivalent to 4 mg/kg busulfan given orally in a single dose. The pharmacokinetic data for this formulation have been published [12]. Fludarabine (medak, Munich, Germany) was infused at 30 mg/m² over 30 minutes from day -6 to day -2. In the unrelated transplants, ATG (Rabbit, Pasteur Mérieux, Lyon, France) was administered at 2.5 mg/kg over 4 hours from day -5 to day -2. In four patients ATG Fresenius (Bad Homburg, Germany) was used at the same dose. No ATG was used in the related setting.

Supportive care

Patients were treated in single or double rooms. All patients received antibacterial and antifungal prophylaxis with ciprofloxacine at 500 mg twice daily and fluconazole at 200 mg/d . Acyclovir was given at 1200 mg daily in patients with positive herpes simplex virus IgG titers. Patients with negative CMV IgG titers received blood products from CMV seronegative donors. Bacterial and fungal surveillance cultures were performed every second week. Broad spectrum antibiotics were begun whenever body-temperature increased beyond 38.5°C, C-reactive protein increased significantly or when a positive finding was made on chest x-ray. PCR for CMV DNA and pp65 antigen testing in peripheral blood were performed once weekly. Patients received filgrastim at 5 μg/kg/d from day + 6 to day +13. Hemoglobin was maintained at a level of > 5 mmol/l and the platelet count was maintained at > 20 x 10^9/L with in-line filtered and irradiated blood products.

GvHD prophylaxis was performed with 3 mg/kg cyclosporine (CsA) starting one day before infusion of the graft. Further intravenous or oral dosage was adapted according to CsA trough blood levels. High-risk AML patients with > 30% blasts in the bone marrow received only CsA (n= 10). Additional Methotrexate (MTX) 5 mg/m^2 was administered in the first 11 recipients receiving unmanipulated grafts on days +1, +3 and +6. Mycophenolate mofetil (MMF) was given orally at 4 x 500 mg from day +1 to day +28 instead of MTX to the subsequent 20 patients because the rate of acute GvHD with MTX still seemed to be quite high (56%) and animal data supposed MMF also to be useful as graft rejection prophylaxis [13]. Patients developing GvHD were maintained at MMF and received 2 mg/kg/d prednisolone in addition which was tapered upon clinical response.

Study endpoints

Engraftment defined as > 0,5 x 10^9/L ANC for 3 days, > 50 x 10^9/L platelets without transfusion and the toxicity of the protocol in this patient cohort were the primary endpoints. Secondary objectives had been the antileukemic effects and the rate of acute GvHD observed. Organ toxicity was documented according to WHO criteria. Acute and chronic GvHD were graded according to consensus criteria [14, 15].

Analysis of chimerism

Chimerism analysis in peripheral blood was performed twice a week during hospital stay. The methods applied were either XY FISH in sex-mismatched donor-recipient pairs [16] or a quantitative multiplex PCR assay with amplification of nine tetranucleotide repeats and the amelogenin locus [17].

Statistical analysis

Most quantitative parameters are provided as median with minimum and maximum. The actuarial overall and event-free survival was calculated as of October 1st, 1999 from the day of transplantation according to the methods of Kaplan and Meier [18].

Table 5. Results

• $CD34^+$ x 106/kg:	5.3 (range, 1.0–16.1)	
• > 0,5 x 109/I ANC:	14 (range, 9–24)	
• > 50 x 109/I plts:	18 (range, 7–38)	
• < 0,5 x 109/I ANC:	8 (range, 2–20)	
• RBC Transfus.:	n=8	(r= 2–28)
• Plt. Transfus.:	n=6	(r=0–25)
• Fever > 38.5°C.:	n=7	(Median 3 days)
• WHO 3–4 Tox.	n=6	3 Mucositis 1 Diarrhea 1 Hyperbilirubinemia 1 Creatinine
• acute GvHD:	n=17	(14 I° + II°, 3 III°)
• Graft-failure unrelated:	n=9/33 (3 $CD34^+$, 2 PBSC, 4 MB) 5 CML, 1 MDS, 2 ALL, 1 AML 6 Rescue with auto-Back-up	
related:	n=0/18	
• Relapse:	n=16 (10 AML, 1 ALL, 2 CML, 2 MH, 1 CMMoL)	
• Causes of death:	n=25 Relapse n=13 GvHD/MOF/Retransplantation n=6 Pneumonia n=6	

Results

The clinical results of both groups are summarized in Table 5.

Toxicity

The maximum WHO toxicity for non hematological parameters observed in 4 patients was grade 4 mucositis or diarrhea. Toxicity grade 3 was observed in additional 2 patients for bilirubine and creatinine, respectively. In 46 patients no toxicity >2 could be documented. No early deaths or severe infectious complications were observed. Only 7 patients experienced fever > 38.5°C for a median of 3 days. (range, 2 to 8 days)

Engraftment

Primary neutrophil engraftment with an absolute neutrophil count (ANC) of greater than 0.5 x 10^9 /L was achieved in 50/51 patients at a median of 14 days posttransplantation (range, 9 to 24 days). Transfusion requirements were moderate with 8 units of RBC (range, 2 to 28) and 6 thrombapheresis products (range,

0 to 25) per patient. A platelet count of > 50 x 10^9/L sustained without transfusion was reached 18 days (range, 7 to 38) after transplantation. The median number of days with an ANC below 0.5 x 10^9 /L was 8 with a range from 2 to 20, dependent on the underlying disease and pretreatment. Non-engraftment was observed in one CML patient. He had received an adequate BM inoculum from a donor with an 1-antigen mismatch in the A-locus. Secondary graft-failure occurred in 8 patients (1 AML, 1 ALL, 2 MDS, 4 CML) receiving grafts from unrelated donors.

GvHD

Acute GvHD was observed in 17 patients. The median day of occurrence of clinical GvHD was + 17. In 15 patients grade I or II GvHD could be controlled with systemic steroids. Two patients experienced grade 3 GvHD of gut and liver and another patient eventually died from acute GvHD. Chronic GvHD was documented in 10 out of 35 patients evaluable after day 100, so far.

Infections and other complications

Varicella zoster reactivation with neuralgic symptoms involving the nervus trigeminus and the cornea occurred in one patient. The same patient had experienced sinusitis colonized by aspergillus fumigatus before. Preemptive therapy for CMV antigenemia had to be started in 9 patients with positive pp65 antigen testing. Invasive CMV pneumonitis was assumed as the cause of death in one patient who had experienced early graft-failure at day +28. All patients with CMV antigenemia or infection had had a positive testing for anti-CMV IgG prior to transplantation. None of the patients with negative CMV serology and a donor positive for anti-CMV IgG experienced CMV reactivation.

Delayed type immune hemolysis occurred in two cases of major blood group incompatibility. The donor isoagglutinin titers decreased spontaneously in one patient whereas the other patient with CML died with signs of relapsing disease. Immune mediated thrombocytopenia occurred in one patient on day +73. Prednisolone 1 mg/kg/d lead to an immediate increase in platelet counts.

Chimerism

Figure 1 compares the increase of donor chimerism in representative patients receiving either related PBSC transplants or unrelated PBSC, BM or CD34 selected PBSC. Although the speed of increase in donor signals was heterogeneous, all patients with stable engraftment eventually developed complete donor chimerism.

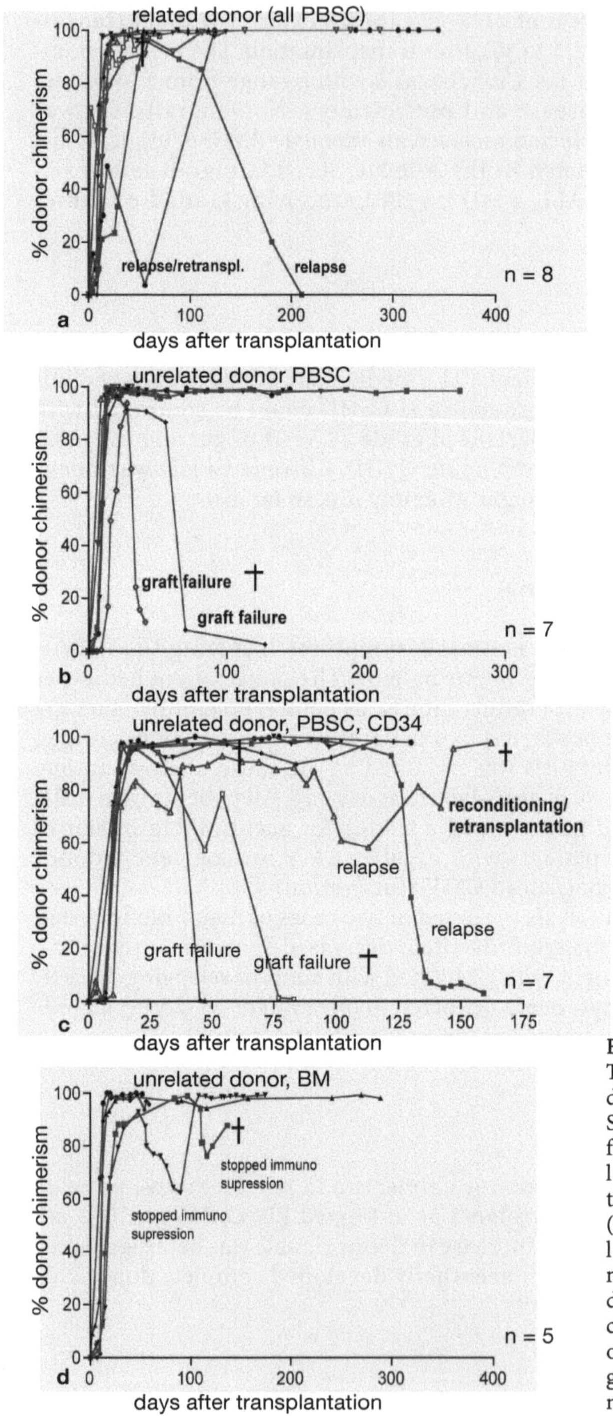

Fig. 1a–d. Over-all chimerism. The figures show the course of donor chimerism measured by STR-PCR after transplantation for patients receiving unmanipulated peripheral blood stem cell transplants (PBSC) from related (**a**) or unrelated (**b**) donors. The lower graphs summarize the dynamics of over-all chimerism during follow-up for patients receiving $CD34^+$ selected PBSC (**c**) or bone marrow (**d**). Cases with graft-failure or relapse are designated

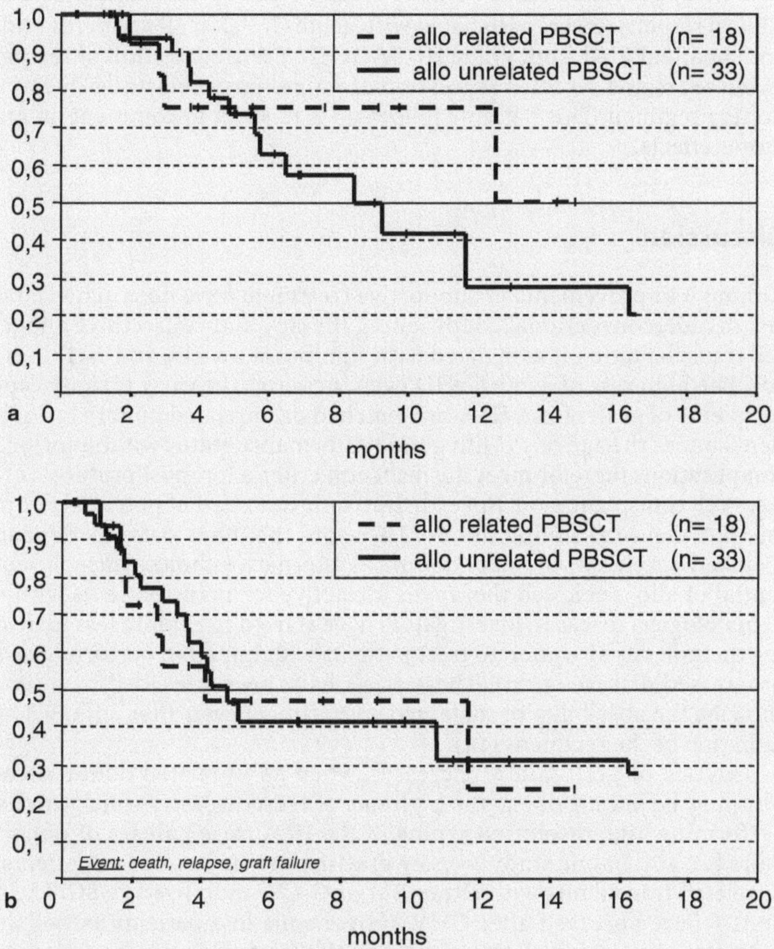

Fig. 2a, b. Survival. The graphs show the Kaplan-Meier estimates for overall (graph A) and event-free (graph B) survival after dose reduced conditioning and allogeneic blood stem cell transplantation from related and unrelated donors

Relapse and survival

Intermittent clinical responses could be documented in most patients. The day 100 overall (OS) and event-free survival (EFS) for all patients is 92% and 75%, respectively. The Kaplan-Meyer Plots for OS and EFS of related and unrelated transplants are depicted in figure 2a and 2b. With a median observation time of 5 months, the expected 12 months OS and EFS for related transplants is 57% and 23%, respectively. The respective figures are 32% and 25% for unrelated transplants. In both patients with progressed renal cell carcinoma and in the patient with metastatic melanoma regression of size of the metastases was observed. The clinical responses were associated with acute GvHD in all 3 patients and the melanoma patient died from grade III-IV GvHD. Early evaluation of the patient with ewing's sarcoma revealed regression of pulmonary metastases due to the conditioning regimen. This patients follow-up is to short to comment on graft-versus tumor effects.

Discussion

Although improvements of supportive treatment have been achieved during the last decade, conventional conditioning therapy and consecutive allogeneic stem cell transplantation is associated with significant toxicity and early morbidity [19, 20]. The high rate of acute GvHD even increases the early toxicity especially for recipients of grafts from HLA mismatched or unrelated donors [21, 22]. Only patients under the age of 50 with good performance status without prior infectious complications therefor meet the inclusion criteria for most protocols of unrelated stem cell transplantation. Nevertheless, only one third of potential recipients have an HLA identical sibling donor. Therefore the other patients depend on HLA matched unrelated volunteer donors as alternative choice. Since the curative potential of allogeneic cell therapy is attractive for many patients with malignant hematological diseases, investigators have started to explore less toxic conditioning therapies as an option to treat patients with impaired performance status and progressed disease [5, 23]. These trials have been preceded by animal models showing the possibility of sustained engraftment even after nonmyeloablative irradiation of the recipient [24].

The rate of graft failure increases, when an unrelated donor is chosen [25]. This may be mainly due to the high rate of HLA disparity which can be found by performing high resolution typing of the HLA class I alleles of donor/recipient pairs [21, 26]. In our study, we saw graft-failure in 9 out of 33 patients receiving unrelated transplants with either BM or G-CSF mobilized PBSC. The secondary graft-failure observed after CMV antigenemia in 2 patients as well as the poor graft function in four CML and three MDS patients may be a sign of unstable hematopoiesis using unrelated stem cell donors after nonablative conditioning. When analyzing engraftment, one has to keep in mind that the leukemic burden had been significant in several patients when chemotherapy was started. Although not statistically definable, graft-failure seemed to occur more often in transplants with HLA-Class I mismatches (n=2) and in patients with myeloproliferative disease or MDS (n=6) where no induction chemotherapy had preceded the transplantation. No graft-failure was observed in the 18 related transplants although ATG had been omitted in contrast to the series reported by Slavin et al [5].

The dynamics of chimerism showed a somewhat slower increase of donor signals when compared with patients after myeloablative conditioning [27]. Predominating donor type chimerism for T and B cells as well as NK cells might be critical for tolerance of the graft [4, 28]. Nevertheless, complete chimerism is obtained in several patients with stable long term engraftment. Infusion of higher doses of CD34 positive cells might possibly further improve engraftment. G-CSF mobilized PBSC have been used for allogeneic progenitor cell transplantation with increasing frequency during the last years. Faster engraftment and similar rates of acute GvHD have been observed [29]. Nevertheless, the amount of CD34 positive PBSC or BM cells available from volunteer donors may stay somewhat limited because the issues of donor safety have to be kept in mind.

Autologous PBSC or BM showed to be useful for rescue of patients with graft failure because there was a significant aplasia even in patients losing their grafts 2–3 months after transplantation. This aplasia may be caused by the occupation of marrow space by donor hematopoiesis when temporary engraftment is achieved [30]. These observations as well as the chimerism analyses showing complete donor chimerism even in CD34 positive progenitors underline the myeloablative nature of these transplants. Therefore we suppose to leave the term 'nonmyeloablative' in this context.

As expected, the low early toxicity of the chemotherapy allowed to treat older patients as well as patients with extensive pretreatment or prior infectious complications. There was no toxic death associated with the chemotherapy applied resulting in an 100 day survival of 92 percent. The dose intensity reached by the use of 3.3 mg/kg busulfan x 2 and 30 mg/m^2 fludarabine x 5 can be regarded to be about 50 percent of that known from conventional conditioning therapy. One has to keep in mind that intensive immunosuppression is induced for several months and acute GvHD might even necessitate intensified immunosuppression and thereby can lead to an increased risk for infectious complications.

The rate of acute GvHD observed was in the range expected. In the group of patients receiving CD34 selected PBSC and delayed T cell add-back only one case of acute GvHD 1 of the skin was observed. Stable engraftment could be reached in patients receiving > 4 x 10^6 CD34/kg positive selected PBSC passively depleted from T cells. It can be argued that the rate of engraftment could have been higher if all patients had received unmodified PBSC. The high rate of acute GvHD observed by Slavin at al. in a cohort of patients receiving PBSC from sibling donors lead us to explore T cell depleted PBSC transplantation with an add-back of a defined dose of T cells in the unrelated setting. Furthermore allogeneic PBSC transplantation was reported to be associated with a higher rate of chronic GvHD compared to BMT in the related setting [31]. So far, chronic GvHD has been observed in 10 patients who had received unmodified BM or PBSC.

CMV antigenemia was observed in 9 out of 51 patients. This rate is similar to the data reported after allogeneic BMT using intensive conditioning therapy [32]. All patients had a positive CMV serology. Subsequent ganciclovir treatment was associated with graft-failure in one patient. Another patient had experienced early graft failure after detection of CMV antigenemia. Residual recipient leukocytes might presumably be the origin of CMV antigenemia in patients receiving less intensive preparative regimens and subsequent immunosuppressive medication. Delayed immunological recovery has been observed after unrelated BMT in adults, especially in recipients of T cell depleted grafts [33]. The same data have to be collected prospectively in patients after less intense conditioning therapy. Whether these patients are at the same risk for invasive CMV infection like myeloablated hosts after T cell depletion is unknown. These knowledge would be important to have more rationales for preemptive treatment strategies like donor leukocyte infusions in this setting.

Although mixed lymphohematopoietic chimerism and subsequent tolerance is the goal of nonmyeloablative conditioning some immunological complications may theoretically occur especially in the unrelated setting. The persistence of recipient T and B cells might lead to delayed erythroid engraftment or pure red cell aplasia in the donor-recipient pairs with major blood group incompatibility [34]. High titers of recipient isoagglutines were observed in 2 patients of the study group. In one CML patient, plasmapheresis had no effect on transfusion requirements. This patient developed pancytopenia and subsequently died with multiorgan failure. A bone marrow aspiration had shown Philadelphia chromosome positive interphases shortly before death. In the second patient, isoagglutinin titers decreased spontaneously and the hemoglobin level increased thereafter. Sudden occurrence of thrombocytopenia was associated with a positive test for platelet associated antibodies (MAIPA). The platelet count rose after prednisolone had been given at a dose of 1 mg/kg/d. Steroids could be tapered subsequently without a second drop in platelet counts. Whether these findings are merely accidental or whether blood group incompatibilities and CMV serostatus are of prognostic importance in this setting has to be studied in a larger cohort.

Unrelated BMT after dose reduced or 'nonmyeloablative' preparative regimens has been described by two groups only recently [35, 36]. The preparative regimen described by Giralt et al. contains melphalan doses of 140 to 180 mg/m^2 which are known to induce prolonged aplasia [37]. Stable allogeneic engraftment has been achieved after conditioning therapy with 240 mg/m^2 melphalan alone [38]. Our data obtained by sequential quantitative analysis of chimerism in cellular subsets show that myeloablation is induced in most patients after 50% of the usual dose of busulfan.

In summary, this study shows that purine analog-containing conditioning therapy can achieve allogeneic engraftment in recipients of stem cell grafts from unrelated volunteer donors. Nevertheless, the rate of secondary graft-failure is still too high (27%). Engraftment can be achieved in the related setting without ATG. The reduced toxicity of the regimen leads to a short hospital stay and a low early mortality compared to intensive conditioning therapy. Nevertheless significant acute and chronic GvHD may occur later after transplantation. Engraftment is possible with BM, PBSC and CD34 positive selected PBSC. Further studies have to explore the leukemia-free survival obtained with this approach compared to standard conditioning therapy. In patients with high risk myeloid leukemia prophylactic donor leukocyte infusion is one way to improve the antileukemic effects of the procedure. Regular quantitative analysis of chimerism is important to detect imminent relapse earlier. As observed in two patients, cessation of immunosuppressive medication offers the possibility to reinduce remission at least in CML patients. Allogeneic immunotherapy seems to be most promising when performed at the stage of minimal residual disease. As described previously, patients with progressive or refractory leukemia are not likely to obtain durable remission [23].

Like other groups, we have observed antitumor responses associated with clinical GvHD in patients with renal cell carcinoma and melanoma [39]. Unfortunately, GvHD was severe in these patients and further attempts have to be undertaken to control GvHD without abrogating Graft-versus-tumor reactions.

Tolerance induction for subsequent organ transplantation might be another potential field of interest. For this purpose, engraftment of HLA mismatched hematopoietic progenitor cells has to be studied. Encouraged by the stable engraftment obtained in one patient with an 1-antigen mismatch, we think this goal might be reached perhaps by modifying the immunosuppressive strategies.

After all, we would like to stress the fact that there are still a lot of unanswered questions in this field which have to be studied in carefully designed trials including patients not eligible for conventional allogeneic blood stem cell transplantation.

Acknowledgments. We thank the 'Deutsche Krebshilfe' for supporting the Bone Marrow Transplantation Unit in Dresden.

References

1. Kolb HJ, Schattenberg A, Goldman JM, et al. Graft-versus-leukemia effect of donor lymphocyte transfusions in marrow grafted patients. European Group for Blood and Marrow Transplantation Working Party Chronic Leukemia. *Blood* 1995; 86, 2041-2050.
2. Slavin S, Naparstek E, Nagler A, et al. Allogeneic cell therapy with donor peripheral blood cells and recombinant human interleukin-2 to treat leukemia relapse after allogeneic bone marrow transplantation. *Blood* 1996; 87, 2195-2204.
3. Colson YL, Wren SM, Schuchert MJ, et al. A nonlethal conditioning approach to achieve durable multilineage mixed chimerism and tolerance across major, minor, and hematopoietic histocompatibility barriers. *J.Immunol.* 1995; 155, 4179-4188.
4. Kimikawa M, Sachs DH, Colvin RB, et al. Modifications of the conditioning regimen for achieving mixed chimerism and donor-specific tolerance in cynomolgus monkeys. *Transplantation* 1997; 64, 709-716.
5. Slavin S, Nagler A, Naparstek E, et al. Nonmyeloablative stem cell transplantation and cell therapy as an alternative to conventional bone marrow transplantation with lethal cytoreduction for the treatment of malignant and nonmalignant hematologic diseases. *Blood* 1998; 91, 756-763.
6. Khouri I, Keating M, Korbling M, et al. Transplant-lite: induction of graft-versus-malignancy using fludarabine-based nonablative chemotherapy and allogeneic blood progenitor-cell transplantation as treatment for lymphoid malignancies. *J.Clin.Oncol.* 1998; 16, 2817-2824.
7. McSweeney PA, Wagner JL, Maloney DG, et al. Outpatient PBSC allografts using immunosuppression with low-dose TBI before, and cyclosporine (CSP) and mycophenolate mofetil (MMF) after transplant. *Blood* 1998; 92 (suppl 1), 519a
8. Ueno NT, Rondon G, Mirza NQ, et al. Allogeneic peripheral-blood progenitor-cell transplantation for poor-risk patients with metastatic breast cancer. *J.Clin.Oncol.* 1998; 16, 986-993.
9. Or R, Ackerstein A, Nagler A, et al. Allogeneic cell-mediated immunotherapy for breast cancer after autologous stem cell transplantation: a clinical pilot study. *Cytokines.Cell Mol.Ther.* 1998; 4, 1-6.
10. Eibl B, Schwaighofer H, Nachbaur D, et al. Evidence for a graft-versus-tumor effect in a patient treated with marrow ablative chemotherapy and allogeneic bone marrow transplantation for breast cancer. *Blood* 1996; 88, 1501-1508.
11. Ottinger HD, Albert E, Arnold R, et al. German consensus on immunogenetic donor search for transplantation of allogeneic bone marrow and peripheral blood stem cells. *Bone Marrow Transplant* 1997; 20, 101-105.
12. Ehninger G, Schuler U, Renner U, et al. Use of a water-soluble busulfan formulation–pharmacokinetic studies in a canine model. *Blood* 1995; 85, 3247-3249.

13. Storb R, Yu C, Wagner JL, et al. Stable mixed hematopoietic chimerism in DLA-identical littermate dogs given sublethal total body irradiation before and pharmacological immunosuppression after marrow transplantation. *Blood* 1997; 89, 3048-3054.
14. Przepiorka D, Weisdorf D, Martin P, et al. Consensus conference on acute GvHD grading. *Bone Marrow Transplant* 1995; 15, 825-828.
15. Sullivan KM, Agura E, Anasetti C, et al. Chronic graft-versus-host disease and other late complications of bone marrow transplantation. *Semin Hematol* 1991; 28, 250-259.
16. Najfeld V, Burnett W, Vlachos A, et al. Interphase FISH analysis of sex-mismatched BMT utilizing dual color XY probes. *Bone Marrow Transplant.* 1997; 19, 829-834.
17. Thiede C, Florek M, Bornhäuser M, et al. Rapid quantification of mixed chimerism using multiplex amplification of short tandem repeat markers and fluorescence detection. *Bone Marrow Transplant* 1999; 23, 1055-1060.
18. Kaplan E and Meier P. Nonparametric estimation from incomplete observations. *J Am Stat Assoc* 1958; 53, 457-462.
19. deMagalhaes SM, Bloom EJ, Donnenberg A, et al. Toxicity of busulfan and cyclophosphamide (BU/CY2) in patients with hematologic malignancies. *Bone Marrow Transplant* 1996; 17, 329-333.
20. Miralbell R, Bieri S, Mermillod B, et al. Renal toxicity after allogeneic bone marrow transplantation: the combined effects of total-body irradiation and graft-versus-host disease. *J.Clin. Oncol.* 1996; 14, 579-585.
21. Nademanee A, Schmidt GM, Parker P, et al. The outcome of matched unrelated donor bone marrow transplantation in patients with hematologic malignancies using molecular typing for donor selection and graft-versus-host disease prophylaxis regimen of cyclosporine, methotrexate, and prednisone. *Blood* 1995; 86, 1228-1234.
22. Hansen JA, Gooley TA, Martin PJ, et al. Bone marrow transplants from unrelated donors for patients with chronic myeloid leukemia. N.Engl.J.Med. 1998; 338 , 962-968.
23. Giralt S, Estey E, Albitar M, et al. Engraftment of allogeneic hematopoietic progenitor cells with purine analog-containing chemotherapy: harnessing graft-versus-leukemia without myeloablative therapy. Blood 1997; 89, 4531-4536.
24. Colson YL, Li H, Boggs SS, et al. Durable mixed allogeneic chimerism and tolerance by a nonlethal radiation-based cytoreductive approach. J.Immunol. 1996; 157, 2820-2829.
25. Madrigal JA, Scott I, Arguello R, et al. Factors influencing the outcome of bone marrow transplants using unrelated donors. Immunol.Rev. 1997; 157, 153-166.
26. Scott I, O'Shea J, Bunce M, et al. Molecular typing shows a high level of HLA class I incompatibility in serologically well matched donor/patient pairs: Implications for unrelated bone marrow donor selection. Blood 1999; 92, 4864-4871.
27. Thiede C, Brendel C, Mohr B, et al. Comparative analysis of chimerism in the early post-transplantation period in cellular subsets of patients undergoing myeloablative and nonmyeloablative allogeneic blood stem cell transplantation. Blood 1998; 92, Suppl. 1, 132a
28. Gyger M, Baron C, Forest L, et al. Quantitative assessment of hematopoietic chimerism after allogeneic bone marrow transplantation has predictive value for the occurrence of irreversible graft failure and graft-vs.-host disease. Exp.Hematol. 1998; 26, 426-434.
29. Bacigalupo A, Zikos P, Van-Lint MT, et al. Allogeneic bone marrow or peripheral blood cell transplants in adults with hematologic malignancies: a single-center experience. Exp.Hematol. 1998; 26, 409-414.
30. Stewart FM, Zhong S, Wuu J, et al. Lymphohematopoietic engraftment in minimally myeloablated hosts. Blood 1998; 91, 3681-3687.
31. Storek J, Gooley T, Siadak M, et al. Allogeneic peripheral blood stem cell transplantation may be associated with a high risk of chronic graft-versus-host disease. Blood 1997; 90, 4705-4709.
32. Bacigalupo A, Tedone E, Isaza A, et al. CMV-antigenemia after allogeneic bone marrow transplantation: correlation of CMV-antigen positive cell numbers with transplant-related mortality. Bone Marrow Transplant 1995; 16, 155-161.
33. Small TN, Papadopulos EB, Boulad F, et al. Comparison of immune reconstitution after unrelated and related T-cell-depleted bone marrow transplantation: Effect of patient age and donor leukocyte infusions. Blood 1999; 93, 467-480.

34. Mizon P, Jouet JP, Vanhaesbroucke C, et al. [Immunohematologic surveillance of patients treated with ABO incompatible bone marrow allografts]. Transfus.Clin.Biol. 1994; 1, 271-277.
35. Giralt S, Cohen A, Claxton D, et al. Fludarabine/melphalan as a less intense preparative regimen for unrelated donor transplants in patients with hematologic malignancies. Blood 1998; 92 (suppl 1), 289a
36. Nagler A, Or R, Naparstek E, et al. Matched unrelated bone marrow transplantation (BMT) using a non-myeloablative conditioning regimen. Blood 1998; 92 (suppl 1), 289a.
37. Tricot G, Jagannath S, Vesole D, et al. Peripheral blood stem cell transplants for multiple myeloma: identification of favorable variables for rapid engraftment in 225 patients. Blood 1995; 85, 588-596.
38. Singhal S, Powles R, Treleaven J, et al. Melphalan alone prior to allogeneic bone marrow transplantation from HLA-identical sibling donors for hematologic malignancies: alloengraftment with potential preservation of fertility in women. Bone Marrow Transplant 1996; 18, 1049-1055.
39. Childs RW, Clave E, Tisdale J, et al. Sucessful treatment of metastatic renal cell carcinoma with nonmyeloablative allogeneic peripheral-blood progenitor-cell transplant: Evidence for a graft-versus-tumor effect. J. Clin. Oncol. 1999; 17, 2044-2049.

Pharmacokinetics of Conditioning Regimens

G. Würthwein, and J. Boos

Department of Pediatric Hematology and Oncology,
Albert-Schweitzer-Strasse 33, University of Münster, 48129 Münster, Germany

High dose chemotherapy

During the last 10 to 20 years, high-dose chemotherapy became a major focus of treatment development. Based on the hypotheses of a dose-effect relationship and the „simple precept that if a little is good, then more is better“ (Kamen et al. 2000) many study protocols included high dose chemotherapy. Improvements of supportive care and autologous bone marrow and/or peripheral blood stem cell support made this escalation of dose-intensity possible.

Which drugs are suitable for high dose chemotherapy?

The employment of drugs for high dose chemotherapy is limited by its toxicity on the primary organ under standard therapy: drugs whose primary organ toxicities are heart-toxicity (anthracyclines), nerve system toxicity (vincristine) or kidney- and ototoxicity (cisplatinum), are not applicable for further dose escalations.

On the other hand, substances showing primary and more or less solely bone marrow toxicity, are suitable drugs for high dose chemotherapy regimens; stem cell transplantation circumvents this factor and enables dose-intensification for the drugs, until other dose-limiting end-organ toxicities occur.

What is „high-dose"?

In *in vitro* assays exponential increase in drug concentration is applied to test for cytotoxic activity of compounds. *In vivo*, however, much lower dose escalations are possible: for the alkylating agents busulfan and thiotepa, about 20-30 fold doses compared to standard low dose regimens are administered, whereas for drugs as melphalan, cyclophosphamide, carboplatinum or etoposide, only 4-5 fold dose increase are considered to be possible before maximum-tolerated doses are reached.

What are the basic pharmacological factors which are responsible for the improved remission rates and disease free survivals associated with high dose chemotherapy?

Etoposide as example

To focus on this question we choose etoposide as example for further discussion.

Etoposide is one of the drugs for which schedule dependency was demonstrated. Clincal studies suggest that low plasma levels (about 0.5-1 mg/l) are associated with cytotoxic activity, whereas higher plasma levels (> 5-10 mg/l) frequently go along with more severe myelosuppression (Greco and Hainsworth 1994, Joel and Slevin 1994). As mentioned above, 4-5 fold dose increase of etoposide is considered to be possible compared to standard dosages with lack of specific organ toxicity. The optimal dose, schedule and duration of high-dose chemotherapy with etoposide in conditioning regimens for BMT remains to be established and should take into account knowledge about dose-response curves and host pharmacokinetics.

To discuss this question in more detail, we apply the proposed schedule dependency of etoposide for a variety of simulated low dose and high dose schedules of etoposide.

Simulation tool for etoposide

A simulation tool for etoposide was developed utilizing published data from children (Lowis et al. 1998) and data from our own group (Würthwein et al. 1999, children as well) who received standard i.v. infusion of etoposide (Würthwein and Boos 2001). Pharmacokinetic parameters of this population were: CL: 23.6 ± 4.5 ml/min/m², Vc: 3.75 ± 0.78 l/m², t½ a: 0.7 ± 0.35 h, t½ ß: 4.1 ± 1.4 h (mean ± standard deviation, n = 27). The model was validated by independently reproducing published data for low-dose as well as high-dose regimens, short time as well as continuous i.v. infusions. Independence of clearance on dose or age could be shown. Pharmacokinetic profiles of the drug reported in literature agreed quite satisfying with the fit of predictions of the tool regarding duration of exposure above predefined concentrations, peak levels, or concentrations at time of BMT after various published schedules.

Therefore, the simulation tool may serve to define concentration-time profiles of high predictive value for different new low dose and high dose etoposide schedules.

Simulation of low dose and high dose regimens of etoposide

As standard low dose regime for etoposide we defined the commonly used schedule of 150 mg/m²/2 h on 3 days, yielding in a total dose of 450 mg/m². 450 mg/m² applied as 96 h continuous infusion was chosen as second low dose schedule. Schedules with 1800 mg/m² (4- fold of standard low dose) applied as 0.5 h, 4 h or 96 h-infusion, respectively, were selected as high dose schedules.

Pharmacokinetic parameters of interest were peak level and duration of exposure above predefined concentrations (>1 mg/l, >10 mg/l) or in the concentration range of 1-10 mg/l. The parameters are expressed in relation to the values evaluated for standard low dose.

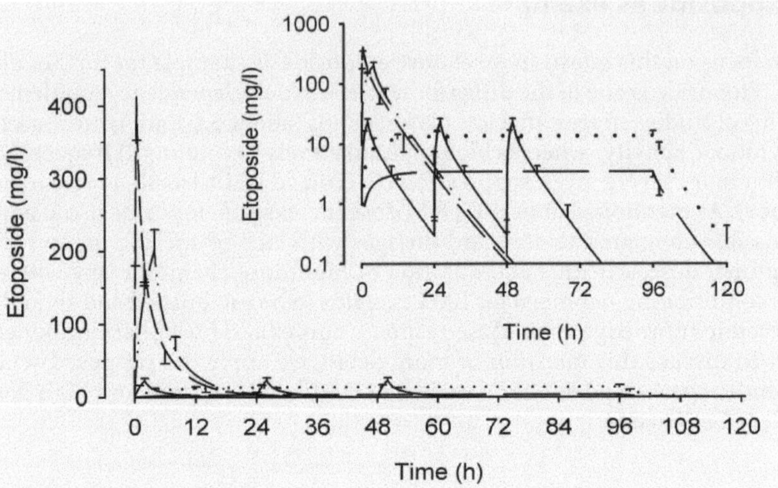

Fig. 1. Concentration-time profiles after different etoposide-schedules, simulations based on a simulation tool (Würthwein and Boos 2001) (mean ± standard deviation):

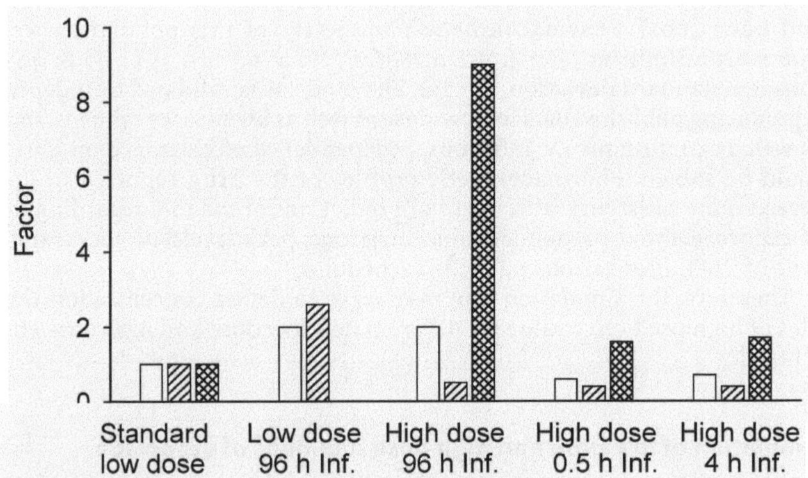

Fig. 2. Simulation of different etoposide schedules: duration of exposure above or within predefined concentration ranges, expressed as factor in relation to standard low dose of etoposide (150 mg/m²/2 h on 3 days). High dose: 1800 mg/m².
exposure > 1 mg/l: ▭, exposure between 1–10mg/L: ▨, exposure > 10 mg/l: ▦.

Concentration-time profiles of the different etoposide-schedules are shown in Figure 1, characteristics of pharmacokinetic profiles are summarized in Figure 2.

Low dose schedules

Standard low dose of 150 $mg/m^2/2$ h on 3 days leads to peak levels of 23.4 mg/l, duration of exposure > 10 mg/l of 10.8 h, > 1 mg/l of 49.2 h and in the range of 1-10 mg/l of 38.4 h.

Applying the same dose, 450 mg/m^2, as continuous i.v. infusions (96 h), the steady-state concentration of 3.4 mg/l is clear below 10 mg/l, thus the possibly critical concentration for myelotoxicity of 10 mg/l is not reached. Duration of exposure > 1 mg/l is 2 fold higher, between 1-10 mg/l 2.6 fold higher than after standard low dose.

High dose schedules

With respect to etoposide high dose regimens we focus on continuous i.v. infusion and short time infusions of the 4-fold dose compared to standard low dose. As etoposide clearance is independent on dose, for all these schedules AUC increases just 4-fold. However, peak levels and results for duration of exposure are quiet different and a function of infusion time:

Continuous i.v. infusion of 1800 mg/m^2 leads to a concentration at steady state of 13.8 mg/l. Therefore, duration of exposure > 10 mg/l is about 9 times, > 1 mg/l still 2 times higher than after standard low dose, exposure between 1-10 mg/l is halve.

The most pronounced change in pharmacokinetic behavior after a short time infusion of high dose etoposide compared to standard low dose is the resulting high peak level (0.5 h-infusion: 18 times higher, 4 h-infusion: still 9 times higher than after standard low dose). Duration of exposure > 10 mg/l is higher, > 1 mg/l and between 1-10 mg/l lower compared to standard low dose (0.5 h-infusion: factors are 1.6, 0.6 and 0.4, respectively; 4 h-infusion: factors are 1.7, 0.7 and 0.4, respectively).

Summary of pharmacokinetic characteristics

High dose schedules offer the alternative to focus on excessive peak concentrations or multifold extension to predefined standard drug concentrations. Extreme schedules of high dose etoposide might result in maximum peak levels of up to 500 mg/l per rapid infusion. On the other hand, maximum time of exposure > 1 mg/l can be achieved by continuous i.v. infusion of 1800 mg/m^2 over about 55 days!

Based on the pharmacological hypotheses, we might choose between quiet different etoposide schedules, depending on whether we intend to get high peak levels or long time of exposure above predefined plasma concentrations. In Table 1 we summarized some of these pharmacological "intention to treat" possibilities.

Table 1. High dose or low dose chemotherapy?: The pharmacological „intention to treat"

What do we intend?	What do we have to do?	for example
high peak level	high dose infusion as short as possible	high dose bolus: peak level = 500 mg/l
high time of exposure > 10 mg/l	high dose continuous iv infusion	high dose 130 h-infusion: steady state level = 10 mg/l
long time of exposure in the range 1-10 mg/l	repetitive short time infusion or repetitive oral administration or continuous i.v. infusion	standard low dose: 2 h infusion / 3 d
high time of exposure to 1 mg/l	continuous i. v. infusion	high dose 55 d-infusion or low dose 14 d infusion: steady state level = 1 mg/l

Conclusions

„High dose" chemotherapy due to the sole principle „more is better" can not be a reasonable strategy. The simulation tool presented allows to predefine pharmacokinetic profiles for new etoposide schedules over a wide range. Based on these profiles, etoposide containing regimens should be designed on the basis of clear pharmacokinetic hypotheses of target levels and exposure times, to allow subsequent development of pharmacokinetic-pharmacodynamic modelling and clinically optimal schedules.

References

1. Greco FA, Hainsworth JD (1994) Prolonged administration of low-daily-dose etoposide: a superior dosing schedule? Cancer Chemother Pharmacol 34 Suppl: S101-S104
2. Joel SP, Slevin ML (1994) Schedule-dependent topoisomerase II-inhibiting drugs. Cancer Chemother Pharmacol 34 Suppl: S84-S88
3. Kamen BA, Rubin E, Aisner J, Glatstein E (2000) High-Time Chemotherapy or High Time for Low Dose. J Clin Oncol 18: 2935-2937
4. Lowis SP, Price L, Pearson AD, Newell DR, Cole M (1998) A study of the feasibility and accuracy of pharmacokinetically guided etoposide dosing in children. Br J Cancer 77: 2318-2323
5. Würthwein G, Boos J (2001) Simulation tool for schedule-dependent etoposide exposure based on pharmacokinetic findings published in literature. Anti-Cancer Drugs; in press
6. Würthwein G, Krümpelmann S, Tillmann B, Real E, Schulze-Westhoff P, Jürgens H, Boos J (1999) Population pharmacokinetic approach to compare oral and i.v. administration of etoposide. Anti-Cancer Drugs 10: 807-814

Megadose Stem Cell Transplantation

M. F. MARTELLI

Hematopoietic Stem Cell Transplant Program, University of Perugia,
06122 Perugia, Italy

One HLA haplotype-mismatched hematopoietic stem cell transplants are being performed more and more often at our Center since we showed the infusion of large numbers of extensively T-cell-depleted hematopoietic stem cells prevents both graft rejection and graft-vs-host disease [1–3].

Over the past 7 years, in an attempt to optimize processing for peripheral blood cells we have changed our T-cell depletion procedure several times. From October 1995 to August 1997, PBPCs were depleted of T lymphocytes by one-step E-rosetting followed by a positive selection of the $CD34^+$ cells with the CellPro device and since January 1999 we have been using the CliniMacs instrument to select $CD34^+$ cells in a one step procedure. All these procedures yield very large numbers of $CD34^+$ cells (10 to 12 x 10^6/kg). When we started using $CD34^+$ positive selection we reduced the number of T lymphocytes by one log (from 22 to 2 x 10^4/kg) (Table 1). Another significant change in our strategy was substituting fludarabine for cyclophosphamide in an effort to reduce the extra-hematological toxicity of our TBI-based conditioning regimen (Fig. 1).

The modifications in the conditioning regimen and in the graft processing did not compromise sustained primary engraftment in a series of 43 high-risk (7 bad-risk CR I, 21 in CR ^{3} II, 15 in refractory relapse) acute leukemia patients we transplanted between October 1995 and August 1997 [3]. As we had hoped, the few T cells we infused successfully prevented GvHD even without any post-transplant immunosuppressive treatment. The extra-hematological toxicity of this innovative conditioning regimen was minimal even in these advanced and heavily

Table 1. The Table summarizes the major changes in processing and composition of the graft since we started the mismatched transplant program in March 1993

Years	1993–95 (n=36)	1995–97 (n=43)	1999–2000 (n=33)
Methods	SBA E-rosette	E-rosette CD34 selection (*Ceprate SC*)	CD34 selection (*CliniMACS*)
$CD34^+$ x 106/kg	10.8	10.5	12
$CD3^+$ x 104/kg	22.4	2.0	1.0

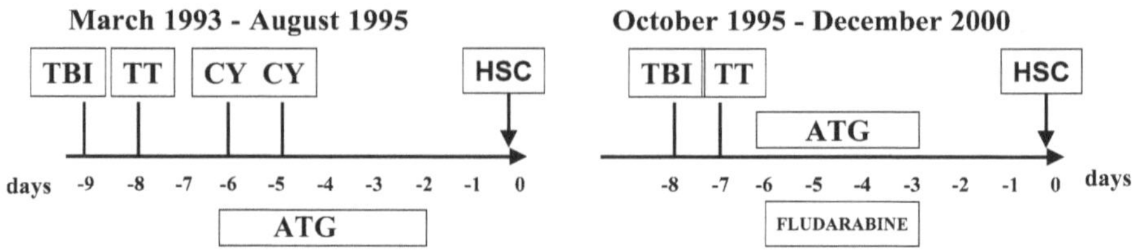

TBI: 8 Gy (7.5 since 1999) in a single fraction at 16 cGy/m (total lung dose 4 Gy)
TT : thiotepa 10 mg/kg
ATG (Fresenius): 5 mg/kg/day x 4
Cyclophosphamide 50 mg/kg/day
Fludarabine 40 mg/sqm/day x 5

Fig. 1. The figure shows the major modifications in the pre-transplant chemotherapy.

pretreated patients. Despite the risk factors at the transplant, 25% of AML and 17% of ALL patients survive disease-free at a median follow-up of 4 years.

These clinical results provide evidence supporting a biological principle which had been observed in vitro and in animal models, i.e. the veto activity of highly purified $CD34^+$ cells. Highly purified $CD34^+$ cells when given in an extremely large dose with no other facilitating cells enhance engraftment. In a mixed lymphocyte culture, Dr. Reisner showed that human $CD34^+$ cells, purified by the same procedure we used, specifically reduced the numbers of CTL precursors against their histocomaptibility antigens but not against third party stimulator cells [4]. In other words, purified $CD34^+$ cells induce specific tolerance and act as veto or facilitating cells.

An analysis of the relapse rate in these high-risk leukemia patients also leads to some interesting obervations. After extensive T-cell depletion, one would expect an increased risk of leukemia relapse in patients who did not develop GvHD. In our two pilot studies the predicted relapse-rate occurred only in ALL patients, who were already in relapse at time of transplant. In those who were not in relapse, leukemia recurrence was similar to the rate after matched transplants. In patients with AML, most of whom were in chemoresistant relapse at transplant, the incidence of relapse was 20%, which is even lower than expected in matched transplants (Fig. 2). The low relapse rate in the AML patients, could be related to potential graft-versus-AML effector mechanisms. We have recently suggested that donor NK cell alloreactivity, a biological phenomenon unique to mismatched transplants, could play a role in this anti-leukemia effect [5].

The last changes we introduced in January 1999 included graft processing with the CliniMACS device which provides a highly purified $CD34^+$ cell population without the need for E-rosetting or any other manipulation of the leukapheresis products. We also decided to stop post-transplant G-CSF administration to recipients because reports on experimental models and in our own preliminary observations have shown it is immunosuppressive [6].

So far 32 high-risk acute leukemia patients have been treated. Ages ranged from 11 to 58 years, with a median of 25. Almost all patients were at very high risk because of the advanced stage of disease at transplant, with 18 patients in relapse. Patients received a median of 12 x 10^6 $CD34^+$ cells/kg and a median of 1 x

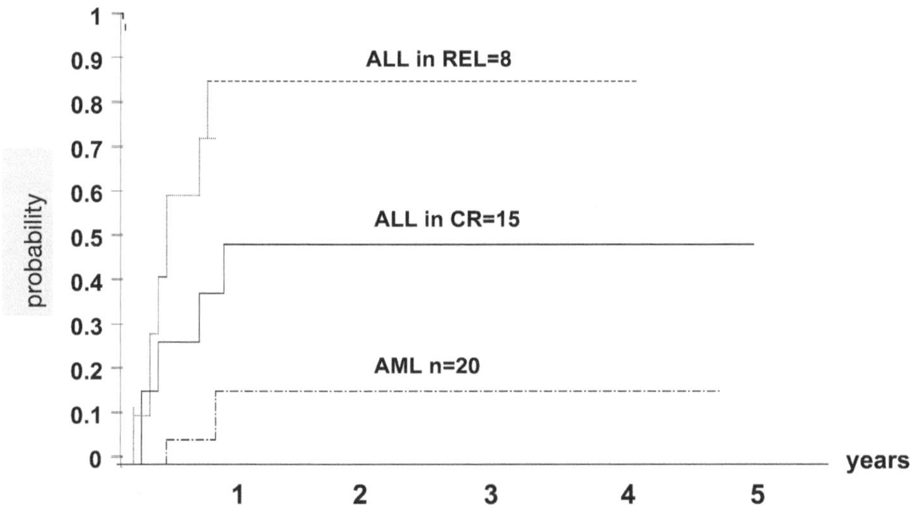

Fig. 2. This is an update of the results in the 43 acute leukemia patients we published in 1998 (3). At a median follow up of 4 years, the probability of leukemia relapse is 0.13 ± 0.08 for the 20 patients with AML, 0.44 ± 0.17 for the 15 patients with ALL in hematological remission at transplant (4 in CR I and 11 in CR ≥ II) and >0.85 for the 8 ALL patients who were already in chemoresistant relapse at transplant.

10^4 $CD3^+$/kg. The engraftment rate was similar to our previous results but as expected neutrophil recovery was four days later than in the 43 patients who received post-transplant G-CSF. Three patients developed acute GvHD which progressed to chronic in two.

Changes in the processing of the leukapheresis products and recipient care significantly influenced the post-transplant immunological reconstitution (Fig. 3). $CD4^+$ cell recovery was greatly improved, but, due to the fact that we still included patients with very poor prognosis, transplant related mortality was only border-line reduced from the 55% of the 43 patients transplanted before January

Fig. 3. Effect of post-grafting G-CSF administration on $CD4^+$ cell recovery in HLA-mismatched hematopoietic transplant recipients. Time kinetics of $CD4^+$ T cell recovery in patients who had received G-CSF vs those who had not . $CD4^+$ cell counts in patients who had not received G-CSF were significantly higher than in those who had ($p<0.0001$) at all time-points from day 60

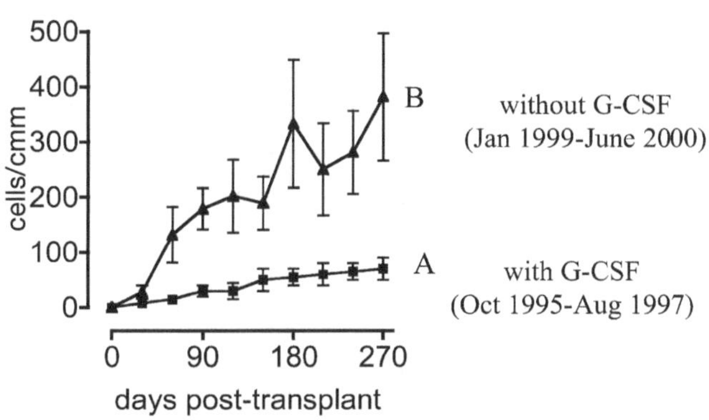

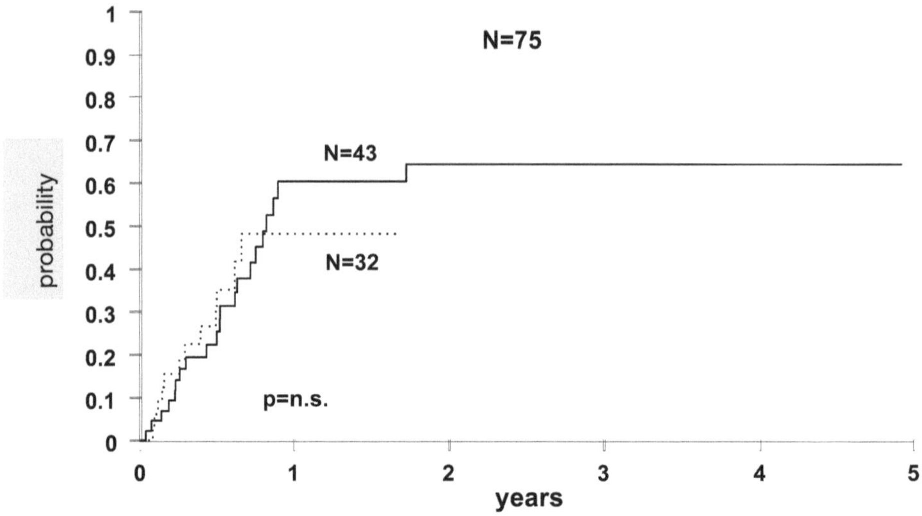

Fig. 4. Probability of transplant-related mortality in the 43 patients who received, between October 1995 and August 1997, Ceprate-separated $CD34^+$ cells and post-transplant G-CSF (solid line), and in the 32 patients who received, between January 1999 and June 2000, CliniMacs-separated $CD34^+$ cells and no post-transplant G-CSF (dashed line).

a
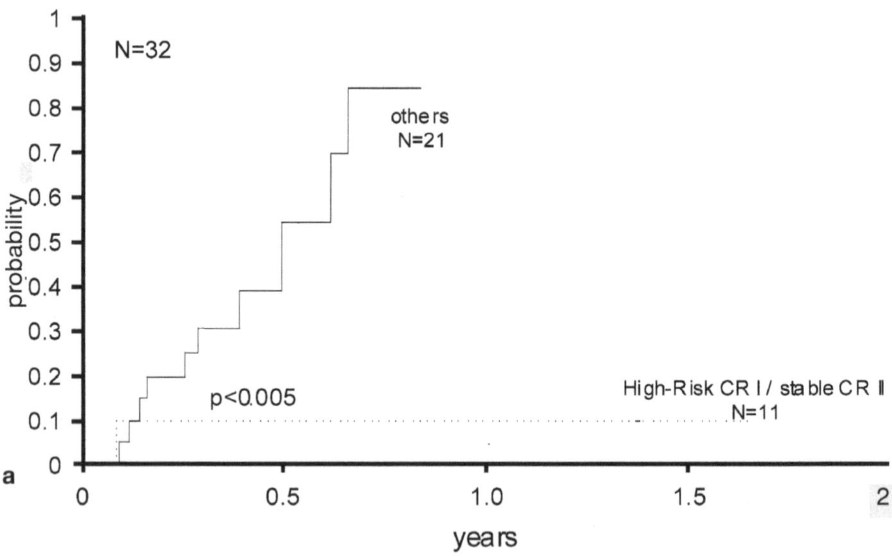

Fig. 5a,b. Effect of the disease status on the probability of transplant-related mortality (panel a) and Event-free survival (panel b) in the 32 patients who received CliniMacs-separated $CD34^+$ cells and no post-transplant G-CSF. The 11 patients who were in either high-risk CR I (n=1) or stable CR II (n=10) have 0.10 probability of transplant-related mortality as compared to 0.85 in the others (a) and 0.70 probability of survival as compared to 0.10 in the others (b).

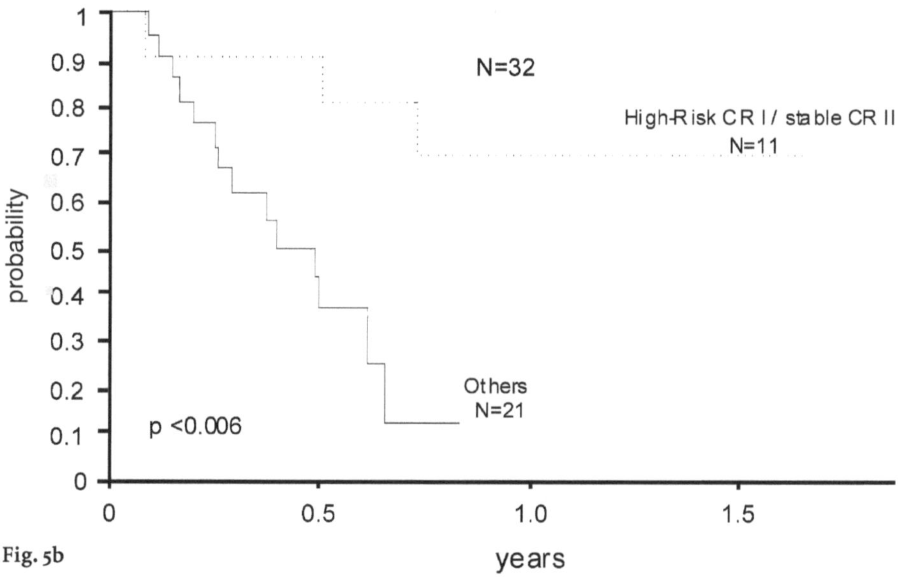

Fig. 5b

1999 to the current 42% (Fig. 4). But if we re-analyze the last 32 patients on the basis of the stages of the disease at transplant (10 patients in second stable CR and one in first CR), TRM is only 10% and 70% of these patients survive event-free at 1.5 years (Fig. 5 a/b).

To conclude, our experience in mismatched transplants demonstrates that engraftment can be achieved without severe GvHD and with low regimen-related toxicity and mortality. The clinal outcome could be improved if transplant candidates were transplanted at a much earlier stage of the disease.

References

1. Aversa F, Tabilio A, Terenzi A, et al.: Successful engraftment of T-cell-depleted haploidentical „three-loci" incompatible transplants in leukemia patients by addition of recombinant human granulocyte colony-stimulating factor-mobilized peripheral blood progenitor cells to bone marrow inoculum. Blood 1994; 84: 3948-3955.
2. Reisner Y, Martelli MF: Bone marrow transplantation across HLA barriers by increasing the number of transplanted cells. Immunol Today 1995;16:437-440.
3. Aversa F, Tabilio A, Velardi A, et al.: Treatment of high risk acute leukemia with T-cell-depleted stem cells from related donors with one fully mismatched HLA haplotype. N Engl J Med 1998;339:1186-1193.
4. Rachamin N, Gan J, Segall R, et al.: Tolerance induction by „megadose" hematopoietic transplants: donor-type human CD34 stem cells induce potent specific reduction of host anti-donor cytotoxic T lymphocyte precursors in mixed lymphocyte culture. Transplantation 1998;65:1386-1393.
5. Ruggeri L, Capanni M, Casucci M, et al: Role of natural killer cell alloreactivity in HLA-mismatched hematopoietic stem cell transplantation. Blood 1999;94:333-339.
6. Volpi I, Perruccio K, Tosti A, et al. Postgrafting administration of granulocyte colony-stimulating factor impairs functional immune recovery in recipients of human leukocyte antigen haplotype-mismatched hematopoietic transplants. Blood 2001;97:2514-2521.

HD-Ara-C in the Conditioning Regimen for BMT in Acute Leukemias

C. Annaloro, E. Pozzoli, V. G. Bertolli, A. Della Volpe, D. Soligo, E. Tagliaferri, and G. Lambertenghi Deliliers

Centro Trapianti di Midollo, Università degli Studi and Ospedale Maggiore IRCCS, Milano Italy.

Introduction

The choice of the most appropriate BMT conditioning regimen depends on whether the BMT is autologous or allogeneic BMT, the characteristics of the underlying disease, its susceptibility to antineoplastic agents, the entity of the expected GVL effect, the risk of GVHD, and the desired level of immunosuppression. Furthermore, there is still no unequivocal evidence concerning the superiority of either of the treatment schedules used in BMT Units (Mineishi et al 1999, Jilella et al 1999).

In acute leukemia patients, high dose cyclophosphamide in combination with hyperfractionated TBI is frequently regarded as the regimen of choice in both autologous and allogeneic BMT, with the busulfan-cyclophosphamide combination sometimes being considered an alternative (Reiffers et al 1996, Cassileth et al 1998). Cyclophosphamide is more rarely replaced by other drugs such as VP-16 and HD-Ara-C (Bassan et al 1998), and only a few Centres add a second drug to the cyclophosphamide-TBI combination (Mineishi et al 1999, Jilella et al 1999, Stein et al 1996).

This paper summarizes our ten-year experience of using HD-Ara-C, in combination with cyclophosphamide and fractionated TBI in the conditioning regimen administerd to patients with acute leukemia.

Materials and methods

Over the last ten years, 146 acute leukemia patients (81 male, 65 female: median age 39 years, range 12-57) have undergone BMT in different disease phases. Forty-four AML (36 in first CR) and 37 ALL patients (16 in first CR) received autografts; thirty-five AML (18 in first CR) and 30 ALL patients (17 in first CR) underwent allogeneic BMT. All of the patients in first CR had been referred to our institution after receiving different treatment programs that always included remission induction and standard dose consolidation/early intensification; the patients not in first CR were heterogeneous in terms of previous treatment and disease phase. In all of the autologous BMT cases, the source of hematopoietic stem cells was unpurged bone marrow that had been harvested and cryopreserved in the same disease phase as that of transplantation. In the case of allogeneic transplants, the source of hematopoietic stem cells was bone marrow in all but ten AML and eight ALL cases.

The conditioning regimen included HD-Ara-C, 3 g/sqm/12 h on days -9/-8, CTX 60 mg/kg/die on days -6/-5 and TBI at a total dosage of 10 Gy fractionated in three equal doses on days -3 through -1. GVHD prophylaxis included cyclosporine-A and MTX at conventional doses.

Only the patients with a minimum post-BMT follow-up of six months were evaluated. Relapse, transplant related mortality (TRM), death during CR and drop-outs were considered events. Event free survival (EFS) curves were calculated according to Kaplan & Meier starting from the date of BMT, and compared by means of the log-rank test.

Results

As of 31 March 2000, 16 patients had died of TRM, 62 had relapsed, three had died in CR (two of a second neoplasm and one of intercurrent disease), and 65 were in continuous CR; the median follow-up of the censored patients was 75 months, range 6–120.

Of the 44 autografted AML patients, 18 had relapsed (2–64 months after autologous BMT), three had died of TRM, one of a second neoplasm, and 22 were in continuous CR; the median EFS was 64 months, and the 10-year chance of EFS was 49.78%. If only the 36 patients autografted in first CR are considered, there were 14 relapses, two TRM and one second neoplasm: 19 patients were in continuous CR; the median EFS had not been reached and the 10-year chance of EFS was 50.2% (Fig. 1).

Of the 37 autografted ALL patients, 21 had relapsed (4–48 months after autologous BMT), two had died of TRM and one of a second neoplasm, and 13 were

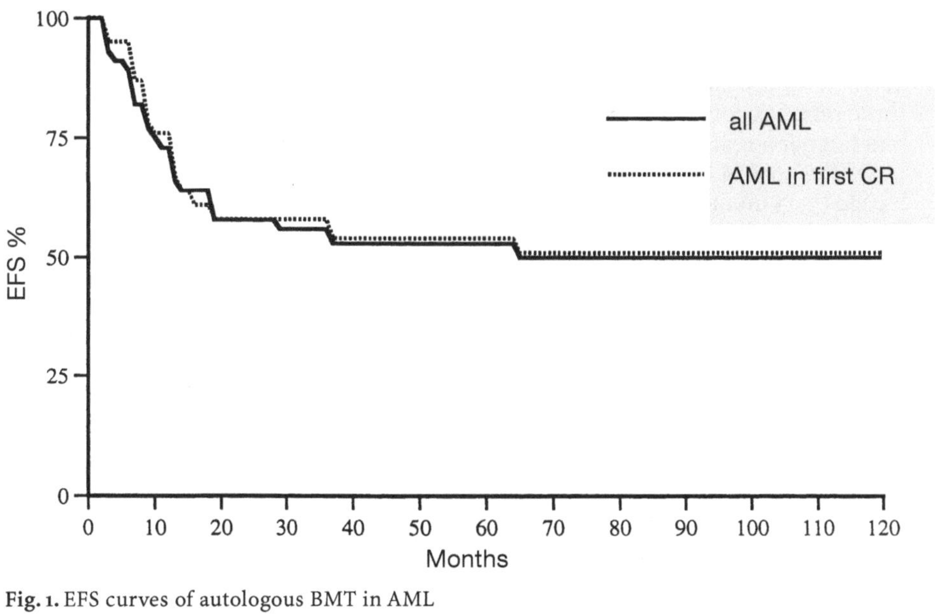

Fig. 1. EFS curves of autologous BMT in AML

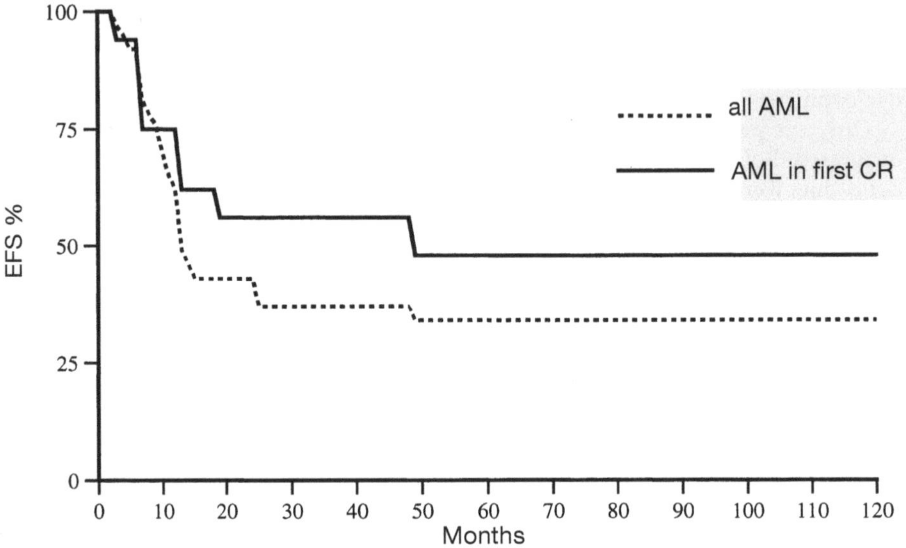

Fig. 2. EFS curves of autologous BMT in ALL

in continuous CR; the median EFS was 13 months, and the 10-year chance of EFS was 34.27%. If only the 16 patients autografted in first CR are considered, there were 6 relapses, one case each of TRM and second neoplasm, and 8 patients were in continuous CR; median EFS was 48 months and the 10-year chance of EFS was 47.58% (Fig. 2).

Of the 35 AML patients undergoing allogeneic transplantation, 14 had relapsed (6-18 months after autologous BMT), eight had died of TRM, and 13 were in continuous CR; the median EFS was 13 months, and the 10-year chance of EFS was 40.78%. If only the 18 patients transplanted in first CR are considered, there were three relapses, four TRM, and 11 patients were in continuous CR; the median EFS had not been reached and the 10-year chance of EFS was 56.96% (Fig. 3).

Of the 30 ALL patients undergoing allogeneic transplantation, nine had relapsed (5–13 months after autologous BMT), three had died of TRM, one had died late in CR, and 17 were in continuous CR; the median EFS had not been reached, and the 10-year chance of EFS was 53.18%. If only the 17 patients transplanted in first CR are considered, there were three relapses, and 14 patients were in continuous CR; the median EFS had not been reached and the 10-year chance of EFS was 83.26% (Fig. 4).

Discussion

The present results refer to a group of acute leukemia patients who received a conditioning regimen consisting of a short course of HD-Ara-C in combination with conventional cyclophosphamide and fractionated TBI. Unlike other studies of conditioning regimens including HD-Ara-C (Kumar et al 1997, Mineishi et al

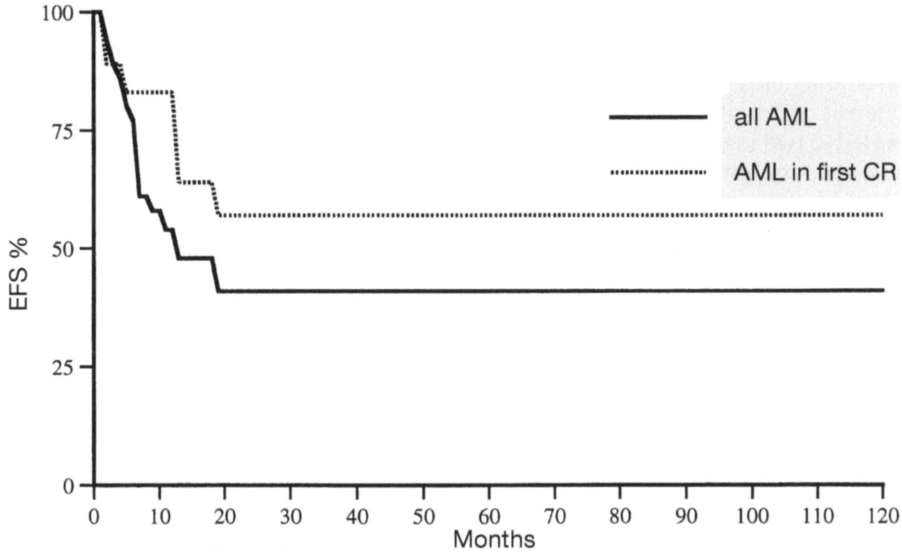

Fig. 3. EFS curves of allogeneic BMT in AML

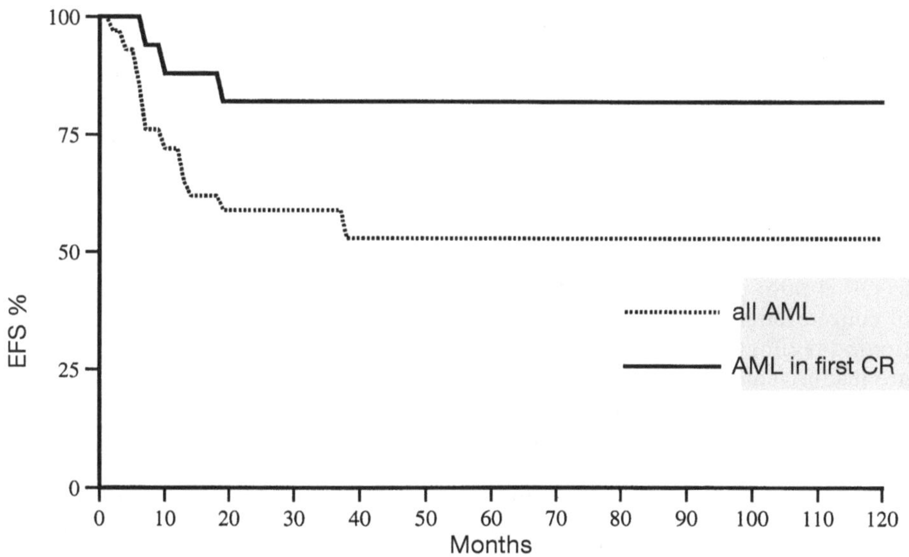

Fig. 4. EFS curves of allogeneic BMT in ALL

1999), the present series is characterized by the presence of only acute leukemia patients and a rather long follow-up.

Despite its well known efficacy in the treatment of acute leukemia and its concomitant immunosuppressive activity (Cassileth et al 1998, Bassan et al 1998, Stein et al 1996, De La Serna et al 1997, Gassmann et al 1988), HD-Ara-C is far less considered in designing conditioning regimens for both autologous and allogeneic BMT. Furthermore, although frequently regarded as promising in terms of antineoplastic activity, HD-Ara-C conditioning regimens are considered disadvantageous in terms of toxicity (Kumar et al 1997, Engelhard et al 1995, Kamani et al 1995). This has led to two major consequences: HD-Ara-C containing regimens are frequently reserved for high risk or advanced-phase leukemic patients (Takahashi et al 1994, Mineishi et al 1999), and, if used at all, HD-Ara-C generally replaces cyclophosphamide and is administered for six consecutive days (Kumar et al 1997, Kamani et al 1995, Takahashi et al 1994). There are relatively few reports concerning the use of short-term HD-Ara-C in combination with cyclophosphamide and TBI (Mineishi et al 1999, Jilella et al 1999). The current opinions concerning the use of HD-Ara-C in BMT may limit its efficacy and increase its toxicity. In our experience, the addition of a short HD-Ara-C course to conventional radiochemotherapy has led to a low rate of TRM despite the fact that many of the patients had advanced disease. Furthermore, early deaths were uncommon in the patients transplanted in first CR, and completely absent in those receiving autologous BMT for AML or allogeneic BMT for ALL in first CR. On the basis of these results, we do not agree that HD-Ara-C can only be cautiously proposed in first CR due to its toxic potential (Kumar et al 1997, Engelhard et al 1995, Kamani et al 1995).

In many studies, the same conditioning regimen has been administered to all acute leukemia patients, regardless of the type of disease or whether they will subsequently receive autologous or allogeneic BMT (Reiffers et al 1996, Cassileth et al 1998). This approach may adversely affect the outcome of an autologous BMT because the long-term chances of EFS exclusively depend on the efficacy of the conditioning regimen (Stein et al 1996), and of an allogeneic BMT for diseases such as ALL, where the GVL effect is expected to be low (Weyman et al 1993, Appelbaum 1997). In our experience, the EFS results of allogeneic BMT for AML were comparable with those commonly reported in the literature (Zittoun et al 1995, Reiffers et al 1996), and it can be inferred that the addition of HD-Ara-C does not confer any significant advantage . The outcome of autografted ALL patients can be regarded as rather poor and may reflect difficulties in achieving good quality CR by means of conventional treatment and in managing residual disease by means of conditioning regimen (Gilmore et al 1991, Lambertenghi Deliliers et al 1993). Our data are insufficient to answer the question as to whether the addition of HD-Ara-C can be recommended as a means of improving the prognosis in these patients. Conversely, the EFS figures of autologous BMT in AML compare favourably with those of allogeneic BMT (Reiffers et al 1996, Cassileth et al 1998), as also reported elsewhere (Mc Millan et al 1990, Schiller et al 1997) and may be due to the achievement of good quality CR even after relapse and the use of autologous BMT as late intensification (Lambertenghi Deliliers et al 1995, Miggiano et al 1996); furthermore, the addition of HD-Ara-C might have increased the antileukemic efficacy of the conditioning regimen without significantly affecting its toxicity . Finally, the most obvious success has been obtained by using allogeneic BMT in the treatment of ALL As only 17 patients were transplanted in first CR, it is necessary to avoid drawing premature conclusions; however, the EFS in this small series is confirmed by the long follow-up. Reinforcement of the conditioning regimen allows a greater reduction in residual disease; it seems to be advantageous because the expected low GVL effect (Weyman et al 1993, Appelbaum 1997) is exerted against a minimized leukemic burden.

Summary

Over the last ten years, we have transplanted 146 acute leukemia patients in different disease (81 males, 65 females; median age 39 years, range 12-57). The conditioning regimen was HD-Ara-C (3g/sqm/12h for two days), followed by HD-cyclophosphamide and fractionated 10 Gy TBI. Fourty-four of the 79 AML patients received autologous BMT (36 in first CR) and 35 allogeneic BMT (18 in first CR); of the 67 ALL patients, 37 received autologous BMT (16 in first CR) and 30 allogeneic BMT (17 in first CR). As of 31-12-99, 61 patients had relapsed (38 after autologous and 23 after allogeneic BMT) and 16 had died of transplant related mortality (five after autologous and 11 after allogeneic BMT), two of second neoplasia and one of an intercurrent event. Twenty-three autografted AML patients (20 transplanted in first CR), 13 autografted ALL (eight in first CR), 13 allografted AML (11 in first CR), and 17 allografted ALL patients (14 in first CR) were still in CR. The respective median EFS and 10-yr EFS chances were as follows: not reached and 52.89% in autografted AML patients (not reached and 54.04% in first CR), 13 months and 34.27% in autografted ALL (49 months and 47.58% in first CR), 13 months and 40.78% in allografted AML (not reached and 56.96% in first CR), not reached and 53.18% in allografted ALL (not reached and 82.36% in first CR). HD-Ara-C is not included in the conditioning regimens of most BMT Units, because it is generally considered not to improve outcome significantly. In our long-term experience, favourable results have been achieved in particular settings, such as autologous BMT in AML and allogeneic BMT in ALL patients. Good quality CR can be achieved even after relapse in AML; the GVL effect is generally low in ALL patients. The addition of HD-Ara-C may have significantly increased the antileukemic efficacy of the conditioning regimen in both cases, thus contributing to the favourable figures.

References

Appelbaum FR (1997) Allogeneic hematopoietic stem cell transplantation for acute leukemia. Semin Oncol 24: 114-23

Bassan R et al. (1998) Outcome assessment of age group-specific (+/- 50 years) post-remission consolidation with high-dose cytarabine or bone marrow autograft for adult acute myelogenous leukemia. Haematologica 83: 627-35

Cassileth PA et al. (1998) Chemotherapy compared with autologous or allogeneic bone marrow transplanattion in the management of acute myeloid leukemia in first remission. N Eng J Med 339: 1649-56

De La Serna J et al. (1997) Idarubicin and intermediate dose ARA-C followed by consolidation chemotherapy or bone marrow transplantation in relapsed or refractory acute myeloid leukemia. Leukemia Lymphoma 25: 365-72

Engelhard D et al. (1995) Cytosine arabinoside as a major risk factor for Streptococcus viridans septicemia following bone marrow transplantation: a 5-year prospective study. Bone Marrow Transplant 16: 565-70

Gassmann W et al. (1988) Comparison of cyclophosphamide, cytarabine, and etoposide as immunosuppressive agents before allogeneic bone marrow transplantation. Blood 72: 1574-9

Gilmore MJML et al (1991) Failure of purged autologous bone marrow transplantation in high risk acute lymphoblastic leukaemia in first complete remission. Bone Marrow Transplant 8: 19-26

Jillella AP et al. (1999) Cyclophosphamide, cytosine arabinoside and TBI as a conditioning regimen for allogeneic bone marrow transplantation in patients with leukemia. Bone Marrow Transplant 23: 1095-100

Kamani N et al. (1995) Fractionated total-body irradiation preceding high-dose cytosine arabinoside as a preparative regimen for bone marrow transplantation in children with acute leukemia. Med Pediatr Oncol 25: 179-84

Kumar M et al. (1997) Toxicity associated with high-dose cytosine arabinoside and total body irradiation as conditioning for allogeneic bone marrow transplantation. Bone Marrow Transplant 19: 1061-4

Lambertenghi Deliliers et al. (1993) Long-term results of autologous bone marrow transplantation in adult acute lymphoblastic leukemia. Leukemia Lymphoma 11: 419-25

Lambertenghi Deliliers et al. (1995) Single-Institution results of autologous bone marrow transplantation in acute myeloid leukemia. Haematologica 80: 136-41

Mc Millan AK et al. (1990) High-dose chemotherapy and autologous bone marrow transplantation in acute myeloid leukemia. Blood 76: 480-8

Miggiano MC et al. (1996) Autologous bone marrow transplantation in late first complete remission improves outcome in acute myelogenous leukemia. Leukemia 10: 402-9

Mineishi S et al. (1999) addition of high-dose Ara-C to the BMT conditioning regimen reduces leukemia relapse withpout an increase in toxicity. Bone Marrow Transplant 23: 1217-22

Reiffers J et al. (1996) Allogeneic vs autologous stem cell transplantation vs chemotherapy in patients with acute myeloid leukemia in first remission: the BGMT 87 study. Leukemia 10: 1874-82

Schiller G et al. (1997) Transplantation of autologous peripheral blood progenitor cells procured after high-dose cytarabine-based consolidation chemotherapy for adults with acute myelogenous leukemia in first remission. leukemia 11: 1533-9, 1997

Stein AS et al. (1996) In vivo purging with high-dose cytarabine followed by high-dose chemoradiotherapy and reinfusion of unpurged bone marrow for adult acute myelogenous leukemia in first complete remission. J Clin Oncol 14: 2206-16

Takahashi S et al. (1994) Recombinant human glycosilated granulocyte colony-stimulating factor (rhG-CSF)-combined regimen for allogeneic bone marrow transplantation in refractory acute myeloid leukemia. Bone Marrow Transplant 13: 239-45

Weyman C et al (1993) Use of cytosine arabinoside and total body irradiation as a condirtioning for allogeneic marrow transplantation in patients with acute lymphoblastic leukemia: a multicenter survey. Bone Marrow Transplant 11: 43-50

Zittoun RA et al. (1995) Autologous or allogeneic bone marrow transplantation compared with intensive chemotherapy in acute myelogenous leukemia. European Organization for Research and Treatment of Cancer (EORTC) and the Gruppo Italiano Malattie Ematologiche Maligne dell'Adulto (GIMEMA) Leukemia Cooperative Groups. N Eng J Med 332: 217-23

TBI-Based Reduced Intensity Conditioning with Allogeneic Hematopoietic Stem Cell Transplantation (SCT) in Patients with High-Risk Hematologic Malignancies

M. J. Kröger[1], A. Schuck[2], M. Kiehl[3], G. Silling[1], R. Leo[1], C. Scheffold[1], W.E. Berdel[1], and J. Kienast[1]

[1] Internal Medicine, Hematology/Oncology, University of Muenster, Germany
[2] Department of Radiotherapy/Radiation Oncology, University of Muenster, Germany
[3] Department of Hematology/Oncology and Bone Marrow Transplantation, Idar-Oberstein, Germany

Conventional chemotherapy is often unsatisfactory in high-risk hematologic malignancies (Carella et al., 1993) while myeloablative chemotherapy followed by allogeneic SCT can produce durable remissions (Forman et al., 1991). Here we studied a novel conditioning regimen including dose-reduced TBI, fludarabine and ATG followed by SCT from an allogeneic donor. Between May, 1999 and December, 2000, 16 patients (14 AML, 1 MDS, 1 CML) refractory to chemotherapy or complicated by severe treatment related events underwent allogeneic SCT from HLA-matched sibling donors (n=11), matched unrelated donors (n=4), or mismatched related donors (n=1). All patients had risk factors precluding them from conventional myeloablative transplantation. Ten of 16 patients had a history of pulmonary aspergillosis.

Preparative regimen

Conditioning therapy consisted of TBI 8 Gy (with the exception of one patient receiving 4Gy), fludarabine (30 mg/m^2/d x 4), and anti-T lymphocyte globuline (rabbit 20 mg/kg/d x 2).

GvHD prophylaxis

GvHD prophylaxis consisted of Cyclosporine A (3mg/kg) and short-course MTX. Cyclosporine was tapered at day +42 and discontinued on day +70.

Engraftment and chimerism

The median number of CD34+ cells infused from an unmanipulated graft on day 0 was 5,93 x 10^6/kg (range: 3,38–9,71). The median times to absolute neutrophil counts greater than 0.5 x 10^9/L was 22 days (range: 17–28 days) and to platelet counts greater than 20 x 10^9/L was 30 days (range: 21–90 days). Chimerism analysis using microsatellite variable-number-of-tandem-repeat (VNTR) or short-tandem-repeat markers revealed complete donor cell engraftment in 10 of 11 evaluable patients. However, 2 of the 11 patients lost evidence of donor hematopoiesis on days +47 and +165 post transplantation coincident with leukemic relapse.

Donor leukocyte transfusions (DLT)

Unmobilized donor leukocytes were obtained by leukapheresis. Indications for DLT were impending or overt leukemic relapse or unstable donor cell chimerism (defined as <85% donor blood cells in the BM biopsy or a decline of 10% in donor cell chimerism between two analyses).

The target number of CD3+ T cells for the first DLT was 5×10^6/kg. In the absence of acute GvHD >grade II, the numbers of CD3+ T cells were escalated from 1×10^7/kg up to 1×10^8/kg. Two patients with AML received DLT starting on days +90 and +141 at escalating doses up to 1×10^8/kg due to overt leukemic relapse. No response was observed in either case. One patient received DLT beginning on day +62 because of incomplete donor cell chimerism and persistent leukemia. No response to DLT was observed.

An additional two patients with AML received DLT beginning on days +91 and +321 because of declining levels of donor cell chimerism and impending leukemic relapse. One of these patients responded with reinduction of complete donor cell chimerism and eradication of the leukemic clone. The other patient is too early to evaluate. The CML patient experienced cytogenetic relapse at day +407 and is currently receiving DLT.

Response

12 of 13 evaluable patients achieved a complete response. 3 patients died early, two of them due to infection, one due to disease progression. In total, 5 relapses occurred: 3 overt leukemic relapses and one impending relapse in AML patients, and a cytogenetic relapse in the CML patient. No response was observed to DLT in patients with overt leukemic relapse (n=3). However, in the AML patient with declining levels of donor cell chimerism and impending leukemic relapse, complete chimerism and remission could be restored by DLT.

GvHD

One patient developed biopsy confirmed grade IV GvHD of the gut after discontinuation of immunosuppressive medication and he died on day +102 in CR. Otherwise, in patients not receiving DLT, no acute GvHD >grade II was observed after a median follow-up of 263 days (range: 81–448 days).

Survival

Eight of 16 patients (50%) are alive at a median of 263 days (range: 82–449 days) post transplant, 6 of them in CR. Two of 16 patients died in CR from treatment-related complications on days +78 (pancreatitis) and +102 (GvHD grade IV). Three patients died early, one from disease progression and the other two due to infections. Three patients died from leukemic relapse after transplantation.

Discussion

Total body irradiation (TBI) in conventional preparative regimens (Clift et al., 1998) or low-dose conditioning (Niederwieser et al.,1999) has been widely used in patients undergoing allogeneic BM transplantation for hematopoietic malignancies. Both approaches prove to be sufficient in achieving engraftment with stable donor cell chimerism. However, full dose TBI may lead to severe toxicity, while low-dose TBI appears to be suitable for patients with controlled disease. We therefore evaluated the role of dose-reduced TBI in 16 patients neither eligible for full dose conditioning nor for conditioning with low dose intensity.

This study shows that dose-reduced TBI is able to induce complete remissions with complete donor cell chimerism in a substantial portion of patients with high-risk hematologic malignancies. The incidence of GvHD >grade II is low (6%). However, the treatment related mortality in this high-risk population is still in the range of 25%. Therefore, consideration is being given to a further dose reduction of TBI to 4–6 Gy. Further, therapeutic intervention with cessation of immunosuppressive medication and early DLT was able to induce remissions in patients with impending relapse. Nevertheless, the response rate of patients receiving DLT for overt leukemic relapse was poor, consistent with data from multicenter studies (Collins et al., 1997). Our protocol has therefore been amended to allow for a more judicious use of DLT based on unstable donor cell chimerism in marrow CD34+ cells.

References

Carella AM, Carlier P, Pungolino E, Resegotti L, Liso V, Stasi R, Montillo M, Iacopino P, Mirto S, Pagano L (1993) Idarubicin in combination with intermediate-dose cytarabine and VP-16 in the treatment of refractory or rapidly relapsed patients with acute myeloid leukemia. The GIMEMA Cooperative Group. Leukemia 7: 196-199

Clift RA, Buckner CD, Appelbaum FR, Sullivan KM, Storb R, Thomas ED (1998) Long-term follow-up of a randomized trial of two irradiation regimens for patients receiving allogeneic marrow transplants during first remission of acute myeloid leukemia. Blood 92: 1455-1456

Collins RH Jr, Shpilberg O, Drobyski WR, Porter DL, Giralt S, Champlin R, Goodman SA, Wolff SN, Hu W, Verfaillie C, List A, Dalton W, Ognoskie N, Chetrit A, Antin JH, Nemunaitis J (1997) Donor leukocyte infusions in 140 patients with relapsed malignancy after allogeneic bone marrow transplantation. J Clin Oncol 15: 433-44

Forman SJ, Schmidt GM, Nademanee AP, Amylon MD, Chao NJ, Fahey JL, Konrad PN, Margolin KA, Niland JC, O'Donell MR, Parker PM, Smith EP, Snyder DS, Somlo G, Stein AS, Blume KG

(1991) Allogeneic bone marrow transplantation as therapy for primary induction failure for patients with acute leukemia. J Clin Oncol 9: 1570-1574
Niederwieser D, Wolff D, Hegenbart U, Mantovani L, Pönisch W, Deininger M, McSweeney P, Edelmann J, Kiefel V, Blume K, Storb R (1999) Hematopoietic stem cell transplants (HSCT) from HLA-matched and 1-allele-mismatched unrelated donors using a nonmyeloablative regimen. Blood 94: 561a (abstract)

Total Marrow Irradiation (TMI), Busulfan, and Cyclophosphamide for Allografting in Multiple Myeloma. A Pilot Study

N. Kröger, G. Derigs[2], H. Wandt[3], K. Schäfer-Eckart[3], G. Wittkowsky[4], R. Kuse[4], J. Casper[5], W. Krüger, T. Zabelina, H. Renges, H. Kabisch, A. Krüll[6], H. Einsele[7], and A. R. Zander

Bone Marrow Transplantation and [6]Dept of Radiotherapy, University Hospital Hamburg-Eppendorf, [2]University Hospital Mainz, [3]Städt. Klinikum Nürnberg, [4]Dept of Hematology A.K. St. Georg, Hamburg, [5]University Hospital Rostock, and [7] University Hospital Tübingen, Germany.

Abstract

To reduce the incidence of severe graft versus host disease (GvHD) and lower the treatment related mortality(TRM) in allogeneic stem cell transplantation from HLA-identical siblings patients with multiple myeloma, we incorporated anti-thymocyte globulin (ATG, Fa Fresenius, Bad Homburg, Germany) in the conditioning regimen of 12 patients. The conditioning regimen consisted of modified total body irradiation, busulfan and cyclophoshamide (n=9) or busulfan and cyclophoshamide (n=3). The median age was 44 years (range, 29–53) and the median time from diagnosis to transplant was 12 months (range, 6 to 56). The stem cell source was bone marrow in 10 , and peripheral blood stem cells in 2 patients. Grade II–IV acute GvHD occurred in 3 patients (27% percent). Severe grade III and IV GvHD developed in only 1 patient. Major toxicity was mucositis. Grad II according the Bearman score was noted in 10 patients, whereas 2 patients experienced grade III , requiring prophylactic intubation. One patient died of severe GvHD grade IV and one patient developed multi-organ failure on day +13, resulting in a TRM of 17%. A complete response in surviving patients after allogeneic transplantation was seen in 4 (40%), and PR in 6 (60%) patients. Two of the patients with PR received a donor lymphocyte infusion (DLI) for further tumor reduction 8 and 14 months after stem cell transplantation, and converted to CR, which increased the rate of CR up to 60%. After a median follow-up of 25 months (range, 5–62), no patient with CR after allogeneic transplantation relapsed during follow-up, while 3 out of 4 patients with P.R. experienced progress within 3 years (p=0.07). The estimated overall survival at three years for all patients is 83 percent (CI 95%: 68%–98%). The estimated progression-free survival at three years is 61 percent (CI 95%: 32%–90%). These results suggest that the incorporation of anti-thymocyte globulin may prevent severe GvHD without obvious increase of relapse. DLI should be administered for patients with incomplete response after transplantation to enhance the rate of complete remission, which results in long term freedom of disease.

Introduction

Allogeneic stem cell transplantation might cure patients with multiple myeloma. In a retrospective study of the EBMT 42% of the patients are disease-free 5 years after allogeneic transplantation [1]. The advantage of allogeneic stem cells to autologous stem cells is a direct anti-tumor activity through the graft versus myeloma effect by allogeneic immunocompetent T-cells [2–4]. However the transplant related morbidity and mortality were up to 40%, resulting in a worse outcome compared to autologous transplantation in a retrospective case matched study, despite a lower progression rate [5]. For this reason , efforts were made to improve the results by more selection of patients and earlier timing of transplant [6], using PBSC as stem cell source [7] and to decrease the transplant related mortality by using more effective methods to prevent severe graft versus host-disease [8, 9]. Recently, the EBMT registry reported a lower transplant related mortality of 20% for patients transplanted after 1995 [10]. To reduce the treatment related mortality and retain the anti-tumor efficacy, we investigated in vivo T-cell depletion with anti-thymocyte globulin as part of the conditioning regimen consisting of total marrow irradiation, busulfan and cyclophosphamide or busulfan and cyclophophamide alone in allogeneic stem cell transplantation with HLA-identical siblings in patients with multiple myeloma. Similiar results showed that ATG as part of the conditioning regimen resulted in a low incidence of severe acute and chronic GvHD in unrelated bone marrow transplantation without obvious increase of relapse rate [11].

Patients and Methods

Between 1995 and 2000 12 patients with a median age of 44 years (range, 29–53) were enrolled in the protocol. A written informed consent was received from each patient, and the study was approved by the local Ethic Committee. Major inclusion criteria were age below 55 years, stage II or III, and the presence of an HLA-identical sibling as donor. There were 9 male and three female patients. All patients had at least minor response to prior induction chemotherapy. 6 out of 12 patients had prior radiation therapy and three of them were therefore not eligible for total marrow irradiation. The median β2 microglobulin serum level at diagnosis was 2.5 mg/dl (range, 1.7 to 7.6). The median time from diagnosis to transplant was 12 months (range, 6 to 56). The characteristics of the patients are shown in Table 1.

9 patients received conditioning with total-marrow irradiation, 900 cGy given over three days in six fractions, followed by busufan 12 mg/kg (n=4) or 9 mg/kg (n=5) and cyclophosphamide (120 mg/kg), and 3 patients with prior radiation therapy received busulfan (14 mg/kg) and cyclophosphamide (120 mg/kg). This modified total body irradiation regimen was delivered by a linear accelerator in 1.5 Gy fractions with lung and liver shielding. After radiation electron beams were given to rib areas that were shielded [12]. Busulfan was administered orally in four divided doses daily for 3,5 days (day -8 to -5) and cyclophosphamide 60 mg/kg was given intravenously over 1 hour for 2 days (day -3 and -2). Phenytoin was

Table 1. Characteristics and outcome of patients with multiple myeloma after allogeneic stem cell transplantation

Patient	Sex	Age	Stage	Pretransplant regimens	Status at transplant	Conditioning regimen	Time from Dx to trans-plant (months)	Response to transplant	Response to DLI	Follow-up (months)
1	F	47	IIIA	7x MP/5xVAD	2.PR	TMI/BU/CY	16	CR	-	CR 27+
2	M	42	IIA	6xVAD	1.PR	TMI/BU/CY	12	PR	CR	CR 43+
3	F	47	IIA	18xMP	3.PR	TMI/BU/CY	58	-	-	Died:organ-failure day13
4	F	42	IIIA	4xMP/3xVAD	2.PR	BU/CY	13	PR	None	Alive with disease: 61+
5	M	45	IIIA	4xVAD	1.PR	TMI/BU/CY	8	PR	PR	DLI after PD: Alive in PR 50+
6	M	53	IIA	14xVCAP	2.PR	TMI/BU/CY	24	CR	-	CR 18+
7	M	49	IIIA	7xVCAP/1xMP	1.PR	BU/CY	10	PR	CR	CR after DLI: CR 18+
8	M	41	IIIB	4xVAD/2xCyclo	1.PR	TMI/BU/CY	12	CR	-	CR 60+
9	M	42	IIA	4xID	1.PR	TMI/BU/CY	6	PR	-	PR 22+
10	M	29	IIIA	4xVAD	m.R.	TMI/BU/CY	8	PR	-	PD, alive27+
11	M	50	IIA	4xID	1.PR	TMI/BU/CY	12	-	-	Died GvHD day 43
12	M	43	IIA	4xID	1.PR	BU/CY	14	CR	-	CR 5+

given to prevent busulfan induced seizure until 2 days after stopping busulfan. Uroepithelial prophylaxis was achieved with hyperhydration and mesna. Bone marrow or peripheral blood stem cells were infused 24–48 h after the last cyclophosphamide administration (day 0).The stem cell source was bone marrow in 10 patients, and peripheral blood stem cells in 2 patients. Regimen related toxicity was graded using the Bearman score [13]. The maximum score for each organ system was recorded. Atempts were made to exclude toxicities due to GVHD from the therapy-related toxicity. Veno-occlusive disease of the liver was graded according the Seattle criteria [14].

GvHD Prophylaxis

Rabbit anti-thymocyte-globulin (Fresenius, Bad Homburg, Germany) was given to all patients within the preparative regimen. 11 patients received a dose of 30 mg/kg over 12 hours on day -3, -2 and –1, and 1 patients received a dose of ATG of 30 mg/kg on day -3. Further GvHD prophylaxis consisted of cyclosporine A, 3 mg/kg, given from day –1 to six months post transplantation. The dose of cyclosporine A was adjusted to cyclosporine A dose level. Cyclosporine A was tapered from day 84 and discontinued at day 180. Methotrexate (10 mg/m^2) was given on day 1, 3 and 6 post transplantation. The standard criteria were used for acute and chronic GvHD [15].

Definition of Response

Complete Response (CR) was defined as lower 5% of plasma cells with normal morphology in bone marrow aspirate and the absence of monoclonal protein on serum electrophoresis and immunofixation analysis, and in case of Bence Jones (BJ) proteinuria by its disappearance in 24 hour urine. A partial response (PR) was defined as decrease of at least 50% of serum paraprotein level or of BJ protein in the urine. Patients with less than partial response were defined as minor responder (mR). An increase of paraprotein > 25% was termed progressive disease and relapse as paraprotein reappearance and/or marrow infiltration.

Results

Engraftment

No graft failure was observed. The median time to reach the leukocyte count of 1.0 x10^9/l was 16 days (range, 11 –5). Platelet count > 20 x10^9/l with platelet transfusion independence was reached at a median of 26 days (range, 16–52)

GvHD

3 patients developed grade I acute GvHD, and grade II–IV acute GvHD occurred in 3 patients (27% percent). Severe grade III and IV GvHD was seen in only 1 patient, who died from acute GvHD. Chronic GvHD was evaluated in 10 patients who survived day 80 post BMT. The incidence of chronic GvHD was only 20 percent, and of these had a limited disease. However, two patients who received DLI for further tumor regression developed acute GvHD grade II and III, respectively and one of them experienced extensive GvHD, and required further immunosuppression consisting of prednisone or cyclosporine A.

Treatment-related toxicity

Major toxicity was mucositis. Grade II according to the Bearman score was noted in 10 patients, whereas 2 patients experienced grade III , requiring prophylactic intubation. Both patients were treated with TMI, cyclophosphamide and busulfan 12 and 9 mg/kg, respectively. Liver toxicity grade II was seen in 6 patients, grade I in 2 patients, whereas 4 patients did not experience liver toxicity. One patient developed EBV associated lymphoma, which resolved completely after anti- CD 20 therapy and T-cell infusion. One patient died of severe GvHD grade IV and one developed multiorgan failure on day +13, resulting in a treatment related mortality of 17%.

Response to BMT

A complete response after allogeneic transplantation was seen in 4 patients (40%), while 6 patients were in partial remission. Two of the patients with partial remission received donor lymphocyte infusion for further tumor reduction 8 and 14 months after stem cell transplantation, and converted to complete remission, which increased the rate of complete remission up to 60%.

Overall and progression-free survival

After a median follow-up of 25 months (range, 5–62), the estimated overall survival at three years for all patients is 83 percent (CI 95%: 68%–98%). The estimated progression-free survival at three years is 61 percent (CI 95%: 32%–90%). The Kaplan-Meier survival curves for overall and event-free survival are shown in Figure 1 and 2. No patient with CR after allogeneic transplantation relapsed during follow-up, while 3 out of 6 patients with only PR after transplantation experienced progress within 3 years ($p=0.07$) (Fig. 3). Two patients with P.R after allogeneic transplantation (positive immunofixation) received a donor lymphocyte infusion (1.5×10^8 and 1×10^7 CD3+ cells/kg) 8 and 14 months after transplanatation, respectively. Both patients developed acute (grade II or III) and chronic GvHD, which resolved after steroid and cyclosporine treatment. Both

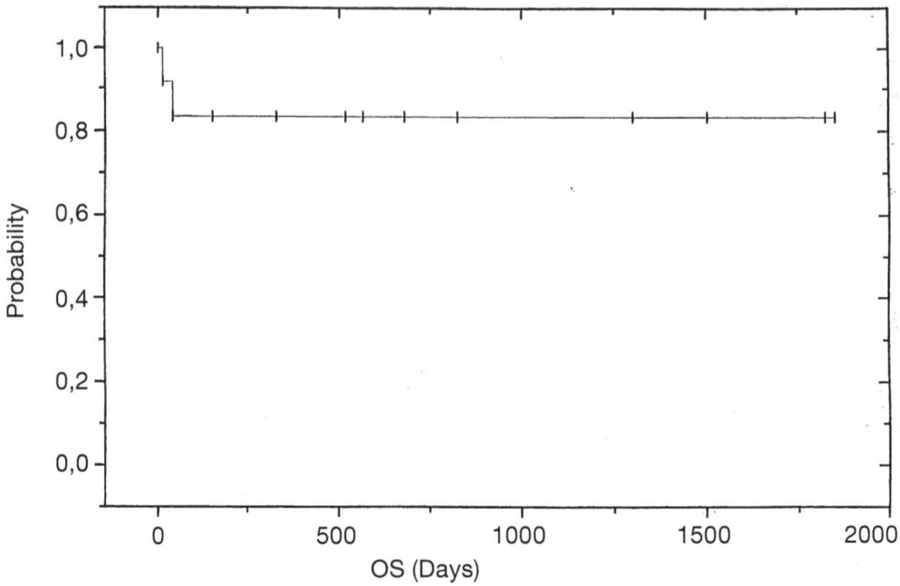

Fig. 1. Overall survival of all patients

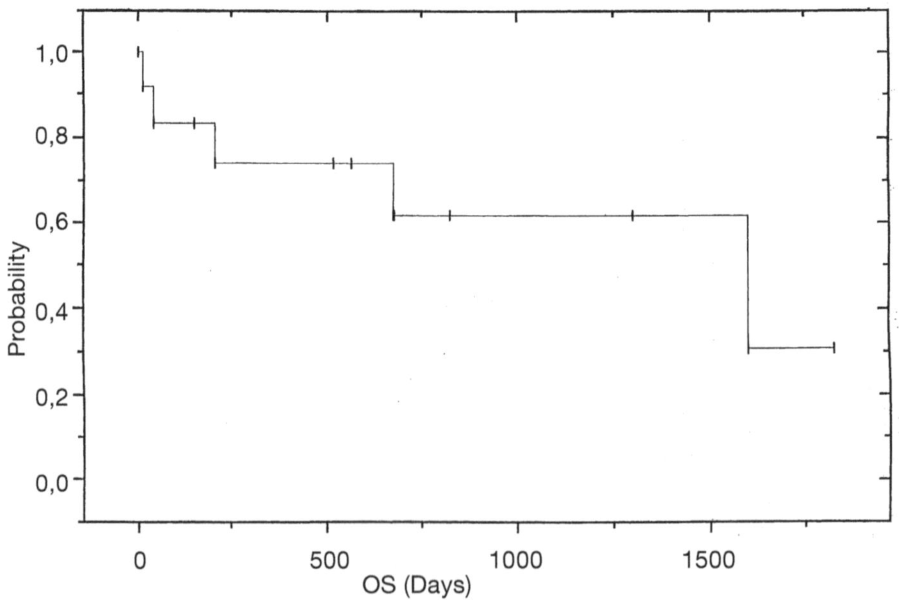

Fig. 2. Event-free survival of all patients

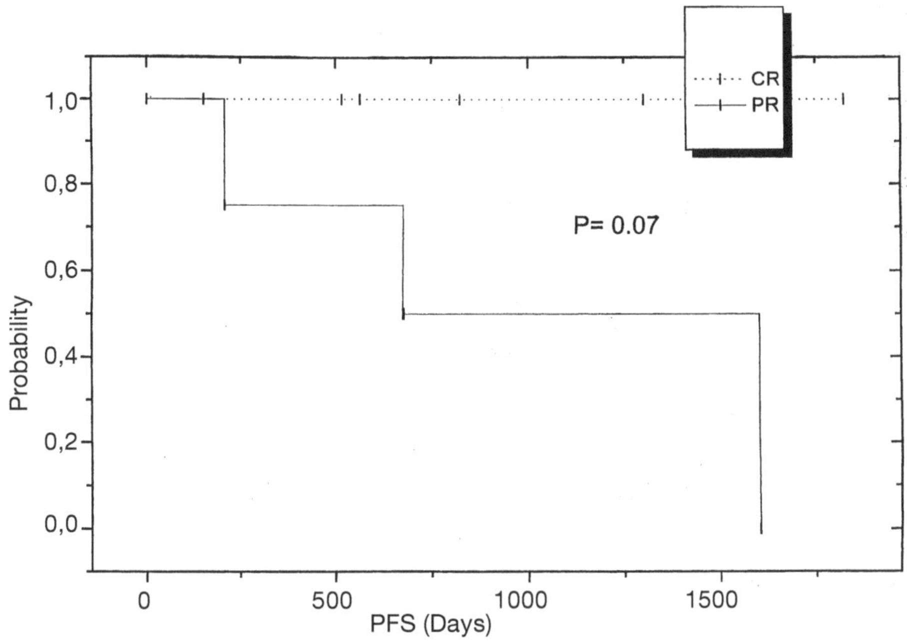

Fig. 3. Progression-free survival of patients with CR or PR after allogeneic transplantation

patients converted from PR to CR after 3 and 4 months, respectively. Two patients with relapse received donor lymphocye infusion (3 x10^7 CD3+ cells/kg). One patients did not respond, the second patient experienced a second PR with limited chronic GvHD.

Discussion

Allogeneic stem cell transplantation is probably the only curable approach in treatment of patients with multiple myeloma. Despite the higher rate of complete remissions and a lower rate of relapse in comparison to autologous transplantation, the treatment related mortality of 35 to 57% reported by the EBMT [5], by the Societe Francaise [16] and by the Seattle group [12] makes the role of allogeneic stem cell transplantation in multiple myeloma heavily disputed. The high treatment related mortality is mainly due to heavily pretreated or refractory patients and to the developement of severe graft versus host disease. Therefore, studies with earlier transplantation, PBSC as stem cell source or T-cell depletion for GvHD prevention resulted in a lower treatment related mortality of about 20% [7, 9]. A recently performed analysis of the EBMT also showed a lower transplant related mortality (20%) for patients transplanted after 1995 in comparison to the patients transplanted before 1995 (40%) [10]. Because of the proven graft versus myeloma effect [3,4], T-cell depletion resulted in less GvHD but higher relapse rate [9]. Our group and others [11,17–19] showed that anti-thymocyte globulin (ATG) as part of the conditioning regimen resulted in a low incidence of severe GvHD without obvious increase of relapse in unrelated stem cell transplantation. Therefore, the first aim of our study was to lower TRM by avoiding severe GvHD. We incorparated ATG in the preparative regimen of modified total body irradiation, busulfan and cyclophosphamide or busulfan and cyclophosphamide. ATG consists of rabbit immunoglobulins. After immunization with cells from a T lymphoblast cell line (Jurkat T cell line), this highly purified immunoglobulin consists of antibodies exerting a direct effect towards lymphoblastic T cells resulting in a T cell depletion via opsonisation and lysis following complement activation. Pharmacokinetic studies of ATG using ELISA techniques and an inhibitory effect on phytohaemagglutinin-induced blastogenesis showed a dose dependent effect of ATG. Rabbit IgG was detectable at least four weeks after administration in the recipient of bone marrow, and the effect of the phytohaemagglutinin-response on normal mononuclear cells lasted up to four days post transplantation [20]. Therefore, the effect of ATG as part of the pretransplant conditioning regimen is likely to be an *in vivo* T cell effect on the donor bone marrow.

The incidence of grade II–IV acute GvHD in our study was only 27%, however one patient developed severe fatal acute grade IV GvHD. The incidence of chronic GvHD was similary low with only 20%. The toxicity of the conditioning regimen was mainly stomatits at least of grade II according the Bearman scale in all patients. Two patients experienced grade III toxicity requiring mechanic ventilation. Both patients died, one of multi organ failure and the other of severe GvHD, resulting in a treatment related mortality of 17%.

The second aim of the study was to achieve a high rate of complete remission which is associated with long term disease free survival [5, 12]. The modified total body irradiation with lung and liver shielding (total marrow irradiation) in combination with busulfan and cyclophosphamide was chosen after a high percentage of complete response was observed in a phase II trial followed by autologous transplantation [21]. 40% of our the patients achieved a complete remission after allogeneic transplantation, while the remaining patients achieved a partial remission. Two of the patients with partial remission received donor lymphocyte infusion for further tumor reduction and converted to continuous complete remission 12 and 28 months after DLI [22], which increased the rate of complete remission to 60%. No patient with CR but 3 out of 4 patients with partial remission experienced progress during follow-up, demonstrating the necessity of further tumor reduction by donor lymphocytes in patients with inomplete remission after allogeneic stem cell transplantation. However the toxicity of DLI with acute and chronic GvHD was considerable and further studies are required to define optimal T- cell dose.

The proven graft versus myeloma effect of allogeneic T-cells and the introduction of less toxic non-myeloablative conditioning regimens for allogeneic transplantation should offer new therapeutic approaches towards a better treatment of multiple myeloma.

We conclude that the conditioning regimen with modified TBI, busulfan and cyclophosphamide is able to induce a high CR rate after allogeneic stem cell transplantation and DLI should be administered in patients with incomplete response after transplantation. The incorporation of anti-thymocyte globulin may prevent severe GvHD without obvious increase of relapse.

Acknowledgement. We thank the staff of the BMT unit for providing excellent care of our patients and the medical technicians for their excellent work in the BMT laboratory.

References

1. Gahrton G, Tura S, Ljungman P et al.: Prognostic factors in allogenic bone marrow transplantation for multiple myeloma. J Clin Oncol 1995; 13: 1312-1322
2. Lokhorst HM, Schattenberg A, Cornelissen JJ, et al. Donor leukocyte infusions are effective in relapsed multiple myeloma after allogeneic bone marrow transplantation. Blood 1997; 90 (10): 4206-4211
3. Tricot G, Vesole DH, Jagannath S, et al. Graft versus myeloma effect: proof of a principle. Blood 1996;87:1196-1198
4. Verdonck L, Lokhorst HM, Dekker AW, et al. Graft versus myeloma effect in two cases. Lancet 1996;347:800-801
5. Björkstrand B, Ljungman P, Svensson H, et al. Allogeneic bone marrow transplanation vs autologous stem cell transplantation in multiple myeloma: a retrospective case matched study from the European Group for Blood and Marrow Transplantation. Blood 1996; 88:4711-4718
6. Reece DE, Shepherd JD, Klingemann HG et al. Treatment of myeloma using intensive therapy and allogeneic bone marrow transplantation. Bone Marrow Transplant 1995; 15: 117-123
7. Majolino I, Corradini P, Scime R, et al. Allogeneic transplanation of unmanipulated peripheral blood stem cells in patients with multiple myeloma. Bone Marrow Transplant 1998; 22: 449-455
8. Anderson KC, Andersen J, Soiffer R, et al. Monoclonal antibody purged bone marrow transplanatation therapy for multiple myeloma. Blood 1993; 82: 2568-2576
9. Schlossman RL, Webb I, Alyea EP, et al. Similar disease free survival after allografting and autografting for multiple myeloma. Blood 1997; 10: (Suppl 1) 994
10. Gahrton G, Svenson H, Apperley J, et al.: Progress in allogeneic hematopoietic stem cell transplantation for multiple myeloma. Bone Marrow Transplant 2000; 25 (Suppl 1): 140
11. Kröger N, Zabelina T, Krüger W, et al. Anti-Thymocyte-Globulin as part of the preparative regimen prevents acute and chronic Graft versus Host disease (GvHD) in allogeneic stem cell transplantation from unrelated donors. Annals of Hematology 2000 (in press)
12. Bensinger W, Buckner CD, Anasetti C, et al. Allogeneic marrow transplantation for multiple myeloma: an analysis of risk factors on outcome. Blood 1996; 88:2787-2793
13. Bearman SI, Appelbaum FR, Buckner CD, et al. Regimen related toxicity in patients undergoing bone marrow transplantation. J Clin Oncol 1988; 6:1562-68
14. McDonald GB, Hinds MS, Fisher LD, et al. Veno-occlusive disease of the liver and multiorgan failure after bone marrow transplantation: a cohort study of 355 patients. Ann Intern Med 1993; 118:255-267
15. Przepiorka KM, Weisdorf D, Martin P. 1994 Consensus Conference on acute GvHD-grading. Bone Marrow Transplantat, 1995; 15, 825-828
16. Marit G, Facon T, Jouet JP, et al. Allogeneic stem cell transplantation in multiple myeloma: a report of the Societe Francaise de Greffe de Moelle. Blood 1997;10 (Suppl 1) 996
17. Kolb HJ, Holler E, Knabe H, et al. Conditioning treatment with Antithymocyte Globulin (ATG) modifies Graft-vs-Host Disease in recipients of marrow from unrelated donors. Blood 1995; 86; (Suppl 1): 952a
18. Finke J, Bertz H, Kunzmann R, et al. Allogeneic transplantation from unrelated donors: improved outcome using in vivo T-cell depletion. Blood 1997; 90 (Suppl1): 451
19. Zander AR, Zabelina T, Kröger N, et al. Use of a five-agent GvHD prevention regimen in recipients of unrelated donor marrow. Bone Marrow Transplantation 1999; 23:889-893
20. Eiermann TH, Lambrecht P, Zander AR. Monitoring anti-thymocyte globulin (ATG) in bone marrow recipients. Bone Marrow Transplantation 1999; 23: 779-781

21. Einsele H, Bamberg M, Zander AR, Kröger N, et al. Total marrow irradiation (TMI), busulfan and cyclophosphamide followed by PBSCT in patients with multiple myeloma. Blood 1998; 92 (Suppl 1) 516
22. Kröger N, Krüger W, Renges H, et al. Donor lymphocyte infusion enhances remission status in patients with persistent disesase after allografting for multiple myeloma. British Journal of Haematolgy 2000 (in press)

Stem Cell Mobilisation, Processing and Characteristics

A „Single" Delayed Application of G-CSF after Autologous Peripheral Blood Stem Cell Transplantation - A Pilot Study

E. Faber, R. Knotková, J. Zapletalová, L. Dušková, J. Kempná, J. Kujícková, Z. Pikalová, Z. Tauber, and K. Indrák

Department of Haemato-oncology, University Hospital Olomouc, I.P.Pavlova 6, CZ 775 20 Olomouc, Czech Republic

Introduction

The engraftment after autologous peripheral blood stem cell transplantation (APBSCT) is influenced by several factors. Among these quality of the graft, scheme used for conditioning, intensity of previous chemo and radiotherapy, diagnosis and age of the patients (PAT) were found to be of importance. The use of growth factors (GF) at the harvesting and after APBSCT could have an impact on the recovery of neutrophils (Lowenthal et al. 1998). However, the exact role of GF after APBSCT is not fully established. They could speed up the recovery of neutrophils by 2–6 days but their influence on neutropenia-related complications (incidence of infection, duration of fever, antibiotic treatment and hospitalization as well as cost-effectiveness) is less well defined (Klumpp et al. 1995, Ojeda et al. 1999, Tarella et al. 1998). Moreover, the optimal schedule for post-transplant application of GF is unknown. We performed a pilot study in order to investigate the safety and the efficacy of delaying the initiation of GF after APBSCT to the point when first neutrophils appear in peripheral blood.

Methods

G-CSF (filgramostim or lenograstim) application after APBSCT in PAT with nonHodgkins (NHL) and Hodgkins lymphoma (HL) was evaluated. GF in the study group were applied from the time neutrophil count reached $0{,}1 \times 10^9/l$. The study group was compared with historical controls who were treated according to the „individual" schedule of GF application - GF were started after the decline of neutrophils under the level of $0{,}5 \times 10^9/l$ (Cetkovský et al. 1997). In both groups GF were applied subcutaneously once a day. There were 4 PAT with HL and 6 PAT with NHL (3 diffuse, 2 follicular and 1 mantle cell) in the study group, while 5 with HL and 5 PAT with NHL (2 diffuse, 2 follicular and 1 marginal zone). Except two PAT in the study group and one PAT in the control group all were in clinical stage III or IV at the diagnosis. Two PAT in the study group had stable disease at the time of APBSCT, all the other PAT were in partial or complete remission. In the study group 3 PAT and in the control group 4 PAT had bone marrow involvement at the time of diagnosis. 3 PAT in the study group and 2 of the controls were irradiated before APBSCT. With one exception (CEI) all PAT were conditioned

Table 1. Characteristics of the patients and grafts.

	Study group	Significance p	Control group
Age: me (range)	43,5 (21–55)	0,87	36,5 (21–63)
Number of previous chemotherapy cycles: me (range)	8 (6–13)	0,69	7 (2–15)
Number of CD34+ cells $x10^6$/kg in the graft: me (range)	8,5 (3,6–27,1)	0,44	10,5 (4,37–45,6)
Number of MNC $x10^8$/kg in the graft: me (range)	2,0 (0,66–7,71)	**0,017**	5,5 (2,64–18,58)

with BEAM chemotherapy. All other information about the PAT is in Table 1. T-test was used for statistical evaluation.

Results

No significant difference between the study and the control group was found with respect to the age, number of previous chemotherapy cycles and the CD 34+ cells content of the grafts. There were significantly more mononuclear cells in the grafts of PAT in the control group (p=0,017). The comparison of CFU-GM was not possible because of different methods used in the PAT.

Table 2. Characteristics of the clinical course, engraftment and complications after APBSCT.

	Study group	Significance p	Control group
Neutropenia <0,5x10⁹/l, days, me (range)	9 (4–10)	**0,003**	6 (5–8)
Engraftment of neutrophils >0,5x10⁹/l, day after APBSCT, me (range)	12 (9–16)	**0,002**	9 (8–11)
Engraftment of platelets >50x10⁹/l, day after APBSCT, me (range)	13 (8–20)	0,64	15 (9–20)
Hospitalization in days, me (range)	20 (18–24)	0,34	21 (17–32)
Febrile days, me (range)	1 (0–6)	0,22	2 (0–8)
Days with iv antibiotics	2,5 (0–11)	0,11	7,5 (0–23)
Dose of G-CSF ug/kg, me (range)	4,15 (2,88–6,58)	0,13	4,9 (2,5–9)
Day of the first application of G-CSF after APBSCT, me (range)	11 (8–15)		3 (2–8)
Duration of G-CSF days, me (range)	1 (1–2)	**0,00001**	7 (3–12)
Dose of G-CSF ug, me (range)	300 (263–789)	**0,00002**	3120 (1365–4800)

The groups were compared with respect to the duration of neutropenia, engraftment of neutrophils and platelets, duration of fever, antibiotic treatment and duration of hospitalization. Significant differences were confirmed in the duration of neutropenia and engraftment of neutrophils only (Table 2). Moreover, the amount of G-CSF was significantly reduced in the study group (p=0,00002). In 6 PAT in the study group a single vial of G-CSF was sufficient to induce the complete recovery of neutrophils within 24 hours. In the rest of the PAT 1 or 2 more applications were needed to induce the recovery within 48 hours. Duration of hospitalization and antibiotic treatment was influenced by different strategies used in the transplant unit at the times when PAT of both groups were treated.

Discussion

G-CSF acts in granulocyte line from the level of determined precursors to mature granulocytes. Its action influences the proliferation, differentiation and maturation of cells. The time necessary for maturation of granulocytes is shortened from 5 to 1 day (Lord et al. 1989). The role of GF in stem cells harvesting and in the improvement of engraftment after autologous bone marrow transplantation has been clearly documented (Linch et al. 1993). Linch demonstrated that the shortening of the time necessary for achieving 1,0 x 10^9/l neutrophils with GF after autologous bone marrow transplantation was more prominent than that of the time necessary for achieving 0,5 x 10^9/l. Linch concluded that the effect of G-CSF is relatively low at the beginning of neutrophil regeneration. However, when the regeneration was initiated, the further application of GF accelerated the neutrophil count exponentially (Linch et al. 1993).

It is obvious, that the knowledge from clinical studies does not suffice to make definite recommendations for the use of GF after APBSCT. The studies performed until present were not comparable with respect to the schemes of dosing GF, age and diagnoses of PAT groups. Some trials were retrospective with only a limited number of PAT included. The addition of GF after APBSCT could speed up the recovery of neutrophils by 2–6 days (Klumpp et al. 1995, Ojeda et al. 1999). In some trials the shortening of hospitalization, reduction of antibiotics use and redution of cost were found (Klumpp et al. 1995, Tarella et al. 1998). In the randomized trial Ojeda confirmed the acceleration of engraftment but had not find any influence on neutropenia-related complications (incidence of infection, duration of fever, antibiotic treatment and hospitalization as well as cost-effectiveness) (Ojeda et al. 1999). In standard PAT with the graft containing more than 5 x 10^6 CD 34+ cells/kg of body weight the effect of GF applied after APBSCT could not be clinically significant (Ojeda et al. 1999).

Our retrospective study within the limited but highly homogenous PAT population demonstrated the clinical safety of the late start of GF after APBSCT. In the control group where GF were started according to the „individual" scheme (Cetkovský et al. 1997) the neutrophil engraftment was in median 2–3 days faster than in the study group. However, no difference between both groups was found with respect to the duration of hospitalization, days with fever, antibiotic use and platelet engraftment. On the other side, the amount of GF applied in the study group was significantly reduced. In 6 PAT the neutrophil count was normalized after single injection of G-CSF and in the rest of PAT 1 or 2 further applications sufficed for full neutrofil recovery. We conclude that the application of G-CSF after APBSCT could be probably safely delayed until the time when first neutrophils appear in the peripheral blood. Using „single" delayed schedule a significant reduction of GF amount could be achieved. The effectiveness of this approach needs to be determined in a prospective randomized trial comparing the standard schedule (start of G-CSF at day +5 after graft reinfusion) with the „single" schedule and the control group without the use of GF after PBSCT. This trial has already been initiated.

References

1. Cetkovský P, Koza V, Jindra P et al. (1997) Individual criteria could be optimal for starting G-CSF application after autologous stem cell transplantation. Bone Marrow Transplant 20: 639-641
2. Klumpp TR, Mangan KF, Goldberg SL et al. (1995) Granulocyte colony-stimulating factor accelerates neutrophil engraftment following peripheral-blood stem-cell transplantation: A prospective, randomized trial J Clin Oncol 13: 1323-1327
3. Linch DC, Scarffe H, Proctor S et al. (1993) Randomised vehicle-controlled dose-finding study of glycosylated recombinant human granulocyte colony-stimulating factor after bone marrow transplantation Bone Marrow Transplant 11: 307-311
4. Lord BI, Bronchud MH, Owens S, et al. (1989) The kinetics of human granulopoiesis following treatment with granulocyte colony-stimulating factor in vivo Proc Natl Acad Sci USA 86: 9499
5. Lowenthal RM, Faberes C, Marit G et al. (1998) Factors influencing haemopoietic recovery following chemotherapy-mobilised autologous peripheral blood progenitor cell transplantation for haematological malignancies: a retrospective analysis of a 10-year singly institution experience Bone Marrow Transplant 22: 763-770
6. Ojeda E, Garcia-Bustos J, Aguado MJ et al. (1999) A prospective randomized trial of granulocyte colony-stimulating factor theryp after autologous blood stem cell transplantation in adults. Bone Marrow Transplant 24: 601-607
7. Tarella C, Castellino C, Locatelli F et al. (1998) G-CSF administration followingy peripheral blood progenitor cell (PBPC) autograft in lymphoid malignancies: evidence for clinical benefits and reduction of treatment costs. Bone Marrow Transplant 21: 401-407

Factors Influencing PBPC Mobilisation and Collection in Haematological Malignancies

J. F. C. Marques Jr., A. C. Vigorito, I. Lorand-Metze, F. J. P. Aranha, G. B. Oliveira, E. C. M. Miranda, E. G. Roveri, and C. A. De Souza

Dept of Internal Medicine, Faculty of Medicine State University of Campinas-SP, Brasil

Introduction

Peripheral blood progenitor cells (PBPC), mobilised by several and collected in apheresis procedures are able to restore hemopoiesis after myeloablative, intensive chemotherapy. This has been currently used in the treatment of several solid tumours as well as haematological neoplasias. Several studies have show tha a safe threshold of PBPS, measured as CD34+ cells, in order to produce a prompt and durable engraftment of autologous marrow is that of 5 x 10^6 $CD34^+$ cells/kg recipient body weight. Values below lead to a risk for delayed peripheral blood count recovery or even engraftment failure [1]. Many factors affect the number of $CD34^+$ cells after mobilisation procedures, such as time from diagnosis to mobilisation, amount of previous chemotherapy regimens received by the patients, specially the cumulative dosis of alkylating agents and fludarabine [2–6].

The aim of the present work was to analyse factors concerning the mobilisation procedure as well as patient's characteristics that influenced the $CD34^+$ cell yield in patients with haematological malignancies that underwent autologous PBPC transplantation (BMT) at our Institution in the last 2 years.

Patients and Methods

Adult patients with confirmed diagnosis of lymphoma, multiple myeloma or chronic myeloid leukemia, treated at the Hematology-Hemotherapy Centre of the State University of Campinas and assigned to autologous BMT according to the Institution Protocols entred the study.

Patients were eligible when they below 60 years old, had a body weight above 30 kg, ECOG performance status 0–2, and normal cardiac, renal, pulmonary and hepatic function. Negative serology for HIV, HTLV-1, hepatites B and C were also requested. All patients gave informed consent.

Patients were mobilised using both chemotherapy and growth factors. Mobilisation chemotherapy was one of the following regimens: cyclophosphamide (CY) 4 g/m² or 7 g/m² [7], DHAP, mini-ICE; VP-16 2g/m². G-CSF or GM-CSF was given 5 mg/kg between day+1 after chemotherapy and the last apheresis.

Leukapheresis began when leukocytes (WBC) reached 1,0 x 10^9/l after nadir. They were made in an automated continous-flow blood cell seperator, collecting large volumes per procedure, in order to concentrate the apheresis during the days of peak of circulating CD34+ cells [8]. The aim was to collect a total of 5 x 10^6 CD34+ cells per kg of patient's body weight.

CD34+ cells were determined in peripheral blood and the apheresis product by a twoplatform protocol (Seattle modification) [9].

Statistical analysis: first we made a descriptive analysis. Then, parameters were adjusted to Gaussian distribution (by goodness-of-fit). Univariate analysis and multivariate analysis were made by ANOVA [10].

Results

During the period between January 1998 and August 1999, 41 consecutive patients were included in the study. The clinical features of the patients as well as the mobilisation regimens are described on Table 1. The majority of the patients had lymphoma. Eigtheen patients were mobilised in the setting of autologous BMT performed as consolidation of a front line chemotherapy.

In the 41 patients, a total of 115 apheresis procedure were performed (Median: 3 per patient, range: 1–6). Blood volume processed by procedure had a median of 9286 ml (4457–13929 ml); median time was 233 min (100–365 min). Final product volume per procedure was 341 ml (50–835 ml).

Table 1. Characteristics o patients and mobilisation regimen (n=41)

Characteristics	
Age-years (range)	35 (12–59)
Sex – (male/female)	26/15
Diagnosis	
non-Hodgkin's lymphoma	21 (51.2%)
Hodgkin's disease	15 (36.6)
Chronic myeloid leukaemia	2 (4.9%)
Multiple myeloma	3 (7.3%)
Previous CT* – median (range)	2 (1–4)
front line	18 (46.2%)
salvage	21 (58.3%)
Previous radiotherapy	27 (65.9%)
Marrow infiltration – number (%)	
non-Hodgkin's lymphoma	4 (19%)
Hodgkin's disease	2 (13.3%)
Mobilisation regimen	
Chemotherapy	
CY 7g/m²	24 (58.5%)
CY 4g/m²	13 (31.7%)
Others	4 (9.8%)
Growth factors	
G-CSF	25 (61%)
GM-CSF	16 (39%)

*excluding CML; CY: cyclophosphamide

Table 2. Clinical and biological mobilisation characteristics

	Median	Range
WBC > 1.0 x 10^9/L (days)*	12	7–19
Platelets > 20.0 x 10^9/L (days)*	10	0–30
Days to discharge ***	17	0–35
Leukapheresis procedures	3	1–6
CD34+ cells (x 10^6/KG) (total)	6.19	0.22–33.78
Nucleated cells (x 10^8/KG)	3.19	0.33–9.84
Mononuclear cells (x 10^8/KG)	1.39	0.16–7.5

* days after CT mobilisation; ** PRBC: packed red blood cells units; *** period between CT mobilisation and last leukapheresis procedure

Factors influencing $CD34^+$ cell yield.

Days to peripheral blood count recovery as well as characteristics of the leukapheresis product are described on Table 2. Eleven patients failed to collect the proposed target of $CD34^+$ cells/kg: 6/21 cases with non Hodgkin's lymphoma and 5/15 had Hodgkin's lymphoma. Their apheresis product had a smilar number of WBC per body weight but a higher number of mononuclear cells (1.25 x 2.13 $p=0.05$).

Age, diagnosis, previous radiotherapy and type of growth factor used in the mobilisation regimen showed no correlation with the number of days to WBC recovery and number of aphereses needed to achieve the target number of $CD34^+$ cells. Patients mobilised with CY 4g/m^2 recovered leukocyte counts in lesss days

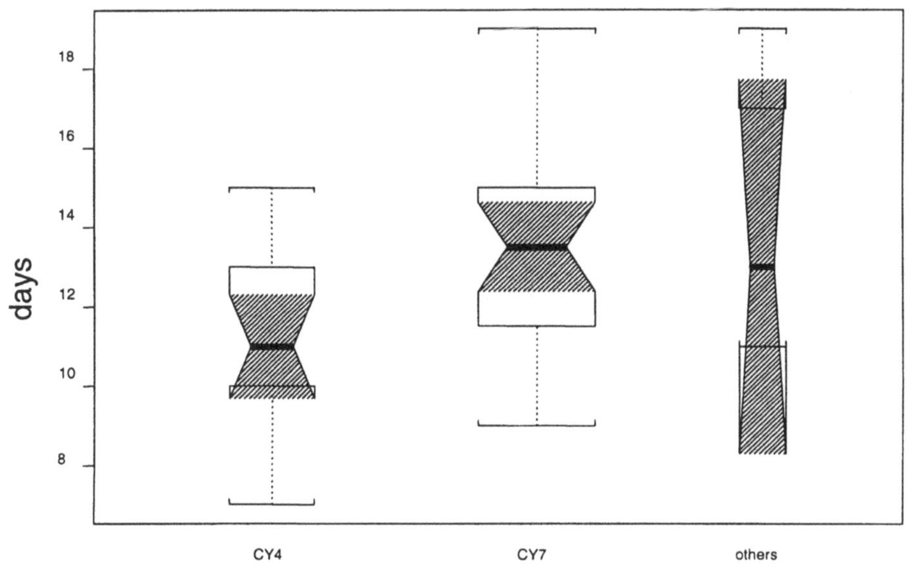

Fig. 1. Boxplot showing the described values of type of mobilisation chemotherapy and leukocyte recovery. The dashed area corresponds to the confidence interval of 95% for the median.

than those who used 7 g/m^2 (Fig. 1). In ANOVA, the number of days needed for leukocyte recovery was a function of the variables „number of aphereses“ and „type of mobilization chemotherapy“ (coefficients: 0.86 and 0.95 respectively). For the pairs of „number of aphereses“ and „days to leukocyte recovery“ a correlation coefficient of 0.36 was obtained. The jointed distribution of both gave a bivariated gaussian distribution.

Discussion and Conclusions

The present study suggests the feasibility to mobilize CD34$^+$ cells in patients that had previous chemotherapy for haematological malignancies. High doses of CY were well tolerated with mild toxicity and no-deaths as has been show by others [4, 7, 11]. The strategy to collect a high volume per apheresis in few procedures was also well tolerated and permitted a good PBPC yield. We found a high interdependence among the number of days to WBC recovery, number of apheresis needed to collect the target number of PBPC and the mobilisation chemotherapy regimen used. Therefore, patients who achieve 1,0 x 10^6 leucocytes in less days have a high probability to have a good CD34$^+$ cell yield with few aphereses.

References

1. Kiss JE, Rybka WB, Winkelstein A et al. (1997) Relationship of CD34$^+$ cell dose to early and late hematopoiesis following autologous peripheral blood stem cell transplantation. Bone Marrow Transplantation 19:303-310
2. Bensinger W, Appelbaum F, Rowley S, Storb R, Sanders J, Lilleby K, Gooley T, Demirer T, Schiffman K, Weaver C, Clift R, Chauncey T, Klarnet J, Montgomery P, Petersdorf S, Weiden P, Witherspoon R, & Buckner C D (1995) Factors that influence collection and engraftment of autologous peripheral-blood stem cells. J. Clin Oncol 13: 2547-2555
3. Ketterer N, Salles G, Moullet I, Dumontet C, ElJaafari-Corbin A, Tremisi P, Thieblemont C, Durand B, Neidhardt-Berard E, Samaha H, Rigal D, Coiffier B (1998) Factors associated with successful mobilisation of peripheral blood progenitor cells in 200 patients with lymphoid malignancies. Brit J Haematol 103: 235-242
4. Gandhi M K, Jestice K, Scott M A , Bloxham D, Bass G, Marcus R E (1999) The minimum CD34 threshold depends on prior chemotherapy in autologous peripheral blood stem cell recipients. Bone Marrow Transplantation 23: 9-13
5. Goldschmidt H, Hegenbart U, Haas R, Hunstein W (1996) Mobilisation of peripheral blood progenitor cells with high-dose cyclophosphamide (4 or 7 g/m^2) and granulocyte colony-stimulating factor in patients with multiple myeloma. Bone Marrow Transplantation 17: 691-697
6. Bolwell B, Gootmastic M, Yanssens T et al. (1994) Comparison of G-CSF with GM-CSF for mobilising peripheral blood progenitor cells and for anhancing marrow recovery after autologous bone marrow transplant. Bone Marrow Transplantation 14: 913-918
7. Santini G, De Souza C, Congiu AM, Nati S, Marino G, Soracco M, Sertoli MR, Rubagotti A, Spriano M, Vassalo F, Rossi E, Vimercati R, Piaggio G, Figari O, Benvenuto F, Abate M, Truini M, Ravetti JL, Ribizzi I, Damasio E (1999) High-dose cyclophosphamide followed by autografting can improve the outcome of relapsed or resistant non-Hodgkin's lymphomas with involved or hypoplastic bone marrow. Leuk Lymphoma 33: 321-330
8. Krause DS, Mechanic SA, Snyder EL (1997) Mobilisation and Collection of peripheral blood progenitor cells. In: McLeod BC, Price TH, Drew MJ, eds Apheresis: Principles and practice. Bethesda, MD: AABB Press.

9. Sutherland DR, Keating A, Nayar R et al (1994) Sensitive detection and enumeration of $CD34^+$ cells in peripheral and cord blood by flow cytometry. Experim Hematol 22: 110-1110
10. Rao Calyampudi Radhakrishna (1995) Linear models: least squares and alternatives. New York (352p). Springer series in statistics
11. DeLuca E, Sheridan WP, Watson D, Szer J, Begley, CG (1992) Prior chemotherapy does not prevent effective mobilisation by G-CSF of peripheral blood progenitor cells. Brit JCancer 66: 893-899

Successful Purging of Stem Cell Products Using CD34 Selection

St. A. Grupp[1], S. Ash[2], J. Donovan[2], J. Temel[2], A. Zuckerman[2], J. Fang[1], G. Pierson[1], A. Ross[3], L. Diller[4], and J. Gribben[2]

[1]Department of Pediatrics, Division of Oncology, Children's Hospital of Philadelphia, University of Pennsylvania, School of Medicine, Philadelphia, PA; [2]Department of Adult Oncology, Dana-Farber Cancer Institute, Boston, MA; [3]Department of Pediatric Oncology, Dana-Farber Cancer Institute and Department of Medicine, Children's Hospital, Boston, MA; [4]Diagnostics Division, Nexell Therapeutics, Inc. Irvine, CA

Abstract

Purging of tumor cells from stem cell products used to support autologous transplant procedures to treat solid tumors may decrease the risk of relapse. Concerns have been raised about the use of the only widely available technique for stem cell purging, CD34 selection, for purging products collected from patients with neuroblastoma (NB), largely because of reports of detection of low levels of CD34 on the surface of some NB cell lines and tumors. We have used 3 approaches to address the issue of purging of NB from stem cell specimens and possible CD34 labeling of NB.

1. *Flow cytometric detection of CD34 on NB cell lines.* We assessed CD34 expression using a panel of anti-CD34 monoclonal antibodies including 9C5, 12.8 and QBend10 and showed no increase in labeling over secondary-only control.
2. *Spiking experiments with the Isolex 50 system.* NB cell lines were used to contaminate aliquots of stem cell collections, after which the products were purified using the Isolex 50. Purging of NB was assessed by quantitative multiplex RT-PCR (Taqman system) using a tumor-specific transcript, GAGE. We demonstrated >2 logs of tumor cell depletion from these specimens.
3. *Analysis of clinical specimens.* Stem cell pre- and post-CD34 selection were analyzed from patients treated on a tandem transplant trial for NB. In nine specimens selected using the Ceprate LC CD34 selection system where tumor was detectable by immunocytochemistry pre-selection, we observed >2.4 to >4.6 logs of NB purging after selection. We then analyzed 23 aliquots of stem

---

This research was supported in part by the University of Pennsylvania Cancer Center (SG), by the Benacerraf/Frei Clinical Investigator Award, Dana-Farber Cancer Institute (LD) and the Fiftieth Anniversary Program for Scholars in Medicine, Harvard Medical School (LD).

The abbreviations used are: FITC, fluorescein isothiocyanate; GAPDH, Glyceraldehyde 3 phosphate dehydrogenase; ICC, immunocytochemistry; MoAbs, monoclonal antibodies; PE, phycoerythrin; RT-PCR, reverse transcriptase-polymerase chain reaction; PBMC, peripheral blood mononuclear cells.

cells infused into patients post-CD34 selection and compared to the product pre-selection. 20/23 specimens showed depletion of NB, although some level of GAGE message was observed in most post-CD34 selection specimens.

These data show that purging of NB from stem cells using CD34 selection is feasible, yielding infused products that are negative at the level of ICC but often positive at the level of RT-PCR.

Introduction

High-dose chemotherapy with stem cell rescue has been shown to improve outcome in patients with high-risk neuroblastoma (NB) [1]. One of the potential limitations of this approach is the possibility that tumor cells may contaminate the stem cell product. Although no clinical trial in autologous transplantation has shown a survival advantage for patients who received stem cell products purged of tumor cells, there is indirect evidence that tumor purging of stem cell products may improve outcome in NB. Gene-marked tumor cells infused with autologous marrow have been found at sites of relapse, suggesting that NB inadvertently collected with autologous marrow can be clonogenic [2]. In other diseases such as lymphoma, patients who receive stem cells in which tumor cannot be detected have a better outcome[3], but whether this phenomenon is due to fewer tumor cells in the stem cell product used to support the therapy or more successful treatment of the disease in the patient is unclear.

A variety of disease or even patient-specific techniques to purge stem cell products of tumor have been developed, depending on recognition of tumor cells to remove them from the product. These approaches are referred to as negative selection. Another, more general approach has been termed positive selection, in which stem and progenitor cells required for both rapid and durable engraftment are purified from the stem cell product. The principal method used for positive selection is selection for the antigen CD34, which is expressed on hematopoietic stem and progenitor cells. CD34 selection devices select for and purify $CD34^+$ cells [4], yielding 2–3 log depletion of $CD34^-$ cells, including possible contaminating tumor cells [5]. This method is appropriate for purging of tumor types which do not express CD34 (including most solid tumors), but not for malignancies which may express CD34 (such as leukemias). CD34 selection has been used to purge stem cell products in patients with neuroblastoma, but concerns have been raised that some NB cells or cell lines may express CD34 or express surface epitopes that cross-react with monoclonal antibodies (MoAbs) that recognize CD34 [6, 7]. In order to further characterize the potential utility of CD34 selection in NB, we have examined the issue of CD34 expression on NB. Using immunocytochemistry (ICC) as well as quantitative RT-PCR detection of tumor-specific RNAs, we demonstrate tumor cell depletion of both NB cell lines and NB contaminating patient stem cell specimens.

Methods

Stem cell sources

Stem cells used in these studies were obtained from one of three sources. Clinical specimens were obtained after informed consent from patients enrolled on the Children's Hospital of Philadelphia/Dana Farber Cancer Institute study of tandem stem cell transplant for high risk NB (entitled CHP-594 or 94-131 at the respective institutions). Patients were eligible for this study if they were over one year of age with INSS Stage 4 [8] disease or INSS Stage 3 with *MYCN* amplification. Stem cell specimens from normal volunteer donors were provided by Nexell (Irvine, CA). For some of the preclinical studies, we utilized stem cell samples collected from patients who did not subsequently undergo transplantation, again after informed consent. Protocols and consent forms were approved by each participating hospital's institutional review board and informed consent was obtained from the parents of each child after the diagnosis was confirmed.

Stem Cell collections

Patients typically underwent their stem cell collection after the third cycle of induction chemotherapy[9]. Products intended for use were collected with a goal of 4×10^6/kg $CD34^+$ cells (minimum of 1×10^6/kg) available for each cycle of HDT/SCR. After cryopreservation of an aliquot of unselected stem cells as a backup, the first day's collection was held overnight and pooled with the second day's collection. The pheresis product then underwent $CD34^+$ selection using the Ceprate SC device (CellPro, Bothell, WA) or the Isolex 300i device (Nexell, Irvine, CA). Samples to assess for neuroblastoma contamination were cryopreserved from both the input and the selected populations.

Immunocytochemical detection of NB

Clinical samples of blood and bone marrow were analyzed by standard ICC at BIS Laboratories (Reseda, CA) using a cocktail of three antibodies specific for neuroblastoma as previously described [10]. Aliquots from daily stem cells collections also underwent high-sensitivity ICC analysis in studies to quantify tumor depletion and has been described elsewhere [9]. Briefly, an aliquot of pheresate was CD34 selected using the Ceprate LC laboratory CD34 selection column (CellPro, Bothell, WA). Both pre- and post-selection fractions were analyzed for NB by ICC in a slide-based assay using a cocktail of four antibodies which recognize NB cells (181.4, ERIC-1, UJ13A, and 5.1H11 [11]). Cell seeding experiments with the NB cell line CCL-127 have shown that this investigational ICC assay has a sensitivity of 10^{-5} to 10^{-6} (data not shown). The positive control CCL-127 line, negative control, pre-selection and post-selection specimens were independently interpreted by two investigators.

RT-PCR detection of NB

RNA was isolated using RNA-STAT-60 (Tel-Test, Friendswood, TX) according to manufacturer's recommendations. 2µg total RNA was reversed transcribed with Superscript II reverse transcriptase (Gibco-BRL, Gaithersburg, MD) and oligo dT primers (PE Biosystems, Foster City, CA). TaqMan PCR using GAGE and tyrosine hydroxylase specific primers and probes was performed in multiplex with primers and probes for GAPDH on an ABI PRISM 7700 sequence detector. The 50 µl quantification reactions contained 2 µl cDNA (10% of RT reaction), 5 µl 10X TaqMan Buffer A (500 mM KCl, 100 mM Tris-HCl, pH 8.3, PE Biosystems), 5 µl 25 mM $MgCl_{2,}$ 200 µM of each of dATP, dCTP, dTTP, dGTP, 1.25 U Platinum Taq DNA polymerase (Gibco BRL), and 100 nM TaqMan probe (PE Biosystems). Primer concentrations were optimized for multiplex PCR. Standard curves for quantification were produced by ten-fold serial dilution of plasmids containing GAGE, tyrosine hydroxylase and GAPDH cDNAs.

Flow cytometry

A panel of NB cell lines was used for these studies, including CHLA-90 and SK-N-RA (kind gift of Dr. P. Reynolds), IMR-5, SY5Y, CHP134 and NLF (kind gift of Dr. A. Evans), PCL 5078, PCL 1771, PCL 4030.2, PCL 4639, PCL 4903.2, PCL 5080, PCL 5282 and PCL 5424. The $CD34^+$ cell KG-1a was used as a CD34+ control. Anti-CD34 monoclonal antibodies (MoAbs) included biotin-12.8 (CellPro, Bothell, WA), 9C5 (Nexell, Irvine, CA), QBend10 (Miltenyi, Auburn, CA), HPCA-1 and HPCA-2 (Becton-Dickinson, San Diego, CA). A positive control for NB staining was provided by MoAb UJ13A (kind gift of Dr. J. Kemshead). These antibodies were detected with phycoerythrin (PE)-streptavidin (in the case of biotin-12.8) or PE- or fluorescein isothiocyanate (FITC)-labeled affinity purified goat anti-mouse IgG (Jackson Immunoresearch, Grove, PA). For staining, 0.3mg (UJ13A), 1 mg (CD34 MoAbs), or 20 mL (HPCA-1 and HPCA-2) of the primary antibody was added to $2x10^6$ cells for 20 min at 4°C, followed by washing and a further incubation with 4 mg of secondary label. Flow cytometry was performed on the FACS Calibur or the FACS Scan (Becton-Dickinson). Secondary-only control was performed for each cell line and fluorochrome.

Results

Detection of CD34 on NB cell lines

Labeling of NB cells with anti-CD34 MoAbs has been seen by one group [6,7], but not by another [13]. In order to further characterize labeling of multiple NB cell lines, we utilized antibodies that are currently used in the major CD34 selection systems, including 12.8 (used in the CellPro Ceprate device), 9C5 (used in the Nexell Isolex 300i) and QBend10 (Miltenyi CliniMACS), as well as MoAbs commonly used for CD34 enumeration (Becton-Dickson HPCA-1 and HPCA-2).

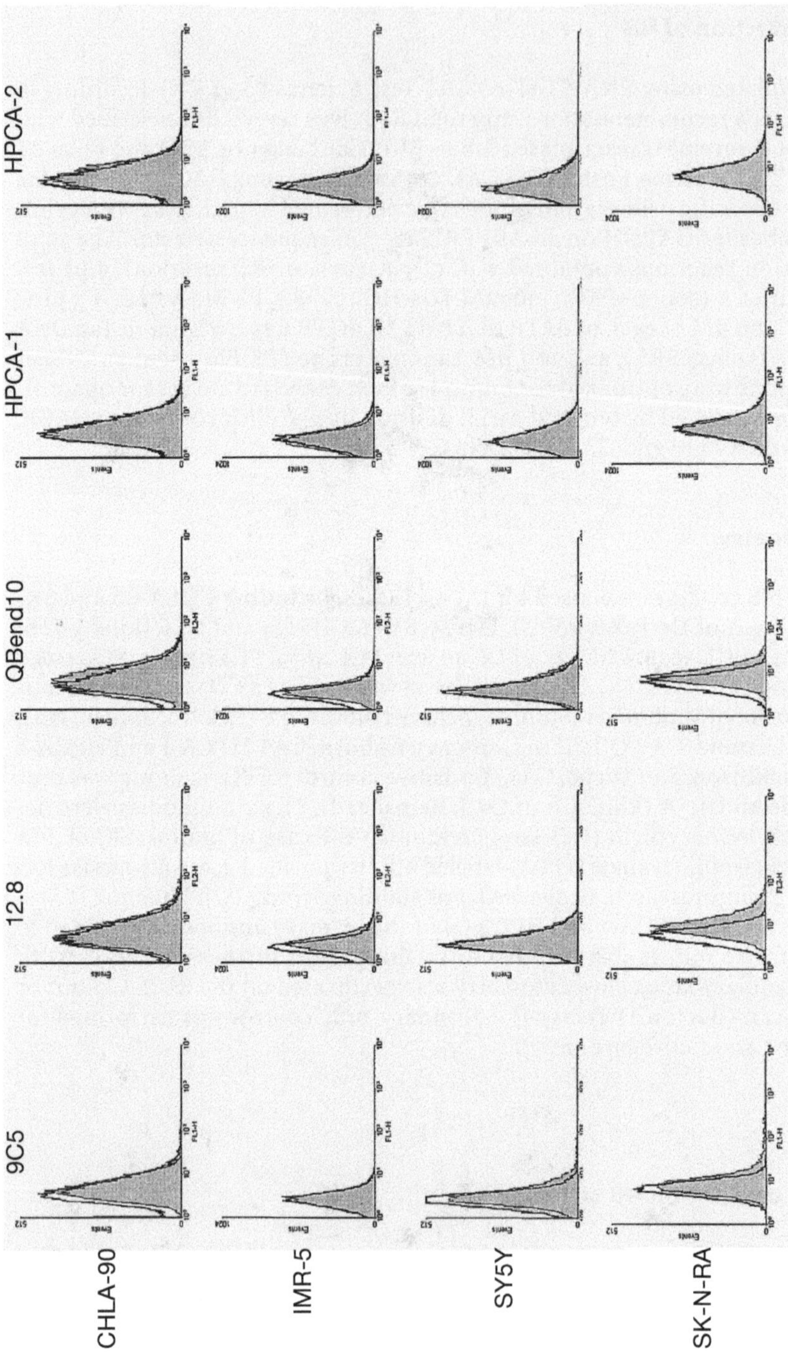

Fig. 1. Staining of NB cell lines by anti-CD34 MoAbs. The shaded curve represents the cell line stained with anti-CD34 plus secondary antibody, while the heavy open curve indicates staining with fluorochrome-conjugated secondary antibody (or streptavidin) alone. HPCA-1, HPCA-2 and 9C5 are mouse MoAb detected by FITC-anti-mouse IgG, 12.8 is biotinylated and detected by PE-streptavidin, and QBEND/10 is directly conjugated to PE.

Each of these MoAbs was detected by the appropriate FITC- or PE- labeled secondary antibody, with the exception of 12.8, which is biotinylated and was detected with PE-steptavidin. Figure 1 shows CD34 labeling of 4 NB cell lines with each of these MoAbs. There was no significant increase in labeling over secondary-only control seen in any of these NB lines using any of the anti-CD34 MoAbs (also demonstrated in two other NB lines, CHP-134 and NLF; data not shown). In order to choose appropriate titrations of the MoAbs and secondary antibodies, we employed as positive controls the CD34+ cell line KG-1a for CD34 staining as well as the anti-NB MoAb UJ13A as a positive control for NB cell line staining (Fig. 2A). Failure to gate out debris and nonviable cells on forward and side scatter resulted in low levels of nonspecific staining, as seen in Figure 2B.

Taqman quantitative RT-PCR assay

Prior experience with ICC detection of tumor cells showed that almost all stem cell products showed no detectable tumor by standard ICC (see below and [12]. We therefore developed a quantitative RT-PCR assay for tumor-specific transcripts

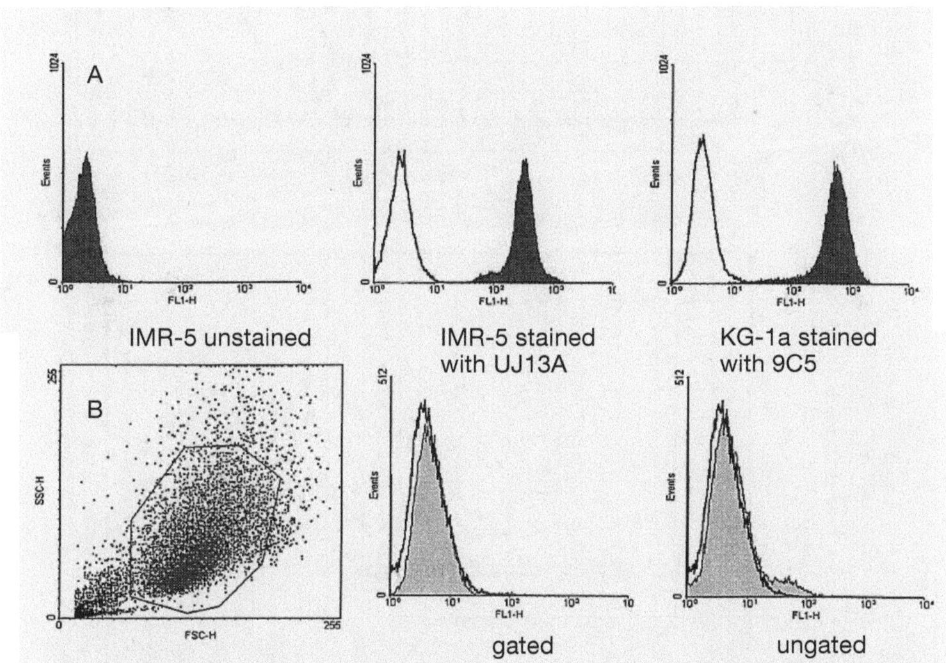

Fig. 2. Cytometric controls. The leftmost flow profile in panel A shows the NB cell line IMR-5 unstained. Positive staining of NB cells is demonstrated with the anti-NB MoAb UJ13A as well as positive labeling of the CD34+ cell line KG-1a with 9C5. Both stains utilize the same antibody titration and goat anti-mouse secondary antibody as Figure 1. Panel B demonstrates the effect of gating on labeling. The gating strategy is shown in the left dotplot. Then, staining of the whole cell population (right histogram) is compared to gated data which eliminates debris and nonviable cells (middle histogram).

using the ABI Prism 7770 (Taqman) sequence detector. Several candidate genes have been used in RT-PCR detection of neuroblastoma, including tyrosine hydroxylase [13, 14] and GAGE [15]. Initial work showed GAGE RT-PCR to be more sensitive in detecting low numbers of NB cells than tyrosine hydroxylase in this system (data not shown). As a result, we chose GAGE for NB detection in the subsequent RT-PCR experiments. 12/12 neuroblastoma cell lines tested for GAGE expression were positive (data not shown). Standard curves were developed to allow for quantitation by 10-fold serial dilution of plasmids containing GAGE and GAPDH (Glyceraldehyde 3 phosphate dehydrogenase) cDNA's (Fig. 3). Correla-

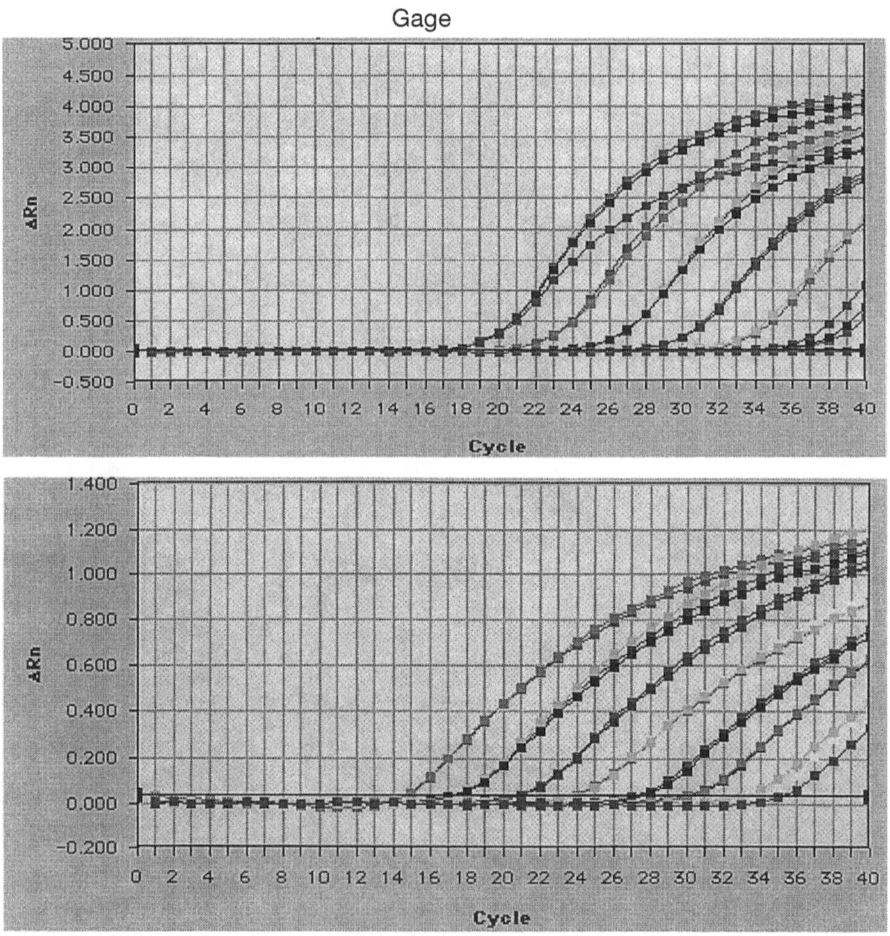

Fig. 3. Standard curves for quantitative RT-PCR. These curves were generated using samples produced by 10-fold serial dilution of plasmids containing GAGE and GAPDH cDNA. Amount of cDNA was quantitated using GAGE and GAPDH-specific probes and primers in the Taqman system. The upper plots show the amplification curves using GAGE and GAPDH. Ct data was then plotted (lower curves) and correlation coefficients calculated.

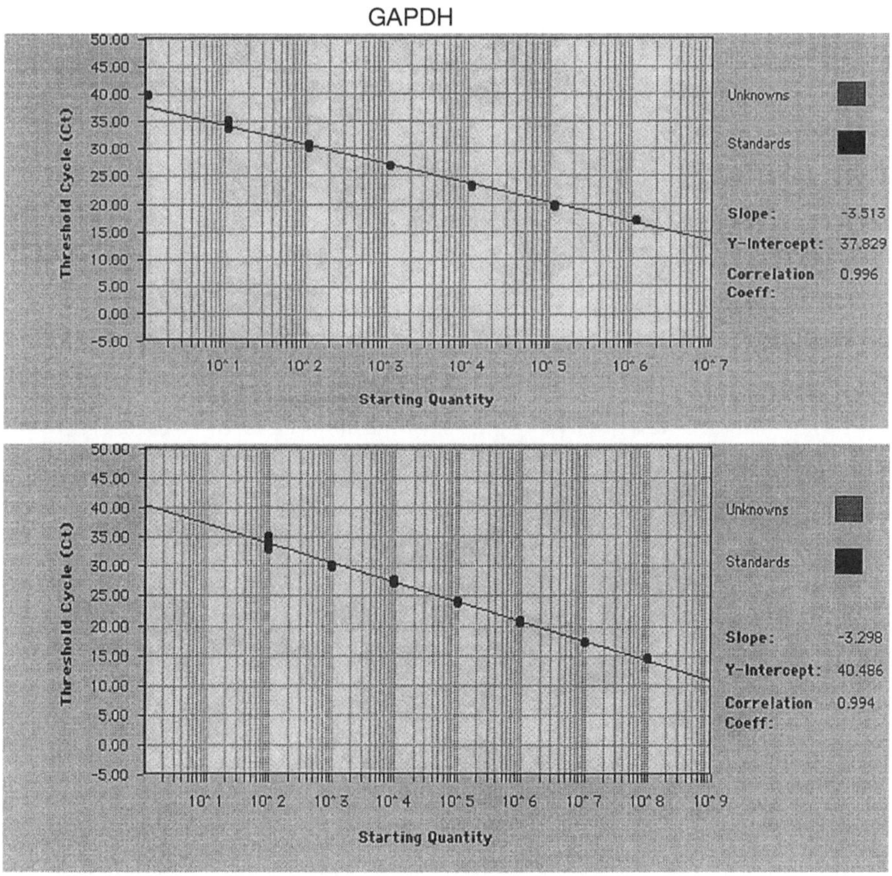

Fig. 3

tion coefficients were calculated from Ct data, r=.996 and .994 respectively) GAPDH was chosen as a housekeeping gene to allow for intra-specimen normalization. To assess the detection threshold using this assay, two cell lines (SKND2 and PCL 5078) were serially diluted into normal peripheral mononuclear cells (PBMC) with percent of NB cells in PBMC ranging from 100% to 0% (Fig. 4). The detection threshold was between 10^{-5} and 10^{-6} using this approach.

In order to demonstrate the reproducibility and intra-assay variability of this quantitative RT-PCR assay, SKND2 cells were diluted 100%, 1% AND 0.01% into PBMC. Seven replicates for each dilution were amplified in multiplex with GAGE and GAPDH (Fig. 5). Amplification curves at each dilution were very reproducible. To examine the inter-assay variability, serial dilutions of SKND2 into PBMC were subjected to quantitative multiplex assay with GAGE and GAPDH in triplicates on 3 separate days. There was no significant day-to-day variability ($p > 0.05$; data not shown).

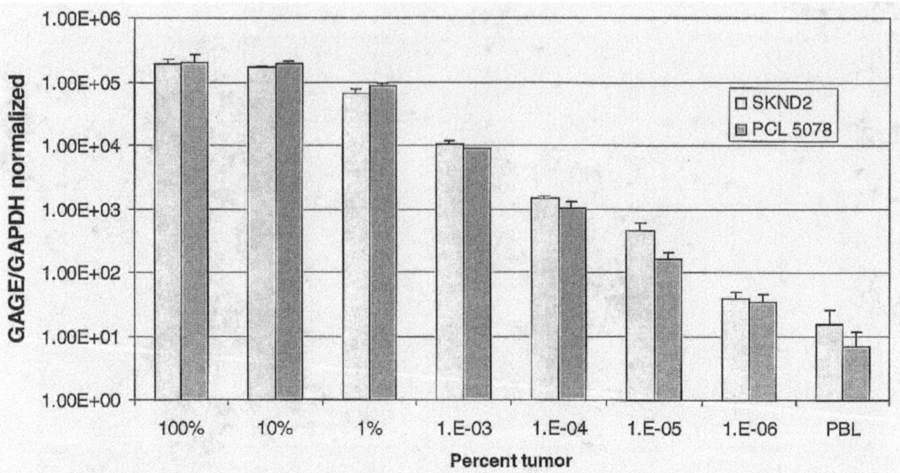

Fig. 4. Detection of low numbers of NB cells by quantitative RT-PCR. Two NB cell lines (SKND2, PCL 5078) were serially diluted in 6 fold increments into PBMC with percent of NB in PBMC ranging from 100% to 0%. The GAGE signal normalized to the amount of GAPDH message for each of the cell lines at the indicated concentrations of tumor cells are shown.

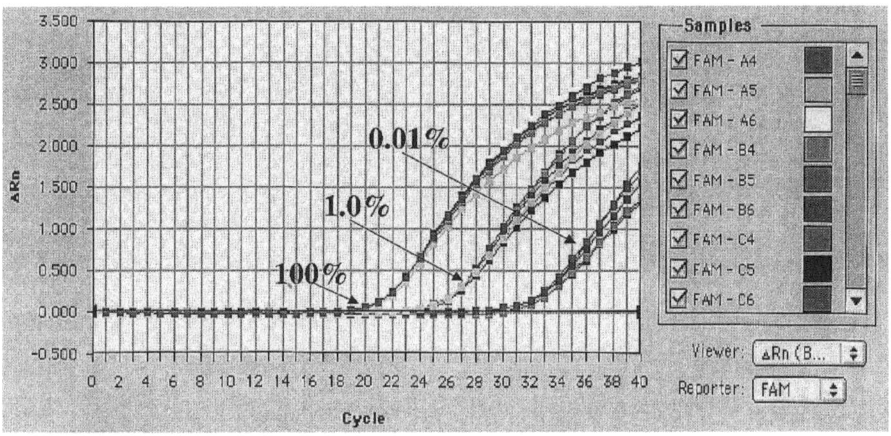

Fig. 5. Intra-assay variability of the GAGE RT-PCR assay. SKND2 NB cells were diluted 100%, 1% and 0.01% into PBMC. Seven replicates for each dilution were amplified in multiplex with GAGE and GAPDH and amplification curves are shown.

Purging of NB from stem cell aliquots

Having failed to demonstrate significant labeling of a panel of NB cell lines with five clinically relevant anti-CD34 MoAb, we then moved to analyze stem cell specimens before and after CD34 selection in the lab. For these experiments, we used either the Ceprate LC or the Isolex 50 laboratory scale CD34 selection devices, both of which use the same MoAb and selection technique as their respective clinical scale devices.

In the experiments utilizing the Ceprate LC, we used aliquots of clinical stem cell specimens collected from patients with NB on a tandem transplant trial (see Methods). These data have been published elsewhere [9] and are summarized here. A minimum of 2.25×10^6 cells from each of 30 stem cell aliquots was assessed by high-sensitivity ICC. This technique has previously been shown to have a sensitivity of NB detection in stem cells between 10^{-5} and 10^{-6} (data not shown). These aliquots, containing a minimum of 10^8 cells, were then CD34 selected on the Ceprate LC and again analyzed by ICC. 1–2 $\times 10^6$ CD34 selected cells were analyzed for each aliquot. 9 of 30 stem cell specimens had detectable NB prior to CD34 selection, ranging from 2.7 to 367 NB cells/10^6 stem cells, while no tumor was detected in the remaining 21 aliquots. After CD34 selection, all of the 21 NB-negative aliquots were still negative. Of the 9 specimens with detectable tumor, 6 were negative by this ICC assay after CD34 selection. The remaining 3 had 0.8–4 NB cells/10^6 stem cells detected. Assuming 1% of total input cells were recovered after CD34 selection (typical for these specimens and the Ceprate LC), tumor cell depletion in the specimens where tumor was detectable was between >2.5 to >4 logs.

In further experiments examining the Isolex technology, we used stem cell aliquots from both patients and normal donors. 2–5 $\times 10^8$ stem cells were contaminated with 0.5–2% NB cells from either the IMR-5, CHLA-90 or SK-N-RA cell lines. The stem cells were then CD34 selected on the Isolex 50 and analyzed using $GAGE^{15}$ RT-PCR. In a total of 12 purifications performed on the Isolex 50, depletion of tumor was seen in each case. 8/12 post-selection samples were negative by RT-PCR for GAGE message. Mean tumor cell depletion (again, adjusted for cell number) was >4.6 logs (Fig. 6).

NB purging from infused products

The majority of the patients treated on the tandem transplant protocol received CD34-selected stem cells in support of tandem courses of high-dose chemo-

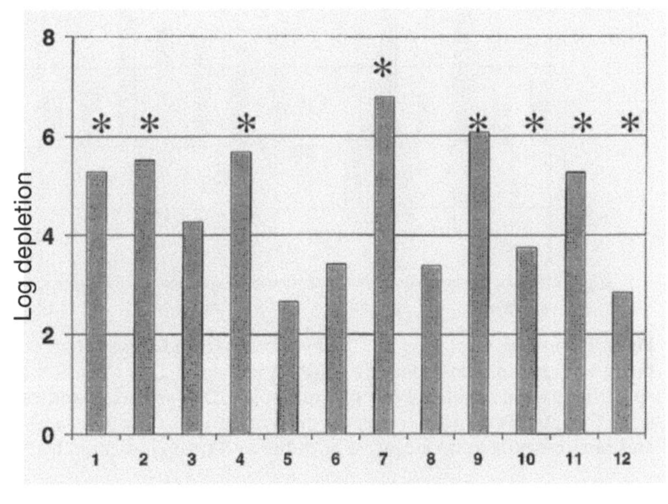

Fig. 6. Depletion of NB cell lines from stem cell specimens using the Isolex 50 system. Minimum log depletion of tumor cells is shown as assessed by quantitative RT-PCR. The starred (*) bars indicate specimens that were RT-PCR negative after purging. In the RT-PCR negative specimens, minimum log purging is estimated based on lower limits of GAGE detection.

therapy. Prior to CD34 selection, specimens were analyzed for NB contamination using standard ICC (BIS Laboratories, Reseda, CA), which has been reported to have a sensitivity of 10^{-5}. Of 29 pooled stem cell collections analyzed by standard ICC, tumor was detected in only one stem cell product, revealing 1 NB cell/10^5 stem cells. Because 10^7 cells are requested for this analysis, representing a large fraction of a CD34 selected graft in a smaller patient, only 5 samples obtained after CD34 selection were assayed for tumor cell contamination, and none of these were positive.

Specimens were also cryopreserved from both the pooled stem cell product and the post-CD34 selection product. These specimens were analyzed for NB contamination using the same Taqman RT-PCR quantitation of GAGE message as described above. 27 specimens were analyzed in triplicate. Of these, 2 were paired (pre and post) specimens from normal donors processed using the Isolex 300i device as negative controls for GAGE expression, 19 were patient specimens processed using the Ceprate SC device (one specimen was run twice; see below), and 5 were patient specimens selected on the Isolex 300i. The two normal donor specimens were negative for GAGE pre and post CD34 selection. Of the patient specimens, 6/25 were RT-PCR negative pre and 11/25 negative post selection. One specimen was negative prior to selection but then became RT-PCR positive after Ceprate SC selection. Enough template existed from the post selection specimen to repeat this triplicate analysis one further time, and the repeat RT-PCR was negative both pre and post (specimens 6 and 7 in Fig. 7). In the 20 specimens in which tumor depletion could be estimated, the mean depletion was >2.9 logs (Fig. 7), and all but specimen 6 showed tumor depletion. These specimens were obtained from patients treated on a tandem transplant trial (see Grupp et al in

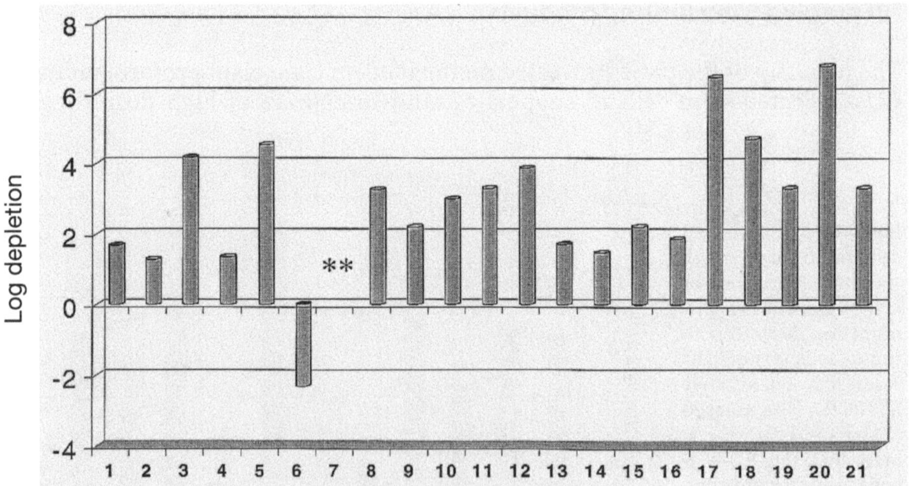

Fig. 7. Tumor cell depletion by CD34 selection from infused stem cell specimens. 21 of 27 specimens with tumor detectable by RT-PCR prior to CD34 selection are included; the remaining specimens were negative both pre and post-CD34 selection and cannot be assessed for depletion. Specimens 6 and 7 are repeat determinations from the same sample, with 6 negative pre and positive post and 7 negative both pre and post (indicated by **).

this issue), and all were treated uniformly. The likelihood of disease progression among the patients receiving GAGE+ stem cells was compared to those who received GAGE- cells, and the event-free survival was essentially the same (p=.5).

Discussion

High-dose chemotherapy with stem cell rescue has contributed to increased event-free survival in several high-risk solid tumors including NB. The toxicity of this intensive treatment modality has been decreased with the near-universal move from bone marrow to support autologous transplant to stem cells. In tumors which have a high likelihood of bone marrow metastasis, there is the possibility that tumor cells may be inadvertently collected with the stem cell product. Again, there is data to suggest that fewer tumor cells may be collected with stem cells than autologous marrow. The extent to which reinfused tumor plays a clinically significant role in the risk of relapse is unknown, and no clinical study has shown an advantage for purging tumor cells from stem cell products in patient outcome.

Negative purging strategies used to remove tumor cells from marrow may significantly delay engraftment, although much of this experience has come in collection of compromised marrow from heavily pretreated patients. In addition, negative purging strategies are dependent upon development and, eventually, FDA approval of tumor-specific antibody „cocktails" which may be cumbersome from a scientific and drug/device development standpoint. The alternative, examined in the studies presented here, is positive selection of $CD34^+$ cells, an approach which has been approved for stem cell purging by the FDA. CD34 selection of stem cells as a purging strategy for patients with NB has three potential advantages. The first is that stem cells may have less tumor cell contamination than marrow. The patients on the tandem transplant study had minimal contamination of the stem cell product even prior to CD34 selection. The second advantage of $CD34^+$ selection is that it causes no delay in engraftment, despite a decrease in the number of stem cells infused [5, 9]).

The third advantage of $CD34^+$ selection of stem cells is that positive selection of stem cells is not dependent on tumor type for depletion, as long as the tumor cells do not express CD34 or an epitope recognized by the anti-CD34 monoclonal antibody used for selection. The extent to which this may be observed is uncertain [6, 7, 16], and we did not observe any labeling of 6 NB cell lines with any of 5 anti-CD34 MoAb. Further, we have examined the depletion of NB from stem cell products using two major CD34 selection technologies in an attempt to determine whether any such labeling is clinically relevant. We find that $CD34^+$ selection depletes neuroblastoma cells from stem cells, as has been shown by others [13, 17–20].

However, though we demonstrate depletion of NB from clinical specimens by CD34 selection, we also find that the majority of stem cell products infused into these patients in support of high-dose chemotherapy still have detectable tumor cells by a GAGE RT-PCR assay developed for this purpose. The clinical relevance of that finding, however, is unknown and, in this relatively small group of patients, did not seem to impact on outcome. To further improve on the purging results obtained by CD34 selection, there is the potential to add negative selection with anti-NB MoAb to the automated CD34 selection process using the Isolex device. Determination of the role of CD34 selection and impact of purging on EFS will require a larger clinical trial. In regard to purging, a phase III randomized groupwide trial to be performed by the Children's Oncology Group has been designed to compare outcome in patients who receive immunomagnetically purged stem cells to patients who receive unselected stem cells.

References

1. Matthay KK, Villablanca JG, Seeger RC, Stram DO, Harris RE, Ramsay NK, Swift P, Shimada H, Black CT, Brodeur GM, Gerbing RB, Reynolds CP. Treatment of high-risk neuroblastoma with intensive chemotherapy, radiotherapy, autologous bone marrow transplantation, and 13-cis-retinoic acid. N Engl J Med 1999;341:1165-73.
2. Brenner M, Rill D, Moen R, Krance R, Mirro J, Anderson W, Ihle J. Gene-marking to trace origin of relapse after autologous bone-marrow transplantation. Lancet 1993;341:85-6.
3. Freedman AS, Neuberg D, Mauch P, Soiffer RJ, Anderson KC, Fisher DC, Schlossman R, Alyea EP, Takvorian T, Jallow H, Kuhlman C, Ritz J, Nadler LM, Gribben JG. Long-term follow-up of autologous bone marrow transplantation in patients with relapsed follicular lymphoma. Blood 1999;94:3325-33.
4. Civin CI, Trischmann T, Kadan NS, Davis J, Noga S, Cohen K, Duffy B, Groenewegen I, Wiley J, Law P, Hardwick A, Oldham F, Gee A. Highly purified CD34-positive cells reconstitute hematopoiesis. J Clin Oncol 1996;14:2224-33.
5. Shpall EJ, Jones RB, Bearman SI, Franklin WA, Archer PG, Curiel T, Bitter M, Claman HN, Stemmer SM, Purdy M, Myers SE, Hami L, Taffs S, Heimfeld S, Hallagan J, Berenson RJ. Transplantation of enriched CD34-positive autologous marrow into breast cancer patients following high-dose chemotherapy: influence of CD34-positive peripheral-blood progenitors and growth factors on engraftment. J Clin Oncol 1994;12:28-36.
6. Hafer R, Voigt A, Gruhn B, Zintl F. Neuroblastoma cells can express the hematopoietic progenitor cell antigen CD34 as detected at surface protein and mRNA level. J Neuroimmunol 1999;96:201-6.
7. Voigt A, Hafer R, Gruhn B, Zintl F. Expression of CD34 and other haematopoietic antigens on neuroblastoma cells: consequences for autologous bone marrow and peripheral blood stem cell transplantation. J Neuroimmunol 1997;78:117-26.
8. Brodeur GM, Pritchard J, Berthold F, Carlsen NLT, Castel V, Castleberry RP, De Bernardi B, Evans AE, Favrot M, Hedborg F, Kaneko M, Kemshead J, Lampert F, Lee REJ, Look AT, Pearson ADJ, Philip T, Roald B, Sawada T, Seeger RC. Revisions of the international criteria for neuroblastoma diagnosis, staging, and response to treatment. J Clin Oncol 1993;11:1466-77.
9. Grupp SA, Stern JW, Bunin N, Nancarrow C, Ross AA, Mogul M, Adams R, Grier HE, Gorlin JB, Shamberger R, Marcus K, Neuberg D, Weinstein HJ, Diller L. Tandem high dose therapy in rapid sequence for children with high-risk neuroblastoma. J Clin Onc 2000;18:2567-75.
10. Moss TJ, Reynolds CP, Sather HN, Romansky SG, Hammond GD, Seeger RC. Prognostic value of immunocytologic detection of bone marrow metastases in neuroblastoma. N Engl J Med 1991;324:219-26.
11. Rogers DW, Treleaven JG, Kemshead JT, Pritchard J. Monoclonal antibodies for detecting bone marrow invasion by neuroblastoma. J Clin Pathol 1989;42:422-6.
12. Donovan J, Temel J, Zuckerman A, Gribben J, Fang J, Pierson G, Ross A, Diller L, Grupp SA. CD34 selection as a stem cell purging strategy for neuroblastoma: pre-clinical and clinical studies. Med. Ped. Oncol. 2000;in press.
13. Lode HN, Handgretinger R, Schuermann U, Seitz G, Klingebiel T, Niethammer D, Beck J. Detection of neuroblastoma cells in CD34+ selected peripheral stem cells using a combination of tyrosine hydroxylase nested RT-PCR and anti-ganglioside GD2 immunocytochemistry. Eur J Cancer 1997;33:2024-30.

14. Burchill SA, Lewis IJ, Selby P. Improved methods using the reverse transcriptase polymerase chain reaction to detect tumour cells. Br J Cancer 1999;79:971-7.
15. Cheung IY, Cheung N-KV. Molecular detection of GAGE expression in peripheral blood and bone marrow: utility as a tumor marker for neuroblastoma. Clin Cancer Res 1997;3:821-6.
16. Greenfield D, Franklin WA, Tyson RW, Giller R, Shpall EJ. CD34 expression on pediatric solid tumors. Proc ASPHO 1996.
17. Tchirkov A, Kanold J, Giollant M, Halle-Haus P, Berger M, Rapatel C, Lutz P, Bergeron C, Plantaz D, Vannier JP, Stephan JL, Favrot M, Bordigoni P, Malet P, Briancon G, Demeocq F. Molecular monitoring of tumor cell contamination in leukapheresis products from stage IV neuroblastoma patients before and after positive CD34 selection. Med Pediatr Oncol 1998;30:228-32.
18. Handgretinger R, Greil J, Schurmann U, Lang P, Gonzalez-Ramella O, Schmidt I, Fuhrer R, Niethammer D, Klingebiel T. Positive selection and transplantation of peripheral CD34+ progenitor cells: feasibility and purging efficacy in pediatric patients with neuroblastoma. J Hematother 1997;6:235-42.
19. Kanold J, Yakouben K, Tchirkov A, Halle P, Carret AS, Berger M, Rapatel C, deLumley L, Vannier JP, Plantaz D, LeGall E, Lutz P, Mechinaud F, Rialland X, Combaret V, Bordigoni P, Deméocq F. Long-term follow-up after CD34+ cell transplantation in children with neuroblastoma. Blood 1998;92:445a (abstr 1842).
20. Kanold J, Yakouben K, Tchirkov A, Carret A-S, Vannier J-P, LeGall E, Bordigoni P, Demeocq F. Long-term results of CD34+ cell transplantation in children with neuroblastoma. Med Pediatr Oncol 2000;35:1-7.

Autologous Transplantation of Non-Cryopreserved HSCs in Oncologic Patients with Poor Prognosis: First Experience in the Ukraine

O. Ryzhak, S. Donska, J. Bazaluk, and N. Genkina

Department of Pediatric Oncology-Hematology,
Kiev Regional Oncologic Hospital, Ukraine

Introduction

High Dose Chemotherapy (HDCT) with hematopoietic stem cell rescue is a curative method for many patients with haematological and non-haematological malignancies who have no chance of cure under conventional chemotherapy [1]. After modern chemotherapy protocols for the treatment of children and adolescents with malignant diseases were introduced in the Ukraine in the early 90s and results comparable with international standards have been achieved [2, 3], the next task was to introduce HDCT for high risk patients.

As the treatment of patients by HDCT is expensive medical technology, its application in a country such as the Ukraine, where resources at the present time are very limited, poses many problems. This is why we initiated a less expensive and better feasible, nonetheless proven effective [4–6], transplantation program at our center, which consisted in the transplantation of non-cryopreserved HSCs following a „short" regime of HDCT. The program was selected for the following reasons:

1. Hematopoietic reconstitution can be achieved by myeloablative CT followed by reinfusion of HSCs which were stored at +4°C for a period of ≤ 72 h [9].
2. 1–2 large volume leukaphereses following mobilization with CT + G(M)-CSF will supply sufficient numbers of PBSCs for engraftment [7, 8].
3. Most high-dose chemotherapy regimens include agents, such as BCNU, melphalan, and etoposide, the therapeutic efficacy of which is not or only partially related to the preriod of their exposition [10, 11].

Patients

From 03.06.1998 to 15.01.2000, 10 patients (5 males, 5 females) with different malignant diseases received 10 autologous HSC transplants at the Department of Pediatric Oncology-Hematology, Kiev Regional Oncologic Hospital. The age range was 4 to 39 years. All patients had a poor prognosis under standard non-myeloablative chemotherapy alone: 4 pts, relapsed or progressive Hodgkin's disease; 1 pt, progressive stage IV non-Hodgkin lymphoma; 1 pt, T-ALL, non-responder to standard chemotherapy; 1 pt, AML relapse; 3 pts, relapsed or progressive solid tumors (Ewing's sarcoma, rhabdomyosarcoma, breast cancer).

The only criterion for the inclusion of patients was achievement of at least partial remission or stable disease prior to transplantation. To this end, all of the

Table 1. Characteristics of patients

No. pts	Sex	Age	Diagnosis	Status on Day 0	Duration of disease	Type of previous cytotoxic therapy	Duration of therapy
1	m.	20 yr	HD III B_S, initially partially resistant to therapy. PR I. Progression in initially involved regions with BM-involv.	PR II	16 months	CT+RT; salvage-CT	13 months
2	f.	19 yr	HD IV B_L. CR I. Late relapse, partially resistant to therapy in initial. involv. regions	PR II	51 months	CT+RT; salvage -CT	19 months
3	m.	15 yr	HD III A_S. CR I. Early relapse in initially involved regions.	CR II	20 months	CT+RT; salvage -CT	8 months
4	f.	18 yr	HD II B_N. PR I. Progression with lung involvement.	PR II	8 months	CT(not adequate) salvage -CT	4 months
5	m.	14 yr	NHL, lymphoblastic, non-T, (initial tumor of bones). SD I. Progression with BM- and CNS-involvement.	CR I	6 months	CT+RT (not adequate) salvage -CT	4 months
6	f.	17 yr	Ewing Sarcoma, stage IV, SD I. Progression (BM+bones)	PR I	14 months	CT+RT (not adequate) salvage -CT+RT	10 months
7	f.	17 yr	AML, M4. CR I. Late combine relapse (BM + CNS)	CR II	70 months	CT+RT+Maint. CT salvage -CT	29 months
8	m.	11 yr	T-ALL, NR to standart CT	CR I	7 months	CT salvage -CT	4 months
9	m.	4 yr	RMS, stage IV (BM) initially partially resistant to CT. PR I. Early BM-progression	CR II	14 months	CT+RT+OP+CT salvage –CT	11 months
10	f.	39 yr	BCR, stage IV, CR I. Late 1st relapse, CR II. 2nd relapse, PR III. Progression.	SD IV	61 months	OP+RT+CT salvage -RT+CT-1st salvage -RT+CT-2nd salvage -CT-3rd	12 months

patients received salvage therapy, i.e. non-myeloablative induction and consolidation chemotherapy (different regimens).

The patients' characteristics are summarized in Table 1.

Methods

Autologous HSC transplants were used as rescue following myeloablative CT intensification: 2 pts had BMT, 2 pts, combined BM/PBSCT, and 6 pts, only PBSCT. The first 2 pts were given BM priming prior to collection, with GM-CSF at a dose of 5 μg/kg/d over 4 days. BM harvesting was done under general anesthesia following established procedures (Thomas and Storb, 1970). After collection, the BM was filtered, placed in autologous plasma, and stored at +4°C (thermostat-controlled).

PBSC mobilization was achieved by different CT regimens + G(M)-CSF in 7 out of 8 pts who received PBSCT, one patient had only G-CSF for mobilization. PBSC collection was performed using cell separators „Fresenius AS 104“ (3 procedures in 3 pts) or „Haemonetics MCS 3p“ (10 procedures in 5 pts). During one collection 2–3 volumes of patient's blood were processed. PBSCs were obtained by central venous subclavicular or femoral catheters. In one patient (4-year-old boy of 16 kg body weight) 2 collections were done by „Haemonetics MCS 3p“, using 500 ml of extracorporal whole autologous blood This blood was collected in three procedures over one week prior to the first collection. No complications during or after collection were registered.

Transplants were stored in autoplasma at thermostat-controlled +4°C, and remained un-processed for 44-69 hours.

In 9 pts, HDCT consisted of two drugs (BCNU 400 (600) mg/m² + VP-16 1000 mg/m² (4 pts) or melphalan 140 mg/m² + VP-16 1000 mg/m² (5 pts)) given over one day. One pt, who showed severe allergic reactions to VP-16, received monotherapy with BCNU 600 mg/m² (one day).

Reinfusion of HSC concentrates followed within 31–37 hours from the end of HDCT. The volume of reinfused BM concentrate was 15–20 ml/kg with 0.51–3.6 x 10^8/kg NCs. Reinfused PBSC concentrate had 0.33–4.5 x 108/kg MNCs (0.33 and 0.4 for BM/PBSCT; 0.8–4.5 for PBSCT). $CD34^+$ cells and CFU-GM were not measured due to the lack of adequate equipment. Nevertheless, based on published data [12–18] we decided to perform the transplantation procedure with calculation of volume and number of NCs for BM concentrates and MNCs for PBSC concentrates. From day +1 to day +8, all pts received G(M)-CSF s.c. at a dose of 5–11 mg/kg/d until the neutrophil count reached 5000/μl. The day of last CSF application ranged between day +17 (minimum) and day +49.

Details of the transplantation procedures are given in Table 2.

Results

Details of the post-transplantation period and patients' outcome are presented in Table 3.

Table 2. Characteristics of Transplantation procedures

No. pts	Date of HSCsT	Type HSCsT	Mobilization	HDCT	Transplantat's characterictics VBM ml/kg	NCs $\times 10^8$/kg	MNCs $\times 10^8$/kg
1	03.06.98	ABMT	prim. BM GM-CSF 5mkg/kg/d No. 4	BCNU 400mg/m^2 VP-16 1000mg/m^2	16	1,6	0,2
2	09.07.98	ABMT	prim. BM GM-CSF 5mkg/kg/d No. 4	Melph. 140mg/m^2 VP-16 1000mg/m^2	15	3,6	1,1
3	20.09.98	ABMT/APBSC	CTX 3 g/m^2 + G(M)-CSF 5 mkg/kg/d No. 10	BCNU 400mg/m^2 VP-16 1000mg/m^2	20	2,6	BM-0,7 PB-0,4
4	24.10.98	ABMT/APBSC	CTX 3 g/m^2 + GM-CSF 5 mkg/kg/d No. 10	BCNU 600mg/m^2	15	0,51	BM-0,04 PB-0,33
5	11.12.98	APBSC	CTX 3 g/m^2 + GM-CSF 9 mkg/kg/d No. 4	Melph. 140mg/m^2 VP-16 1000mg/m^2	—	—	1,4 (fibrinization under storage)
6	22.01.99	APBSC	EVAIA+GM-CSF 6,5 mkg/kg/d No. 14	BCNU 600mg/m^2 VP-16 1000mg/m^2	—	—	0,8
7	04.11.99	APBSC	VP-16 600mg/m^2 + GM-CSF 5 mkg/kg/d No. 7	Melph. 140mg/m^2 VP-16 1000mg/m^2	—	—	0,9
8	19.11.99	APBSC	CTX 3 g/m^2 + GM-CSF 6 $\rightarrow$ 12 mkg/kg/d No. 13	Melph. 140mg/m^2 VP-16 1000mg/m^2	—	—	1,3
9	06.01.00	APBSC	ICE + GM-CSF 10 mkg/kg/d No. 13	Melph. 140mg/m^2 VP-16 1000mg/m^2	—	—	4,5
10	15.01.00	APBSC	G-CSF 5 mkg/kg $\times$ 2/d No. 6	BCNU 400mg/m^2 VP-16 1000mg/m^2	—	—	2,9

Table 3. Characteristics of Posttransplantation period

No. pst	G(M)-CSF	Engraft Neutr. ≥ 500/mkl	PLT ≥ 20000/mkl	Status on D.+30	Status on D.+100	Status on 6.04.2000	Therapy after the transplantation
1	G-CSF 8mkg/kg/d d.+5 → +17	d. +13	d. +22	CR	CR	alive in PR IV 22 months after 2 relapses	palliative OP+CT+RT palliative-CT
2	G-CSF 8mkg/kg/d d.+4 → +22	no d. +22 WBC 400/mkl	no	died d. +22	—	died on d. +22 TR complic.	—
3	G-CSF 5-10mkg/kg/d d.+5 → +24	d. +19	d. +38	CR	CR	alive in CCR 19 months	no
4	GM-CSF 5mkg/kg/d d.+1 → +37	d. +19	d. +27	CR	Relapse d. +100	LFU	no
5	GM-CSF 9mkg/kg/d d.+1 → +49	d. +37	d. +107	CR	CR	alive in CCR 16 months	α-IFN 3mln ED × 3/weekly 4 weeks
6	GM-CSF/GM-CSF 6mkg/kg/d d.+3 → +25	d. +17	no	CR	died d. +60	died on d. +60 TR complic.	no
7	GM-CSF 5mkg/kg/d d.+3 → +28	d. +19	d. +160	CR	CR	alive in CR 5 months	no
8	GM-CSF 11mkg/kg/d d.+1 → +30	d. +16	no	CR	Relapse d. +87	died on d. +124 disease progres.	Salvage-CT
9	G-CSF 10mkg/kg/d d.+4 → +18	d. +11	d. +19	CR	—	alive in CR d. +91	RgT on primary tumors region + maint.CT-Melph. + +VP-16 p. o.
10	G-CSF 5mkg/kg/d d.+4 → +5	—	—	died d. +5	—	died on d. +5 TR complic.	—

Eight out of 10 transplanted pts achieved engraftment between day +11 and day +37 (median, 19 days).

Two patients died before engraftment, i.e. at days +5 (acute cardiopulmonary failure) and +22 (pneumonia with acute respiratory distress syndrome – ARDSS); both of these patients had received pulmonary irradiation for pulmonary metastases.

At day +30 all of those 8 pts who achieved engraftment were in CR.

One patient died after engraftment at day +60 due to pneumonia with ARDSS; this girl had received very intensive pre-treatment and had pulmonary fibrosis. One patient relapsed at day +88 and died at day +124 from disease progression despite post-transplant salvage therapy. One patient, who relapsed at day +100, refused further treatment and was lost to follow-up.

Thus, at day +100, 6 pts were alive; 4 of these pts were still in CR, 2 had relapsed. One of the transplanted pts, who had not gone beyond day +91 at the day of the analysis (06.04.2000), was in CR.

One patient, who had a first relapse at day +120, received palliative treatment (OP+CT+RT) and achieved partial remission (PR III), then relapsed again at day +600, again received palliative CT and achieved another partial remission (PR IV).

At the day of the analysis, 5 out of 10 transplanted pts were alive with complete engraftment after observation periods of 22 to 3 months; 4 of these pts have been in CR for 19 to 3 months, and 1 pt was in PR IV after two post-transplant relapses. Two pts relapsed and 3 pts died from transplantation-related complications.

Discussion and Conclusion

At the day of the analysis, 5 of the transplanted patients were alive, with 4 of them in CR. Those 4 pts in CR were the same ones who had CR at the beginning of the transplantation procedure and had not undergone intensive pre-treatment.
On the other hand, only 1 among 6 pts with unfavorable events after transplantation had been in CR at day 0; 3 pts who died and 2 of 3 who relapsed had only PR. Looking at the transplantation-related mortality in our small group of patients, it is seen that very long and intensive pretreatment before the transplantation procedure, especially when followed by lung dysfunction/fibrosis, is the most important risk factor for very serious post-transplant complications (Table 4).
Based on our findings with the introduction of non-cryopreserved autologous HSC transplantation in poor prognosis cancer the following conclusions can be drawn:

- This method is an inexpensive, simple and feasible variant of transplantation procedure.
- The described procedure is effective in patients with complete remission at the beginning of the transplantation procedure.
- The most important risk factor for post-transplant complications and mortality is very intensive and long pretreatment, especially when combined with lung irradiation and the occurrence of pulmonary failure.

Table 4. Results of HSCsT according to remission-status on Day 0 and in connection with „very intensive pretreatment" (VIP) before HSCsT

No. pts.	Diagnosis	Status Day 0	VIP	Result (06.04.2000)
3	HD	CR	no	alive 19 months in CCR
5	NHL	CR	no	alive 16 months in CCR
7	AML	CR	no	alive 5 months in CR
9	RMS	CR	no	alive 3 months in CR
1	HD	PR	no	alive 22 months in PR IV after 2 posttransplant. relapses: on Day +120 and Day +600
4	HD	PR	no	relapse on Day +100 ? LFU
8	T-ALL	CR	no	relapse on Day +87 ? Death on Day +124
2	HD	PR	yes with RT on lungs	death on Day +22 (ARDSS) without engraftment
6	ES	PR	yes pulmonal fibrosis	death on Day +60 (ARDSS) after engraftment
10	BRC	SD	yes with RT on lungs	death on Day +5 (acute heart-lung disfunction)

Acknowledgements. We are very grateful to Prof. Dr. med. A.M. Carella (Ospedale S. Martino, Genova) for professional training, permanent consultation and advice.

We would like to thank very much Prof. Dr. med. G. Schellong (Univ.-Kinderklinik, Münster) for continuous methodological and material support.

Finally, we wish to express our thanks to Frau Irmgard Buhr, chairlady, and to the members of the International charity organization „Tchernobyl Kinderhilfe, Munich" – Dr.med. F. Snigula, Frau H. Eggi, Frau L. Telkyeva, and others for continuous support with equipment, drugs and materials for performing transplantation procedure.

References

1. Santos G.W. Historical background to hematopoietic stem cell transplantatuon. In: Atkinson K., eds. Clinical Bone Marrow and Blood Stem Cell Transplantation. 2nd ed. Cambridge University Press; 2000.
2. Donska S., Polischuk R., Trojanovska O. et al. Results of first multicentric study of therapy children and adolescents with acute lymphoblastic leukemia in Ukraine. EJC. 1999; 35 Suppl. 4; 112.
3. Ryzhak O., Donska S., Korenkova I. et al. Preliminary results of therapeutical multicentric study for treatment children and adolescents with AML in Ukraine. Annals of Hematology. 1999; 78 Suppl. II; 43.

4. Koppler H., Pfluger KH., Havemann K. High-dose chemotherapy with autologous bone marrow rescue: haemopoietic recostitution by non-cryopreserved marrow. Bone Marrow Transplant 1991; 7 Suppl 2; 143.
5. Taylor P.R., Jackson G.H., Lennard A.L. et al. Autologous transplantation in poor risk Hodgkin's disease using high dose melphalan/etoposide conditioning with non-cryopreserved marrow rescue. Br J Cancer. 1993; 67 (2); 383-387.
6. Jones N., Williams D., Broadbent V. et al. High-dose melphalan followed by autograft employing non-cryopreserved peripheral blood progenitor cells in children. EJC. 1996; 32A(11); 1938-1942.
7. Diaz M.A., Alegre A., Benito A. et al. Peripheral blood progenitor cell collection by large-volume leukapheresis in low-weight children. J of Hematotherapy. 1998; 7; 63-68.
8. Hillyer C.D., Tiegerman K.O., Berkman E.M. et al. Increase in circulating colony-forming units-granulocyte-macrophage during large volume leukapheresis: Evaluation of a new cell separator. Transfusion. 1991; 31(4); 327-332.
9. Rowley S.D. Techniques of bone marrow and stem cell cryopreservation and storage. In: Smith D.M., Sacher R.A., eds.Peripheral Blood Stem Cells. Bethesda. Maryland: American Association of Blood Banks; 1993.
10. Dorr R.T., Von Hoff D.D. Drugs Monographs. In Dorr R.T., Von Hoff D.D., eds. Cancer Chemotherapy Hanbook. Appelton & Lange, Connecticut, 1993.
11. Illiger H.J., Bornmann L., Herdrich K. Drug Interactions in the Therapy of Malignat Diseases. W. Zuckschwerdt Verlag, Munchen-Bern-Wien-New York, 1995.
12. King C.R. Periferal stem cell transplantation: past, present and future. In: Buschel P.C., Whedon M.B., eds. Bone Marrow Transplantation: Administration and Clinical Strategies. Boston^ Jones and Barlett; 1995.
13. Shpall E.J., Jones R.B. Mobilization and collection of peripheral progenitor cells for support of high dose cancer therapy. In: Forman S.J., Blume KGm Tomas E.D., eds. Bone Marrow Transplantation. Boston; Blackwell Scientific Publication; 1994.
14. Williams S.F., Bitran J.D., Richrds J.M. et al. Peripheral blood-derived stem cell collections for use in autologous transplantation after high dose chemotherapy: An alternative approach. Bone Marrow Transplantation 1990; 5: 129-133.
15. Kiesel S., Pezzutto A., Korbing M. et al. Autologous peripheral blood stem cell transplantation: Analisis of autografted cells and lymphocyte recovery. Transplantation Procedures,1989; 21: 3084-3088.
16. Cantin G., Marchand-Laroche D., Bouchard M.M., Leblond P.F. Blood- derived stem cell collection in acute nonlymphoblastic leukemia: Predictive factors for a good yield. EXP. Hematol. 1989; 991-996.
17. To L.B., Juttner C.A. Peripheral blood stem cell autografting: A new therapeutic option for AML? Br. J Hematol. 1987; 66: 285-288.
18. Dreger P., Gluckman E., Schmitz N. Source of Haemopoietic Stem Cells. In Apperley J.F., Gluckman E., Gratwohl A., eds. Blood and Marrow Transplantation (The EBMT Handbook). 2000 Revised Edition.

A Randomized Comparison of Once Versus Twice Daily rhG-CSF (Filgrastim) for Stem Cell Mobilisation in Healthy Donors for Allogeneic Transplantation

N. Kröger[1], H. Renges[1], W. Krüger[1], K. Gutensohn[2], C. Löliger[2], I. Carrero[2], B. Cortez[1], and A. R Zander[1]

Department of Bone Marrow Transplantation[1] and Transfusion Medicine[2], University Hamburg/Germany

Abstract

To evaluate the schedule dependency of G-CSF (filgrastim) for stem cell mobilisation we conducted a randomized trial in 50 healthy donors, with one subcutaneous daily injection of 10µg/kg G-CSF (n=25) compared to twice injections daily of 5µg/kg G-CSF (n=25). The two groups were well balanced for age, bodyweight, and gender. G-CSF application was performed on an out-patient basis and leukapheresis was started in all donors on day 5. The most frequent side effects of G-CSF were mild to moderate bone pain (88%), mild headache (72%), mild fatigue (60 and 48%) and nausea (8%) without differences between the two groups.

The $CD34^+$ cell count in the first apheresis was 5.4 x 10^6/kg donor weight (range, 2.8 to 13.3) in the 2 x 5µg/kg group compared to 4.0 x10^6/kg (range, 0.4 to 8.8) in the 1 x 10µ/kg group (p=0.007). The target of collecting >3.0 x10^6 $CD34^+$ cells/kg donor weight with one apheresis procedure was achieved in 24/25 (96%) patients in the 2 x 5µg/kg group and 17/25 (68%) patients in the 1 x 10µg/kg group. The target of collecting >5.0 x10^6 $CD34^+$ cells/kg in the first apheresis was achieved in 64% in the 2 x 5µ/kg group, but only in 36% in the 1 x 10µg/kg group. The progenitor cell assay for CFU-GM and BFU-E was higher in the 2 x 5µg/kg than in the 1 x 10µg/kg group (7.0 vs 3.5 x 10^5/kg; p= 0.01, and 6.6 vs 5.0 x 10^5/kg; p=0.1).

Administering G-CSF (filgrastim) at a dosage of 5µg/kg twice daily rather than once 10µg/kg daily is recommended, leading to a higher $CD34^+$ cell yield and requiring fewer aphereses procedures without increasing toxicity or cost.

Introduction

Peripheral blood progenitor cells (PBSC) instead of bone marrow can be used for allogeneic transplantation [1,2]. Despite the fact that mobilized PBSC contain 10 times more T-cells than bone marrow the incidence of acute GvHD in allogeneic PBSC is similiar to allogeneic bone marrow transplantation [1,3]. However, there might be a higher incidence and severity of chronic GvHD after allogeneic PBSC transplantation [4]. Mobilization of progenitor cells in healthy donors is achieved with cytokines such as granulocyte colony stimulating factor (G-CSF) or granulocyte-macrophage colony stimulating factor (GM-CSF). G-CSF is preferred because of less side effects and higher mobilization efficacy [5].

The possible advantage for the donor of PBSC includes the avoidance of general anaesthesia, the less invasive procedure and the lack of hospitalisation [6].

Although the mobilization kinetics of CD34+ progenitor cells after G-CSF have been studied [5, 7, 8], neither the optimal dosage nor the optimal schedules have been established so far.

Recent data in healthy donors as well as in cancer patients show a dose response effect to G-CSF- dosages between 3μg/kg and 30μg/kg body weight (BW) [2, 9-11]. In our retrospective analysis of progenitor cell mobilisation in breast cancer patients with G-CSF from steady state hematopoesis we found a significantly higher cell harvest after stimulation with daily 2x5μg/kg compared to daily 1x10μg/kg Filgrastim [12]. To confirm this schedule dependency of G-CSF administration we conducted a prospective randomized trial in normal donors comparing peripheral blood progenitor cell mobilization applying daily subcutaneously either a single injection of 10μg/kg G-CSF or two injections of 5μg/kg G-CSF for allogeneic transplantation.

Patients and Methods

Between January 1998 and Dezember 1999 50 healthy donors were enrolled in this prospective randomized comparison. Donors were randomized to receive either 5 μg/kg G-CSF (Filgrastim, Neupogen, Amgen, Munich, Germany) twice per day with a time interval of 12 hours (n=25) or 10μg/kg G-CSF (Filgrastim; Neupogen, Amgen, Munich, Germany) once daily in the morning (n=25). Donors for patients who were treated within the ongoing EBMT protocol comparing ABMT versus PBSCT received one dose of 10μg/kg Filgrastim daily. G-CSF dosage were rounded to standard size ampoules of 300 or 480μg rhG-CSF, resulting in a median of 10.1μg/kg filgrastim in the 10μg/kg (range, 8.8 to 10.8) and of 9.8μg/kg (range,

Table 1. Donor characteristics

Variables	1 x 10μg/kg	2 x 5μg/kg	p-value
No. of donors	25	25	
Gender: male/female	14/11	15/10	
Median age (range)	37 (21-64)	48 (27-56)	0.27
Median kg body weight (range)	76 (50-98)	87 (56-110)	0.07
Median daily dose of G-CSF (range)	10.1 (8.8-10.8)	9.8 (8.8-10.8)	1.0
Median ml processed blood volume (range)	11146 (7645-14351)	11899 (7658-14447)	0.2

Table 2. CD34+ cell harvest and progenitor cell assay

Variables	1 x 10µg/kg	2 x 5µg/kg	p-value
WBC /nl prior to 1.LP	42 (21-67)	51 (31-78)	0.018
CD34+ x 10^6/kg in 1.LP (range)	4.0 (0.4-8.8)	5.4 (2.8 –13.3)	0.007
CFU-GM x 10^5/kg in 1.LP (range)	3.5* (0.7-8.6)	7.0** (3-12.5)	0.001
BFU x 10^5/kg in 1.LP (range)	5.0* (0.5-10.9)	6.6** (3.1-10.8)	0.15

* n=10; ** n=13

8.8 to 10.8) in the 2 x 5µg/kg group. G-CSF application was performed on an outpatient basis. Leukapheresis was started in all donors on day 5. G-CSF application was continued until completion of leukapheresis, depending on the required cell dose of the recipient. For this study the $CD34^+$ cell harvest of the first apheresis was calculated on the donor body weight. The mobilisation protocol was approved by the local ethics commission.

The collection of PBSC was performed after G-CSF stimulation identically in all donors on day +5 with a Cobe Spectra using a 250 ml volume collection chamber. A total of 8 to 14 l blood per apheresis was processed at a flow rate of 50 to 70 ml/min; a mean volume of 250 ml was collected.

The number of heamatopoietic progenitor cells in leukapheresis product was assessed using a methylcellulose culture assay as described before [13].

For determination of CD34 positive cells the method published by Sutherland et al. [14] was used. A minimum of 50,000 events was counted.

Statistic analysis was performed using WinSTAT software (Kalmia Co. Inc.). For comparison of the two different G-CSF groups the independent t-test was used. A p-value of < 0.05 was considered to be significant.

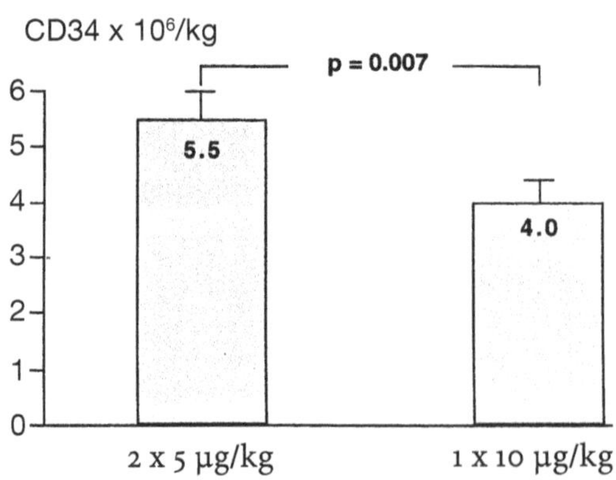

Fig. 1. $CD34^+$ cell harvest in first aphersis product per kg body weight of the donor after after stimulation with 2 x 5µg/kg or 1 x 10µg/kg G-CSF.

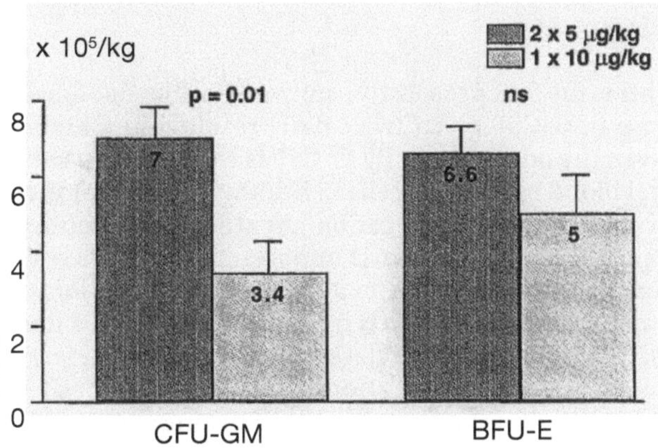

Fig. 2. CFU-GM and BFU-E in first apheresis product after stimulation with 2 x 5µg/kg or 1 x 10µg/kg G-CSF.

Results

Tolerance of G-CSF

In both groups cytokine priming as well as collection of peripheral blood stem cells (PBSC) were well tolerated: 60% in the 2 x 5µg/kg group and 48% in the 1 x 10µg/kg group experienced mild fatigue (grade 1 CTC); 88% of the donors in both groups complained of bone pain (grade 1 or 2), whereas headache (grade 1 or 2) and mild nausea (grade 1) were noted in 72% and 8% in both groups, respectively. No severe grade 3 or 4 toxicity was observed.

PBSC collection

For all donors the median collected CD34 cell count in first apheresis was 4.9 x 10^6/kg (range, 0.4 to 13.3). The median leukocyte-count before the first apheresis was 46/nl (range 21 to 78) and correlated with the CD34+ cell yield (r:0.4; p =0.0026). The median leukocyte count beforethe first apheresis was higher in the 2 x 5µg/kg than in the 1 x 10µg/kg group (51/nl vs 42/nl; p= 0.018). The CD34+ cell count in the first apheresis was 5.4 x 10^6/kg (range, 2.8 to 13.3) in the 2 x 5µg/kg group and 4.0 x10^6/kg (range, 0.4 to 8.8) in the 1 x 10µ/kg group (p=0.007).

The target of collecting >3.0 x10^6 $CD34^+$ cells/kg with one apheresis procedure was achieved in 24 out of /25 patients (96%) in the 2 x 5µg/kg group and in 17 out of /25 patients (68%) in the 1 x 10µg/kg group. The target of collecting >5.0 x10^6 $CD34^+$ cells/kg in the first apheresis was achieved by 64% in the 2 x 5µ/kg group, but only by 36% in the 1 x 10µg/kg group.

Progenitor cell assays were performed in 10 donors of the 10µg/kg group and in 13 donors of the 2 x 5µg/kg group. The median number of CFU-GM was higher in the 2 x 5µg/kg group than in the 1 x 10µg/kg group (7.0 vs 3.5 x 10^5/kg; p= 0.01). Additionally, the median number of BFU-E was higher in the 2 x 5µg/kg group, however the difference did not reach statistical significance (6.6 vs 5.0 x 10^5/kg; p=0.1).

Discussion

This is the first prospective study in healthy donors demonstrating that the same dose of G-CSF given twice daily resulted in a higher CD34+ cell harvest than given the dose once daily. G-CSF is extensively used for mobilization of peripheral blood progenitor cells in healthy donors, but the optimal schedule and dose of growth factor application has still to be established [5–8]. A higher allogeneic PBSC mobilisation is important for donors resulting in less apheresis procedures and less G-CSF exposure and for recipients leading to a rapid hematopoietic engraftment. Several studies suggested a dose response effect to G-CSF [5, 9, 11]. However there are only few reports referring to the schedule dependency of G-CSF application. A retrospective study of different G-CSF dosages in healthy donors suggested that splitting the G-CSF dosage into two injections with a 12 hour intervall might lead to a higher $CD34^+$ cell harvest [15]. Recently, we could demonstrate in breast cancer patients that splitting the dosage of G-CSF into twice daily resulted in a significant higher $CD34^+$ cell harvest than applying the whole dosage in a single injection once daily [12]. In a small comparative study of 11 healthy donors the twice-daily schedule was not more effective than the once daily schedule, however due to the high interindividual range of $CD34^+$ cell mobilization in healthy volunteers, probably more donors are needed to find significant differences [16, 17]. We therefore started a prospective randomized trial in healthy donors comparing stem cell mobilization with filgrastim applied either once daily as 10µg/kg s.c. or twice daily 5µg/kg with a 12 hour intervall given for 4 consecutive days. Apheresis was started on day 5, because several investigators reported a peak number of circulating $CD34^+$ cells after filgrastim stimulation on day 5 [5–7, 16]. We compared the once daily 10µg/kg schedule as standard regime, which has been recommended by the EBMT group [18], with the splitted dose based on several considerations. First, the pharmacological profile of G-CSF in healthy donors and cancer patients shows a maximum serum concentration after subcutaneous application within 2-8 hours [19] and due to the short elimination half-time of G-CSF (Filgrastim) of only about 3 to 4 hours regardless of the route of administration the twice daily schedule might improve the CD34+ cell yield. Second, kinetic studies of G-CSF serum levels in healthy volunteers after stimulation with G-CSF indicate a higher level after the twice daily schedule compared to the once daily schedule [16]. In our study, the $CD34^+$ cell count of the first apheresis in the 2 x 5µg/kg group was 5.4 x 10^6/kg (range, 2.8 to 13.3) compared to 4.0 x 10^6/kg CD34+ cells (range, 0.4 to 8.8) in the 1 x 10µ/kg group (p=0.007).

Additionally, the number of CFU-GM and BFU-E were higher in the apheresis product of the 2 x 5µg/kg group. The intervall between G-CSF administration and apheresis is unlikeley to be the cause of the observed differences, because previous studies indicate a higher $CD34^+$ cell yield when cell harvesting is performed 12-18 hours after G-CSF application [20].

The short-term side effects of G-CSF like bone pain, headache and fatigue were predominantly minor and transient with no differences between the two groups.

In summary, this study indicates that priming with 10μg/kg G-CSF for healthy donors is safe, well tolerated and effective in mobiliziation of PBSC. Adminstering G-CSF 5μg/kg twice daily rather than once 10μg/kg daily is recommended, leading to a higher $CD34^{+}$ cell yield and requiring fewer apheresis procedures without increasing toxicity or cost.

References

1. Bensinger WI, Weaver CH, Appelbaum FR, Rowley S, Demirer T, Sander J, Storb R, Buckner CD (1995) Transplantation of allogeneic peripheral blood stem cells mobilized by recombinant human granulocyte colony-stimulating factor. Blood 85: 1655-1658.
2. Körbling M, Przepiorka D , Huh YO, Engel H, van Besien K, Giralt S, Andersson B, Kleine HD, Seong D, Deisseroth AB, Andreef M, Champlin R (1995) Allogeneic blood stem cell transplantation for refractory leukemia and lymphoma: potential advantage of blood over marrow allografts. Blood 86: 2842-2848.
3. Schmitz N, Bacigalupo A, Hasenclever D, Nagler A, Gluckman E, Clark P, Bourquelot P, Greinix H, Frickhofen N, Ringden O, Zander AR, Apperley JF, Gorin C, Borkett K, Schwab G, Goebel M, Russell NH, Gratwohl A. (1998) Allogeneic bone marrow transplantation vs filgrastim-mobilised peripheral blood progenitor cell transplantation in patients with early leukemia: first results of a randomised multicentre trial of the European Group for Blood and Marrow Transplantation. Bone Marrow Transplantation 21: 995-1003.
4.. Brown RA, Adkins D, DiPersio J, Goodnough T. (1997) Allogeneic peripheral blood stem cell transplantation is associated with an increased risk of chronic graft versus host disease. Blood 90: 225a.
5. Grigg AP, Roberts AW, Raunow H, Houghton S, Layton JE, Boyd AW, McGrath KM, Maher D. (1995) Optimizing dose and scheduling of filgrastim for mobilization and collection of peripheral blood progenitor cells in normal volunteers. Blood 86: 4437-4445.
6. Anderlini P, Przepiorka D, Seong D, Miller P, Sundberg J, Lichtiger B, Norfleet F, Chan KW, Champlin R, Körbling M (1996) Clinical toxicity and laboratory effects of filgrastim mobilization and blood stem cell apheresis from normal donors and analysis of charges for the procedures. Transfusion 36: 590-595.
7. Tanaka R, Matsudaira T, Tanaka I, Muraoka K, Ebihara Y, Ikebuchi K, Nakahata T. (1994) Kinetics and characteristics of peripheral blood progenitor cells mobilized by G-CSF in normal healthy volunteers. Blood 84: 541a.
8. Dreger P, Haferlach T, Eckstein V, Jacobs S, Suttorp M, Löffler H, Müller-Ruchholtz W, Schmitz N. (1994) G-CSF mobilized peripheral blood progenitor cells for allogeneic transplantation: safety, kinetics of mobilization, and composition of the graft. British Journal of Haematology 87: 609-613.
9. Engelhardt M, Bertz H, Afting M, Waller CF, Finke J. High-versus standard dose filgrastim (rhG-CSF) for mobilization of peripheral blood progenitor cells from allogeneic donors and CD34+ immunoselection. (1999) J Clin Oncol 17: 2160-2172.
10. Weaver CH, Birch R, Greco FA, Schwartzberg L, McAneny B, Moore M, Oviatt D, Redmond J, Gearge C, Alberico T, Johnson P, Buckner CD.(1998) Mobilization and harvesting of peripheral blood stem cells: randomized evaluations of different doses of filgrastim. British Journal of Haematology 100: 338-347.
11. Zeller W, Gutensohn K, Stockschläder M, Dierlamm J, Kröger N, Köhne G, Hummel K, Kabisch H, Weh HJ, Kühnl P, Hossfeld DK, Zander AR. (1996) Increase of mobilized CD34-positive peripheral blood progenitor cells in patients with Hodgkin's disease, non-Hodgkin's lymphoma, and cancer of the testis. Bone Marrow Transplant 17, 709-713.
12. Kröger N, Zeller W, Hassan HT, Krüger W, Löliger C, Zander AR. (1998) Schedule dependency of granulocyte colony stimulating factor in peripheral blood progenitor cell mobilisation in breast cancer patients. Blood; 91:1828.
13. Hassan HT, Zeller W, Stockschläder M, Krüger W, Zander AR (1996) Comparison between bone marrow and G-CSF mobilized blood allografts undergoing clinical scale CD34 positive cell selection. Stem Cells 14:419-429.

14. Sutherland DR, Anderson L, Keeney M. (1996) The ISHAGE guidelines for CD34+ cell determination by flow cytometry. J Hematotherapy 5:213.
15. Arbona C, Prosper F, Benet I, Mena F, Solano C, Garcia-Conde J. Comparison between once a day vs twice a day G-CSF for mobilization of peripheral blood progenitor cells in normal donors for allogeneic PBSC transplantation. Bone Marrow Transplantaton 1998; 22:39-45.
16. Yano T, Katayama Y, Sunami K, Deguchi S, Nawa Y, Hiramatsu Y, Nakayama H, Arakawa T, Ishimaru F, Teshima T, Shinagawa K, Omoto E, Harada M. (1997) G-CSF induced mobilization of peripheral blood stem cells for allografting: comparative study of daily single versus divided dose of G-CSF. Int. J Hematology 66: 169-178.
17. Brown RA, Adkins D, Goodnough LT, Haug JS, Todd G, Wehde M, Hendricks, Ehlenbek C, Laub L, DiPersio. (1997) Factors that influence the collection and engraftment of allogeneic peripheral blood stem cells in patients with hematologic malignancies. J Clin Oncol 15:3067-3074.
18. Russel N, Gratwohl A, Schmitz N. (1996) The place of blood stem cells in allogeneic transplantation. Br J Haematol 93: 747-753.
19. de Haas M, Kerst JM, van der Schoot C, et al. (1994). Granulocyte colony-stimulating factor administration to healthy volunteers: analysis of the immediate activating effect on circulating neutrophils. Blood 84:3885
20. Fujisaki T, Otsuka T, Harada M, Ohno Y, Niho Y. (1995) Granulocyte colony stimulating factor mobilizes primitive hematopoietic stem cells in normal individuals. Bone Marrow Transplantation 16, 57-62.

CD133/CD34 Expression on Hematopoietic Stem-/Progenitor Cells and Acute Leukemic Blasts*

U. Ebener[1], S. Wehner[1], A. Brinkmann[1], V. Zotova[2], T. Azovskaja[3], E. Niegemann[1], J. Sörensen[1], and D. Schwabe

[1] J.W. Goethe University, Centre of Pediatrics Hematology and Oncology, D-60590 Frankfurt/M., Germany; [2] Clinic of Pediatrics of Medical University Rostov-on-Don, Russia, [3] Pediatric Oncological Center, Ekaterinburg, Russia

Abstract

CD133, a recently discovered antigen on human progenitor cells, demonstrating 5-transmembra-neous domains is expressed by 30–60% out of all $CD34^+$ cells. Our aim therefore was to investigate the extent of human stem-/progenitor cells expressing CD133 antigen in umbilical cord blood, peripheral blood without or following an application of granulocyte-colony stimulating factor (rhG-CSF). The main task was the investigation of bone marrow aspirates derived from children suffering from newly diagnosed acute leukemias, as well as from patients with a relapse or during a complete remission. The determination of antigen expression was done by application of flow cytometry (FACScan analyses) and the usage of newly developed monoclonal antibodies (CD133/1 and CD133/2; Miltenyi Biotec GmbH) in combination with monoclonal antibody directed against CD34-antigens (HPCA-2; BD).

Our studies till now show average percentages in umbilical cord blood derived from 43 newborns about 0.294±0.165% $CD133^+$ *vs.* 0.327±0.156% $CD34^+$ hematopoietic stem-/ progenitor cells (HSPC). In peripheral blood from 11 healthy donors we verified up to 0.15% $CD34^+$ as well as $CD133^+$ HSPC's. The concentration of progenitor cells was found to be obviously higher in peripheral blood from children with various diseases (neuroblastoma, rhabdomyosarcoma, ALL/AML) and undergoing application with rhG-CSF in order to be prepared for PBSC-transplantation. In those cases we found up to 3.51% $CD133^+$ cells as well as slightly higher values (3.94%) for CD34 antigens.

Additionally we quantified 180 bone marrow (BM) samples for $CD133^+$ and $CD34^+$ cells. In 20 BM samples, derived from patients without any neoplasia, the $CD34^+$ cells were about 0.03% and 1.49%, whereas CD133 values were up to 0.64%. Bone marrow aspirates from 69 children with acute leukemias at time of diagnosis (ALL: n=55 / AML: n=14) have been immunophenotyped and leukemic blast cells have been proved for CD133- and CD34 antigen expression. 40/55 (73%) of lymphoblastic leukemic cells showed to be positive for CD34 antigen and 27/55 (49%) demonstrated CD133 antigens. Interestingly there were 3 ALL patients with pathological blast cells positive for CD133 but lacking of any CD34 antigens. 43%

*Dedicated to Professor Dr. med. Dr. h. c. Bernhard Kornhuber

(6/14) of investigated AML patients showed $CD34^+$ phenotype, on the other hand there were only 29% (4/14) with $CD133^+$ phenotype. Similar values were found in relapsed patients (n=27). In BM samples from patients during complete remission (n=64) we could detect percentages up to 5.70% for CD34 and up to 1.25% for CD133 positive stem-/progenitor cells. Such quite high data may be explained by occasionally application of rhG-CSF therapy.

Our results till now lead to the conclusion, that it seems to be useful, to recruit quantification of $CD34^+$ HPSC by additionally detecting CD133 antigens. This new stem cell marker (CD133) maybe of great value in case of autologous peripheral blood stem cell transplantation (PBSCT) because it could be an alternative to the usual $CD34^+$ *MACS* selection system.

Introduction

The majority of patients suffering from various malignancies (e.g. leukemias, Non-Hodgkin-tumors) are undergoing a high dosis chemotherapy. The stressing of the body following the various cellular chemotherapeutics results in a persistent damage of the hematopoietic system. Additional side effects may be infections and hemorrhagous bleedings and can be overcome by transplantation of peripheral blood stem cells, i.e. $CD34^+$-progenitor cells.

The treatment of patients with solid tumors and hematological diseases applying highdosis-chemotherapy is nowadays often combined with the transplantation of autologous peripheral blood stem cells (PBSC). In contrast to autologous bone marrow transplantation (BMT) PBSCT is less burdening for the patients and leading to an accelerated recovery of hematopoiesis, especially by simultaneously application of growth factors, f.e. rhG-CSF [1].

Autologous transplantation of cells may be associated with danger. The risk to transfer tumor cells has to be taken in one's mind, specially when those cells can infiltrate to peripheral blood as usually given in acute leukemias. Several technical possibilities are available, to remove such tumor cells from transplants by various „purging" strategies. At time best results are achieved using immunomagnetic beads in combination with column-systems. This technique profits from the knowledge referring to the expression of classical stem cell markers (CD34) on hematopoietic stem cells and therefore enables one to isolate such cells by positive selection and achieving purities up to 95% [2].

However application of this purging-strategy is predominantly limited to diseases, with malignant cells not demonstrating CD34-phenotype. In contrast to most solid tumors, with the exception of neuroblastomas [3, 4], acute childhood leukemias are characterized to express stem cell antigen CD34 in high percentages [5–7]. Therefore at the present time very rare high risk patients with ALL or AML can profit from an autologous peripheral blood stem cell transplantation (PBSCT). In order to minimize the danger of tumor cell contamination, at time various modifications of established isolation-procedures are proved applying specific antibodies directed against additional stem cell antigens, e.g. CD117 [8].

Development of new hematopoietic stem cell antigen, named CD133 and demonstrated by 30 - 60% of all stem- and progenitor cells positive for CD34-antigen

[9–10]), reveals additional possibilities and alternative purging strategies. Two monoclonal antibodies, recognizing different epitopes of 5-transmembraneous CD133-antigens, are commercially available and are examined by us and other researchers for significance in progenitor cells as well as in leukemic blast cells [11–14].

In the present study we therefore were interested, if and in which content acute leukemic blast cells at time of diagnosis and during a relapse coexpress the newly developed stem cell marker CD133 and the classical stem cell antigen CD34. Furthermore we investigated the frequency of CD34-positive stem-/progenitor cells in umbilical cord blood, in peripheral blood of healthy donors and in bone marrow (BM without any tumor cells) and coexpressions applying anti-CD133. The results presented shall contribute to describe the value of CD133 with respect to autologous peripheral blood stem cell transplantation (PBSCT).

Material and Methods

Patients and Controls

Material included to the present study as well as numbers of flow cytometric analyses are given below. Patients' material was derived from children treated in our department of Pediatric Hematology and Oncology (Clinic III). Bone marrow aspirates (BM) from 20 children without any hematological disease, and investigated to exclude any neoplasias, served as controls. Additionally flow cytometric analyses were done with PB from oncological patients following various long lasting application with rhG-CSF (n=39). BM aspirates from patients with acute leukemia (ALL/AML) were analyzed at different times of disease (newly diagnosed: n=69 (ALL: n=55, AML: n=14); during remission: n=64, in relapse: n=27; (ALL: n= 20, AML: n=7). The immunological subtyping was done according to the criteria of the EGIL-Group and based to the consensus protocol [15, 16].

As a control we investigated additional peripheral blood (PB) from hematological healthy donors (n=11) and umbilical cord blood (UCB; n=43) derived from the centre of Gynecology, University of Frankfurt/Main.

Reagents

Immunoreagents used in the present study were subscribed by following sources: anti-CD45 FITC, anti-CD45 PerCP, anti-HPCA-2 FITC and HPCA-2 PE, isotypic-controls mouse IgG1 FITC / IgG2a PE, isotypic-controls mouse IgG1 PE [Becton Dickinson/Heidelberg, Germany]; anti-CD117 RPE [DAKO/Hamburg, Germany]; anti-CD133/1 PE, anti-CD133/2 PE [Miltenyi Biotec GmbH/Bergisch Gladbach, Germany]. FACS™ Lysing Solution and FACS-Flow™ Sheat-Solution have been purchased from Becton Dickinson / Heidelberg, Germany.

Quantitative evaluation of CD34 and CD133 positive HSPC was done in detail according to the recommendations of Gutensohn and Serke [17].
The determination of antigen expressions on leukemic blast cells during immunophenotyping, was done following the suggestions of the EGIL-Group [15].

Phenotyping was done on a flow cytometer FACScan [Becton Dickinson/ Heidelberg, Germany]. Data acquisition and -evaluation was performed on a Macintosh Quadra 650 applying CELLQuest software.

Flow cytometry

Flow cytometric cell marker analyses were done as „whole lysed blood"-procedure. At first the amount of cellular content in materials was estimated using a cell counter [CellDyn 1700 / Abbott / Wiesbaden, Germany] and respectively 2 x 10^6 leukocytes were tested in each reaction. Concentrations of antibodies have been selected according to the recommendations of the companies. Subsequently following an incubation time about 15 minutes at room temperature in darkness we lysed erythrocytes by incubating 2 ml FACS™ Lysing Solution. Subsequently samples were washed out using phosphate buffered saline (PBS) at 248 *g* and resuspended in 500 µl PBS for data acquisition on a FACScan instrument. Flow cytometer (FACScan) is equipped with a 488 nm argon laser. For adjustment of FACScan and compensation of fluorescence channels we applied CaliBRITE Beads [Becton Dickinson / Heidelberg, Germany] following the companies' recommendations. Additionally we proved compensation for individual samples by labeling the containing T-lymphocyte subpopulations (CD4-FITC, CD8-PE, CD3-PerCP). In every case we estimated between 10.000–50.000 cells applying FACScan technology.

Evaluation

Flow cytometric quantification of $CD34^+$- and $CD133^+$-stem- / progenitor cells (HSPC) was done according to the recommendations of consensus protocol referring to CD45 positive leukocytes [17]. In BM aspirates from newly diagnosed leukemia patients or suffering from a relapse percentages of $CD34^+$- and/or $CD133^+$-cells were estimated for mononucleated cellular compartment. In BM aspirates derived from leukemia patients content of pathological leukemic blasts was between 72% and 97%. In BM samples from patients with acute leukemia, where percentage of $CD34^+$- and/or $CD133^+$-cell was < 10%, estimated results were not assigned to leukemic blast cells. In those cases the result was given to be negative for leukemic cell population.

Results

Antigenic Pattern of CD133 vs. CD34 Expression on Stem-/Progenitor Cells

Results of flow cytometric marker analyses in order to quantify stem-/progenitor cell antigens CD34 and CD133 in various blood- and bone marrow aspirates are summarized in Table 1.

Table 1. Expression of CD34 *vs.* CD133 in Various Specimens

Specimens	number [n]	CD34 [%] range	AD133 [%] range
Umbilical Cord Blood (UCB)	43	0.05 – 0.67 (0.327 ± 0.156)[a]	0.06 – 0.65 (0.294 ± 0.165)[a]
Peripheral Blood from healthy donors (PB)	11	0–0.15	0–0.10
PB (rh-G-CSF Application)	39	0.10–3.94	0.10–3.51
Bone Marrow (BM)[b]	20	0.03–1.49	0.09–0.64
BM (Leukemia-Remission)	64	0.13–5.70[c]	0.19–1.25[c]

Flow cytometric quantification referring to CD45-positive leukocytes. [a] (x ± SD); [b] Bone marrow from children without any haematological neoplasia; [c] th-G-CSF treatment in order to overcome an aplasia

In Table 1 we compare our results of CD133 and CD34 expressions in non-mobilized, rhG-CSF mobilized peripheral blood (PB, PB/rhG-CSF), umbilical cord blood (UCB) as well as in bone marrow (BM) derived from patients without any hematological disease and BM from patients with acute leukemias at time of complete remission.

We were able to estimate CD34 positive cells in all samples given, in some cases in very small amounts. Performing double staining procedures we could demonstrate, that the predominant compartment of CD34-positive cells simultaneously show the newly developed stem cell antigen CD133.

In peripheral blood from healthy donors we found only very rare concentrations (<0,15%) of $CD34^+$ HSPC and predominantly coexpression of CD133.

An evident increase in values found in peripheral blood is achieved following mobilization with growth factor rhG-CSF, dependent on the duration of application. Determined maxima were about 3.94% $CD34^+$ or 3.51% $CD133^+$ cells in mobilized PB. Compared to results from peripheral blood from donors (< 0,15%) even umbilical cord blood (UCB) showed higher average percentages of about 0.327 ± 0.156% $CD34^+$ or rather 0.294 ± 0.165% $CD133^+$ hematopoetic stem-/ progenitor cells as demonstrated in Table 1.

In bone marrow from patients, where neoplasias had been ruled out and with diseases that are not tumor-associated (i.e. aplastic anemia)- percentages ranged between 0.64% $CD133^+$- and 1.49% $CD34^+$- cells.

Participation of HSPC -characterized by CD34 and CD133 antigens- in bone marrow from children with acute leukemias during complete remission is very variable. In remission-BM we could estimate between 0.02% and up to 5.7% positive for CD34 antigens and up to 1.25% for CD133.

Antigen Expression of CD34 and CD133 in BM in Acute Leukemias (newly diagnosed and at time of relapse)

In our study we were interested in the relative frequency of CD34 and CD133 antigen expression in acute leukemias at time of diagnosis.

We recorded as summarized in Table 2 by immunophenotyping altogether 69 BM-samples from children with newly diagnosed acute leukemias (55 ALL and 14 AML). 67% of analyzed leukemias demonstrated $CD34^+$-Phenotype, however only 45% expression of CD133 antigen.

Separately evaluation of ALL-group and AML-group assigns 73% of cases to acute lymphoblastic leukemias with $CD34^+$ phenotype and 43% of all to AML's with $CD34^+$ phenotype.

Comparing both groups with respect to CD133 expression, we likewise found distinct differences. 49% of ALL-patients showed $CD133^+$ blast cell population in contrast to 29% of AML-patients.

Table 2 summarizes CD34 *vs.* CD133 values found in bone marrow samples from altogether 55 children, who had been immunophenotyped and diagnosed as acute lymphoblastic leukemia (ALL).

Heterogeneous pattern of stem cell antigens CD34 and CD133 in acute leukemic blasts could be demonstrated by double staining procedures as shown in Figure 1.

In our investigations we proved leukemic blasts in bone marrow aspirates from 14 children with AML diagnosis for antigenic pattern of both stem cell markers CD34 and CD133.

Even this cohort does not show an homogeneous behavior in antigen expressions, too.

Our results for 27 children with ALL and AML suffering from a relapse are demonstrated in Table 3.

Table 2. CD34 *vs.* CD133 Antigenexpression in Childhood Acute Leukemia at Time of Diagnosis

BM-Aspirates at time of Diagnosis	number [n]	$CD34^+$-AL [%]	$AD133^+$-AL [%]
ALL	55	*73*	49
AML	14	*43*	29
total	69	*67*	45

Table 3. CD34 *vs.* CD133 Antigenexpression in Childhood Acute Leukemia at Time of Relapse

BM-Aspirates at time of Relapse	number [n]	$CD34^+$-AL [%]	$AD133^+$-AL [%]
ALL	20	*60*	25
AML	7	*100*	71
total	27	*70*	37

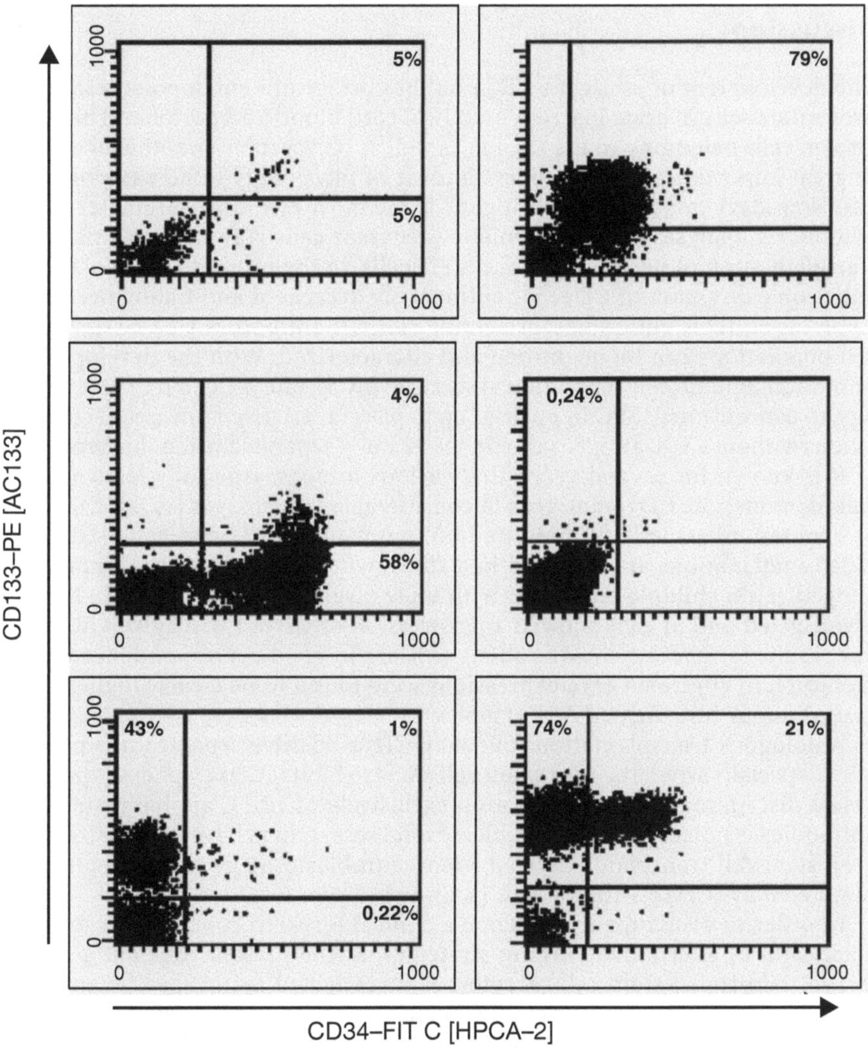

Fig 1. Demonstration of flowcytometric analyses of various bone marrow samples following gating strategy due to size and granularity of mononucleated cells (MNC). X-axis shows logarithmic amplification of anti-CD34-FITC [HPCA-2 FITC] vs. CD133-PE [AC133 PE] labelling on y-axis. Dotplots (Diagrams 2–6) represent leukemic blasts characterized by distinguishable CD133 and CD34 antigen expressions.
Dotplot-1: demonstration of FACS-analysis of bone marrow during complete remission. In this dotplot there is seen a small frequency of $CD34^+/CD133^+$ cells, and however a small part of cells showing only CD34 expression. Because pathological blasts could not be detected by the usage of morphological and immunological techniques, those cells have to be assigned to be hematopoetic precursor cells. 2nd quadrant (upper right); 4th quadrant (lower right).
Dotplot-2: shows the analysis of common ALL subtype in case of first relapse. Leukemic blasts (79%) are described by double-positivity of fluorescence labelling ($CD34^+/CD133^+$) as given in 2nd quadrant (upper right).

Discussion

The development of antigens CD34 on the surface of hematopoietic stem- and progenitor cells in bone marrow, umbilical cord blood and peripheral blood, but also on cells belonging to the stroma as well as on vascular endothelial cells, was of great importance for the understanding of physiology in hematopoiesis [18-20]. Nowadays this „stem cell antigen“ is the most common parameter for flow cytometric analyses of hematopoietic precursor cells [16] and essential for the transplantation of peripheral blood stem cells. In the progress of cellular differentiation expression of CD34 is continuously decreased and finally perfect lost. Applying suitable antibodies, preferring class III antibodies [16], CD34-positive cell populations can be quantified and characterized. With the development of immunomagnetic cell separation systems *(MACS)*, one is in charge of a technology, to concentrate HSPC in purities up to 98% [2, 21]. Even unwanted cell populations without CD34 antigens can be successfully separated using this procedures.

It is known for several years, that various tumors, especially leukemic blast cells demonstrate CD34-antigens in considerable percentages [19, 20, 22, 23]. 40–60% out of all acute leukemias are immunophenotyped positive for CD34. Detailed informations are acquired in a study, where bone marrow samples from altogether 481 children and adults with acute myeloid leukemias (AML) had been investigated and in 44% showed an expression of CD34 [7]. As given in Table 2, our results for pediatric AML's about 42% are in good correspondence with the literature. In contrast CD34-expressions were found to be clearly higher in 78% (32/41) of our investigated ALL samples.

Autologous transplantation following CD34-positive separation is problematical, specially when the malignant cell clone exhibits „CD34“-phenotype. In this case a discrimination and separation exclusively of HSPC applying anti-CD34-antibodies is not any longer possible. Several researchers have demonstrated that even stem cell transplants derived from neuroblastoma patients are often contaminated by ($CD34^+$)-tumor cells [3, 21, 24].

In order to overcome this dilemma, clinical research concentrates to the development of alternative purging-strategies. At the present time antigenic pattern of additional stem cell receptors is investigated using specific antibodies and to prove their effectiveness for positive separation. Neu et al. [8] recently published a successful isolation and immunophenotypic characterization of CD117-positive cells.

Dotplot-3: demonstration of FACS-analysis of bone marrow from a patient with AML. The pathological blast cells are identified by the expression of CD34 and the absence of CD133 antigen (<5%).

Dotplot-4: represents again a sample derived from a child with AML. In this case leukemic blasts are characterized because of the absence of both, CD34 as well as CD133 antigens. 1st quadrant (upper left) shows in a small frequency (0.24%) a population, obviously CD133+ stem-/precursor cells.

Dotplots-5–6: illustrate acute leukemias, showing pathological blasts either expressing CD133 exclusively (Dotplot-5) or as given in Dotplot-6 leukemic blast cells are predominantly [74%] of $CD133^+/CD34^-$-phenotype, however coexpressing in a small amount [21%] additionally CD34 antigen.

At the end of 1997 *Miraglia et al.*, and *Yin et al.* [9, 10] described a newly developed stem cell antigen, called CD133. Since the commercially availability of two monoclonal antibodies (CD133/1 and CD133/2) this antigen has become across great interest of immunologists and hematooncologists.

CD133 is a glycoprotein and is a newly identified cellular surface molecule, composed of a 5-transmembranous structure (5-TM) with C-terminal intracellular aminoacid-loops as well as N-terminal loops in extracellular area [9]. Molecular weight of CD133 is about 120 kD and demonstrates homologue with mouse protein prominin [13, 24]. The function of CD133 is not known yet, but the murine antigen could play a role in transferring signals of neuroepithelial and epithelial cells [9, 10, 13].

In literature [9] it is known, that CD133 is expressed by 30–60% of human hematopoietic stem- / and progenitor cells, showing classical marker CD34 and CD90 (Thy-1) as well as being positive for CD117 (c-kit), but negative for HLA-DR and mostly negative for CD38. Therefore $CD133^+$-cells seem to represent a subtype of early HSPCs [26, 27].

First indications, that leukemic blasts with $CD34^+$-phenotype coexpress CD133, too, are from *Miraglia et al.* [9]. This observation was the reason for us to include the immunophenotypic analyses of acute leukemias for the expression of CD133 in our study [12].

The evaluation of altogether 69 BM samples from children with acute leukemias at time of diagnosis showed, that nearly half of those leukemias had CD133-positive blast cells (Table 2). Comparing estimated values of ALL group and AML group it turned out that only 29% of AML's in contrast to 49% of ALL's exhibited newly stem cell marker CD133.

Applying double staining procedures with monoclonal antibodies HPCA-2-FITC (anti-CD34) and CD133-PE we could demonstrate heterogeneous behavior in antigen expression in ALL's as well as in AML's. In most cases relative values were higher for CD34 than those for CD133. In 10 ALL samples with CD34-positive phenotype we could not find any expression of CD133, in 3 other cases we in contrast found an expression of CD133 without simultaneously expression of CD34. This unusual differentiation till now was observed only in very single cases. The announcement of such -indeed very rare- cases are published by other researchers as well, i.e. Kratz-Albers [28] and Snell et al. [29] in AML's, as well as Baersch et al. [30], reporting a child with common ALL (cALL) and high expressions of CD133 but missing any CD34 expression of leukemic blasts ($CD133^+/CD34^-$). If those rare marker constellations are of prognostic value, has to be proved by long term investigations.

At the present time in numerous centers the concepts of stem cell transplantation is proved and following long term observations will be modified if necessary. Our results make sure even now, that the quantification of $CD34^+$- hematopoietic stem- and progenitor cells should be completed by additional verifying CD133 antigen expression. Additionally the quantification of CD34 and CD133 expression of leukemic cell clone at time of diagnosis is just as important.

Acute leukemias with „$CD34^+/CD133^-$" phenotype and no or only few response to therapeutic regimens, could profit from an autologous peripheral blood stem cell transplantation especially following purging of $CD133^+$-stem-/precursor cells.

Based upon first experiences [12, 31] *MACS*-technology in combination with CD133-Microbeads could be developed to be an alternative to established CD34-positive selection system.

Acknowledgements. For cooperation with university clinic of pediatrics in Heidelberg we are grateful to Dr. H. Sieverts. Special thanks to „Hilfe für krebskranke Kinder Frankfurt/M. e.V." and „Frankfurter Stiftung für krebskranke Kinder" for finacial supports.

References

1. Siena, S., M. Bregni, M. Gianni: Estimation of peripheral blood $CD34^+$ cells for autologous transplantation in cancer patients. Exp. Hematol 21 (1993) 203-205
2. Miltenyi, S., W. Müller, W. Weichel, A. Radbruch: High gradient magnetic cell separation with MACS. Cytometry 11 (1990) 231-238
3. Häfer, R., A. Voigt, B. Gruhn, F. Zintl: Neuroblastoma cells can express the hematopoietic progenitor cell antigen CD34 as detected at surface protein and mRNA level. J. Neuroimmunology 96 (1999) 201-206
4. Lode, H.N., R. Handgretinger, U. Schuermann, G. Seitz, T. Klingebiel, D. Niethammer, J. Beck: Detection of neuroblastoma cells in CD34+ selected peripheral stem cells using a combination of tyrosine hydroxylase nested RT-PCR and ganglioside GD2 immunocytochemistry. Eur. J. Cancer 33 (1997) 2024-2030
5. Ebener, U., S. Wehner, A. Brinkmann, E. Niegemann, V. Zotova, B. Kornhuber: Comparison of the Expression of AC133 and CD34 in childhood acute leukemia. Onkologie, 22 suppl 1 (1999) 106, [abstract no. 0391]
6. Pui, C.H., M.L. Hancock, R. David, G.K. Rivera, A.T. Look, J.T. Sandlund, F., F.G. Behm: Clinical Significance of CD34 Expression in Childhood acute lymphoblastic Leukemia. Blood 82 (1993) 889-894
7. Sperling, C., T. Büchner, U. Creuzig, J. Ritter, J. Harbott, C. Fonatsch, C. Sauerland, M. Mielcarek, G. Maschmeyer, H. Löffler, W.D. Ludwig: Clinical, morphologic, cytogenetic and prognostic implications of CD34 expression in childhood and adult *de novo* AML. Leuk. and Lymph. 17 (1995) 417-426
8. Neu, S., A. Geiselhart, S. Kuci, F. Baur, D. Niethammer, R. Handgretinger: Isolation and phenotypic characterization of CD117-positive cells. Leuk Res. 30 (1996) 963-971
9. Miraglia, S., W. Godfrey, A.H. Yin, K. Atkins, R. Warnke, J.T. Holden, R.A. Bray, E.K. Waller, D.W. Buck.: A novel five-transmembrane hematopoietic stem cell antigen: isolation, characterization, and molecular cloning. Blood 90, 12 (1997) 5013-21
10. Yin, A. H., S. Miraglia, E.D. Zanjani, G. Almeida-Porada, M. Ogawa, A.G. Leary, J. Olweus, J. Kearney, D.W. Buck: AC133, a novel marker for human hematopoietic stem and progenitor cells. Blood 90, 12 (1997) 5002-5512
11. Baersch, G., M. Baumann, J. Ritter, H. Jürgens, J. Vormoor: Expression of AC133 and CD117 on candidate normal stem cell populations in childhood B-cell precursor acute lymphoblastic leukaemia. B.J. Haematol. 107 (1999) 572-580
12. Ebener, U., S. Hakuba, S. Wehner, M. Stegmüller, E. Niegemann, B. Kornhuber, D. Schwabe,: Phenotypic characterization of various CD34+ cell populations using anti-AC133. Annals Hematol, Supplement II, 77 (1998) 153 [abstract no.606]
13. Miraglia, S., W. Godfrey, D.W. Buck: A response to AC133 hematopoietic stem cell antigen: human homologue of mouse kidney prominin or distinct member of a novel protein family? Blood 91, 11 (1998) 4390-4391 [Letter]
14. de Wynter, E.A., D. Buck, C. Hart, R. Heywood, L.H. Coutinho, A. Clayton, J.A. Rafferty, D. Burt, G. Guenechea, J.A. Bueren, D. Gagen, L.J. Fairbairn, B.I. Lord, N.G. Testa: CD34(+) AC133(+) cells isolated from cord blood are highly enriched in long-term culture-initiating cells, NOD/SCID-repopulating cells and dendritic cell progenitors. Stem Cells 16, 6 (1998) 387-396

15. Bene, M.C., G. Castoldi, W. Knapp, W.D. Ludwig, E. Matudes,, A. Orfao, M.B. van't Veer: Proposals for the immunological classification of acute leukemias. European group for the immunological characterization of leukemias (EGIL). Leukemia 9 (1995) 1783-1786
16. Rothe, G., G. Schmitz, D. Adorf, S. Barlage, M. Gramatzki, H. Hanenberg, H.G. Höffkes, G. Janossy, R. Knüchel, W.D. Ludwig, T. Nebe, C. Nerl, A. Orfao, S. Serke, R. Sonnen, A. Tichelli, B. Wörmann: Consensus protocol for the flow cytometric immunophenotyping of hematopoietic malignancies. Leukemia 10 (1996) 877-895
17. Gutensohn, K., S. Serke: Durchflußzytometrische Analyse CD34-exprimierender hämatopoetischer Zellen in Blut und Zytaphereseprodukten. Infusionsther. Transfusionsmed. 23, Suppl. 2 (1996) 1-23
18. Civin , C.I., L.C. Strauss, C. Brovall, M.J. Fackler, J.F. Schwartz, J.H. Shaper: Antigenic analysis of hematopoiesis. III. A hematopoietic progenitor cell surface antigen defined by a monoclonal antibody raised against KG1a cells. J. Immunol., 133 (1984) 157-165
19. Katz, F., R.W. Tindle, D.R. Sutherland, M.D. Greaves: Identification of a membrane glycoprotein associated with hemopoietic progenitor cells. Leuk. Res. 9 (1985) 191-198
20. Krause, D.S., M.J. Fackler, C.I. Civin, W.S. May: CD34: Structure, biology, and clinical utility. Blood, 87 (1996) 1-13
21. Handgretinger, R., P. Lang, M. Schumm, C. Tailor, S. Neu, E. Koscielnak, D. Niethammer, T. Klingebie: Isolation and transplantation of autologous peripheral CD34+ progenitor cells highly purified magnetic-activated cell sorting. Bone Marrow Transpl. 21 (1998) 987-993
22. Aiba, S., N. Tabata, H. Ishii, H. Ootani, H. Tagami: Dermatofibrosarcoma protuberans is a unique fibrohistiocytic tumour expressing CD34. Br. J. Dermatol. 127 (1992) 79-84
23. Westra, W.H., W.L. Gerald, J. Rosai: Solitary fibrous tumor. Consistent CD34 immunoreactivity and occurrence in the orbit. Am. J. Surg. Pathol. 18 (1994) 992-998
24. Moss, T.J., D.G. Sanders, L.C. Lasky, B. Bostrom: Contamination of peripheral blood stem cell harvests by circulating neuroblastoma cells. Blood 76 (1990) 1879-1883
25. Corbeil, D., K. Röper, A. Weigmann, W.B. Huttner: AC133 hematopoietic stem cell antigen: human homologue of mouse kidney prominin or distinct member of a novel protein family? Blood 91, 7 (1998) 2625-2626 [Letter]
26. Bühring, H.J., M. Seiffert, T.A. Bock, S. Scheding, A. Thiel, A. Scheffold, L. Kanz, W. Brugger: Expression of novel surface antigens on early hematopoietic cells. Ann N Y Acad Sci 872 (1999) 25-38
27. Pettengell, R., D. Pearce, E.C. Gordon-Smith, C. McGuckin, J.C.W. Marsh: AC133 selects an earlier haematopoietic subset than CD34. 40th Annual Meeting of the American Society of Hematology (1998), [abstract no. 1830]
28. Kratz-Albers, K., M. Zühlsdorf, R. Leo, W.E. Berdel, H. Serve.: Expression of AC133, a novel stem cell marker, on human leukemic blasts lacking CD34(-) antigen and on human CD34(+) leukemic cell line: MUTZ-2. Blood 92, 11 (1998) 4485-4487, [Correspondence]
29. Snell, V., E. Jackson, D. Buck, M. Adreeff: Expression of the AC133 antigen in leukemic and normal progenitors. 40th Annual Meeting of the American Society of Hematology (1998) [abstract no. 483]
30. Baersch, G., M. Baumann, J. Ritter, H. Jürgens, J. Vormoor: Asynchronous expression of AC133 on CD34-negative leukemic blast cells in childhood B-cell precursor ALL. In: Hematology and Blood Transfusion, Acute Leukemias VIII: Prognostic Factors and treatment Strategies (ed. by T. Büchner,, W. Hiddemann, W. Wörmann and J. Ritter) Springer-Verlag, Berlin (2000), [in press]
31. Yin, A. H., J. Phi-Wilson, Y. Zeng, B. Ware, K. Sheehan, D. Recktenwald, P. Law: Large scale AC133+ cell selection with MACS technology, (1998), [abstract no. 1820]

Identification of Minimal Residual Leukemia Applying Continuous Gating

S. WEHNER, H.-D. KLEINE*, B. KORNHUBER, and U. EBENER

J.W. Goethe University, Clinic of Pediatrics-III, Dept. of Hematology and Oncology, Theodor-Stern-Kai 7, D-60590 Frankfurt/M.; *University of Rostock, Clinic of Internal Medicine; Germany

Abstract

Clonal expansion of hematopoietic progenitor cells arrested at various differentiation steps demonstrating defined antigen expressions are characteristic for acute leukemias. The detection of hyperdiploid leukemic blast cells are an independent prognostic factor strongly associated with favorable clinical outcome. Therefore a combination of immunophenotype and aneuploid DNA-index may be of great benefit for the detection of minimal residual disease in acute leukemias.

In the present study we therefore used „Continuous Gating“ (medac Hamburg/ Germany) for identifying minimal involved tumor cells in bone marrow of acute lymphoblastic leukemia.

Following application of immunophenotyping leukemic blast cells by characteristic marker profile (i.e. CD10 in cALL) and subsequently staining of cellular DNA using propidium iodid, we, applying FACS-analysis, were able to simultaneously demonstrate both: antigen expression and DNA content. Following data acquisition maintained list mode files were analyzed applying a new software, able to automatically identify an-euploid tumor cells with unknown DNA-index. Primarily we discriminate doublets from the data set and then identify diploid G0/G1-peak by means of immunophenotyped remaining hematopoiesis as an internal standard. Subsequently the software itself creates a 200 x 200 channel-gate (out of 1023 x 1023 channels) in order to scan the whole SSC/FITC dot plot 10.000 times. This gate is moved by the program itself to higher channel numbers with a certain step size and the evaluation is done repeatedly with increasing DNA-indices. The cells, defined by the 10.000 different dot plot gates, were investigated for percentage of cells within the DNA-gate. The results are displayed in up to 25 „Continuous-Gating“-contour-plots attached with the tested DNA-indices. Enrichments of G0/G1-phase cells together with the tested DNA-index are shown in the contour plot as well.

Simultaneously performing both, establishing immunophenotype supported DNA-analysis and automatically detection of aneuploid tumor cells with unknown DNA-index in a standardized manner, profits from the different tech-

Supported by „Hilfe für Krebskranke Kinder Frankfurt e.V.“ and „Frankfurter Stiftung für krebskranke Kinder“.

niques' advantages. The described method may be an useful tool for identifying minimal residual leukemic blast cells with known marker profile as well as an aneuploid DNA-index.

Introduction

In patients suffering from acute leukemias a high complete remission rate is currently achieved. Nevertheless patients will eventually relapse due to the persistence of low numbers of residual leukemic cells, which are undetectable using conventional cytomorphologic criteria. This condition is known as minimal residual disease (MRD). The most common techniques suitable for detecting MRD are polymerase chain reaction (PCR) analysis and immunophenotyping of aberrant combinations of leukemic markers [2, 8].

Through the progress of flow cytometric techniques we in the present publication want to proof the applicability of simultaneous immunophenotype-supported detection of an-euploid DNA-content using flow cytometry in combination with new software „Con-tinuous Gating“ (medac GmbH / Hamburg) in order to identify minimal residual leukemia in bone marrow aspirates of childhood acute leukemia.

Material and Methods

Investigations were applied to bone marrow aspirates or peripheral blood samples derived from patients with acute leukemia (n=49) at time of diagnosis / relapse or during remission. To prove sensitivity of applied combined procedure serial dilution experiments were prepared. For this purpose mononucleated cell population was isolated by Ficoll-Paque gradient centrifugation from bone marrow of acute leukemia patients with blast cell concentrations about 95%. Subsequently separated cell suspension have been diluted with peripheral blood lymphocytes derived from healthy donors. By this way pathological blast cells have been diluted down to 0,00001 %.

Immunophenotype supported DNA-analyses

The main basics of flow cytometric simultaneous immunological DNA-analysis are described examplarily for bone marrow aspirate of newly diagnosed cALL. Hematological specimen, as usual for diagnosis of leukemias, especially bone marrow includes a multitude of heterogeneous subpopulations, different not only quantitative but also in proliferating activity. The analysis of malignant cells within hematological probes therefore should exclude normal hemopoiesis from estimation of ploidy status. We therefore at first applied immunophenotyping characteristic marker profile of leukemic blast cells or normal hemopoiesis with fluorescein isothiocyanate (FITC) conjugated monoclonal antibodies (i.e. CD10 in cALL) to enable distinguishing tumor cells from normal bone marrow cells.

Afterwards cellular DNA was stained stoechiometrically by intercalating DNA-dye propidium iodide [5, 7].

Data acquisition was done on FACScan (Becton Dickinson / HD) using CELLQuest-software and Doublet Discrimination module. At least between 10.000 and 50.000 single cell events have been acquired.

„Continuous Gating"

Estimation of aneuploidy and for studying minimal residual disease in childhood acute leukemia via immunophenotype supported DNA-analyses, we applied commercially available new software "Continuous Gating®" (medac GmbH, Hamburg) to automatically identify aneuploid tumor cells with unknown DNA-index. The procedure of CG is illustrated in (Fig. 1–5). Results, this means aneuploidies, are expressed as DNA-indices in combination with certain defined cellular attributes.

Definition of DNA-index

DNA-index (DI), flow cytometric parameter for estimation of cellular DNA-content, was defined according to the current nomenclature for DNA cytometry. DNA ploidy levels are expressed as DI, representing the ratio of relative fluorescence intensities of G0/G1 peaks of pathological blast cell population and diploid hemopoietic reference standard. A DI of 1.0 is set as the DNA content of normal non-proliferating lymphocytes and defining diploid DNA. Aneuploidy is characterized by the presence of two or more different peaks of cells in the G0/G1 cell cycle phase. In childhood acute leukemia hyperdiploidy with DI > 1.16 is of prognostic value [6].

Preparation of data sets

The basic adjustments of data sets are illustrated in Figure 1. The upper series demonstrate the essential preparation of list mode files of newly diagnosed cALL, the lower series those of a beginning cALL-relapse. Respectively at first following gating residual diploid hemopoiesis by means of immunophenotyping, the position of G0/G1-phase-peak of normal BM-cells is defined in DNA-histogram. In case of immunophenotyping leukemic blasts, normal hemopoiesis can be identified by fluorescence-negativity (CD10-FITC negative population; white frames), whereas common ALL blasts are positive for CD10. As shown in the lower series in case of beginning cALL-relapse -as expected- the remaining hemopoiesis is more dominant. This is reflected in DNA-histogram as well: an an-euploid G0/G1-peak can be identified only difficult.

The final evaluation will admit again all datas, only cellular conglomerates are excluded by gating in DNA-parameter dot plot (FL2-W vs. FL2-A). Thereby only such results are considered, that are created by single cells simultaneously be-

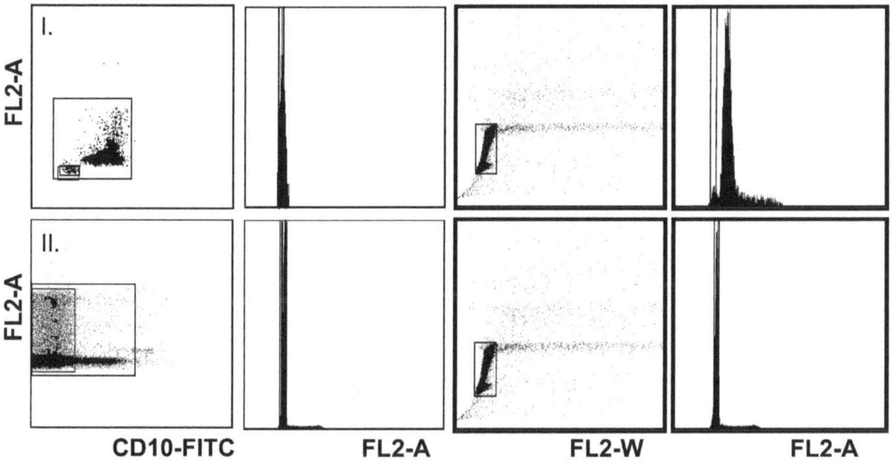

Fig. 1. Criterions for Evaluation

longing to certain populations. Subsequently mentioned adjustments, the actual analysis, so called „Continuous Gating" is started in SSC vs. FL1-Dotplot.

The main principle of „Continuous Gating" (CG) is illustrated in Figure 2. As the softwares' name impresses, CG itself creates an analysis gate of defined size (i.e. 200x200 out of 1023x1023 channels) in order to scan automatically the complete SSC/CD10-FITC dot plot 10.000 times for the presence of suspected aneuploidy. Thereby the previously determined position of diploid G0/G1-peak of normal hemopoiesis in DNA-histogram is used as a reference. The analysis-gate is moved by the program itself to higher channel numbers with a certain step size

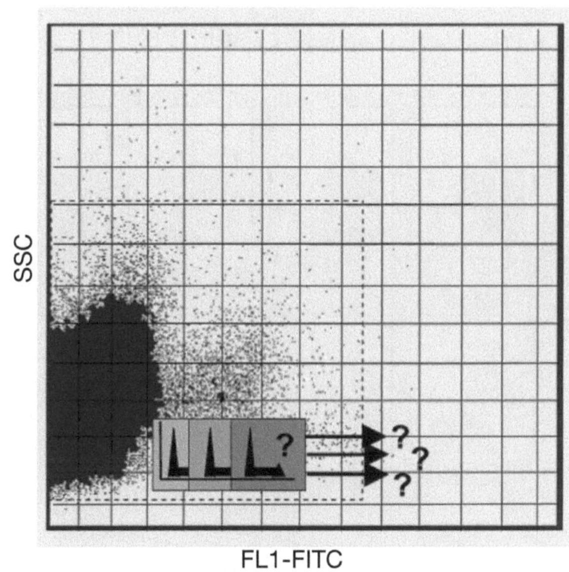

Fig. 2. Summary of CG-plots at time of dianosis

and the evaluation is done repeatedly with increasing DNA-indices. By this way several 10.000 overlapping gates are maintained. Each single gate enables the demonstration of DNA-content and estimation of percentage of affected cells for each intensity of antigen expression of previously chosen parameters [4].

Results

The results are displayed in up to 25 „Continuous-Gating"-contour-plots attached with individual DNA-indices. Enrichments of aneuploid G0/G1-phase cells together with the tested DNA-index are visualized in the CG-plots using a colour code (Fig. 3, 4).

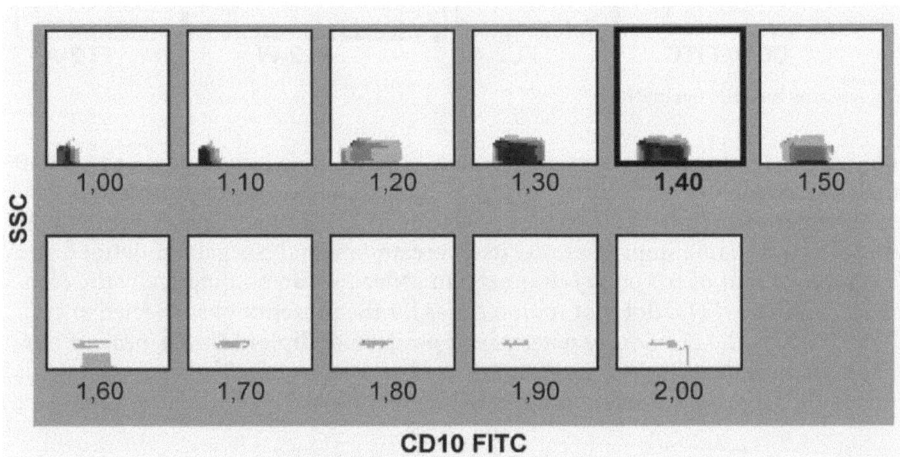

Fig. 3. Principle of „Continuous Gating"

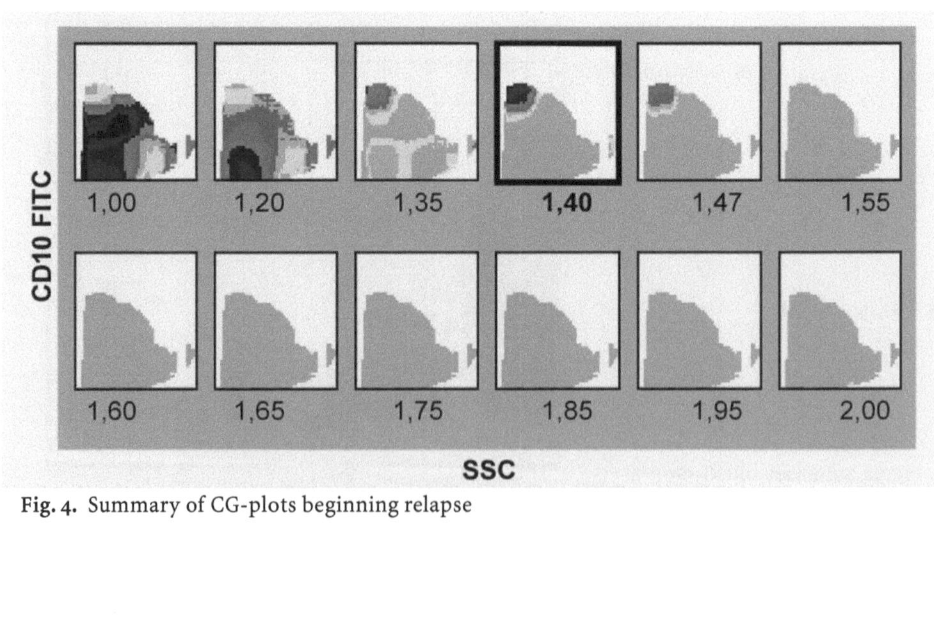

Fig. 4. Summary of CG-plots beginning relapse

The CG-plots derived from newly diagnosed cALL are demonstrated in Figure3. CG-plots 1 and 2 show Go/G1-phase cells of normal BM with diploid DNA-content, whereas all following plots show the position of CD10 positive cALL-blast cells. The colour code demonstrates most high concentration of aneuploid leukemic blast cells in 5th CG-plot and DI = 1.40.

In Figure 4 such a result-window is given in case of beginning relapse, with high concentrations of diploid hemopoiesis. In this example the 4th CG-plot colourizes a small population with DNA-index of 1.40. These cells are defined by specific granularity and antigen expressions. This special CG-plot can be chosen in order to be reanalyzed in detail.

As demonstrated in Figure 5 a simple mouse-click in any region of this interesting plot is sufficient to automatically show results of selected areas. This means, distribution of an-euploidies of cells, can be visualized and proved via individual DNA-histograms. As shown, the coloured area covers hyperdiploid cells, so Go/G1-phase cells of pathological blast population, and can be discriminated from normal hemopoiesis.

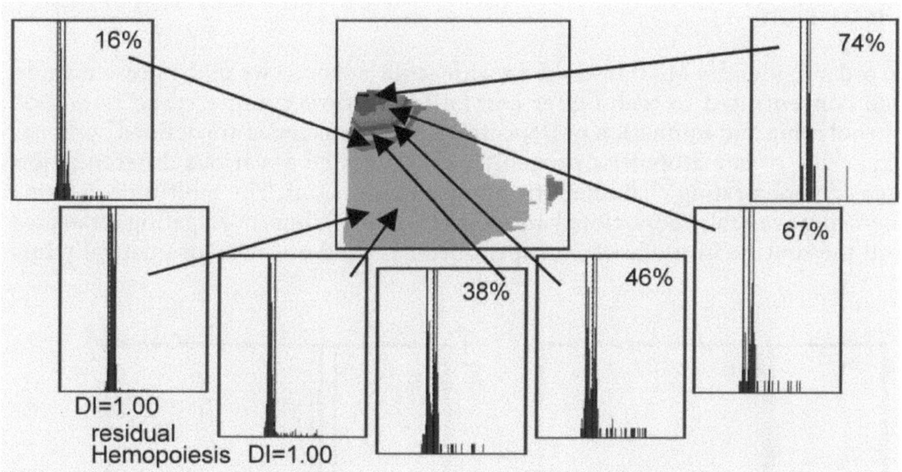

Fig. 5. CG Enables Verifying of Results

Table 1. Results of Immunophenotype-Supported Determination of DNA-Ploidy

Patients	number [n]	Ploidy-Status diploid	*vs.*	aneuploid
pre-B-ALL	32	14		18
T-ALL	9	7		2
AML	8	5		3
total	49	26		23

Distribution of DNA-ploidy in Acute Leukemias

Our results are summarized in Table 1. To the present study 49 pediatrics suffering from acute leukemias (pre-B ALL: n=32; T-ALL: n=9; AML: n=8) were comprised. In 56% of analyzed pre-B-ALLs we found aneuploid DNA-content. Hyperdiploidy could be eva-luated in 2/9 T-ALLs, respectively in 3/8 AMLs.

Sensitivity of Continuous Gating

Based on dilution experiments, the detection limit of combined techniques ranged between 10^{-4} to 10^{-5}. Figure 6 summarizes the way CG achieves such sensitivities. The left DNA-histogram is obviously derived from diploid sample. Subsequently applying CG has resulted in the right DNA-histogram, identifying an aneuploid G0/G1-peak. The patients sample therefore could be verified to be contaminated by obviously invisible aneuploid leukemic blast cells.

Discussion

In order to identify MRD in children with acute leukemia we in the present study had concentrated to techniques committed to flow cytometry, so immunophenotyping and estimation of DNA-index. Acute leukemias are defined by clonal expansion of hematopoietic progenitor cells arrested at various differentiation steps demonstrating characteristic antigen expressions. The multitude of commercially available monoclonal antibodies (MoAbs), improved gating strategies and the routine in usage of multiparameter procedures have dramatically im-

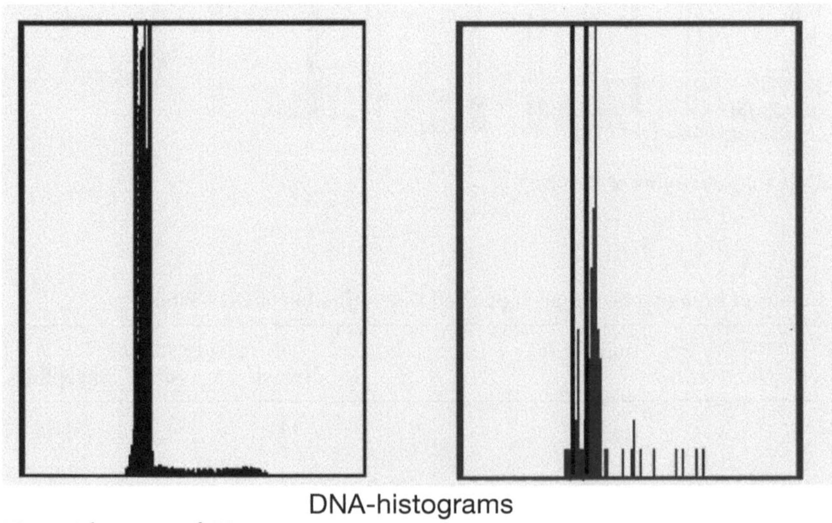

Fig. 6. Advantages of CG

proved the diagnostic utility of flow cytometry. On the other hand an abnormal nuclear DNA-content, thus aneuploidy has proved to be a conclusive marker for malignancy [3, 6].

In contrast to mitotic karyotyping, estimation of DNA-ploidy by FACS-analysis is performed directly on Go/G1 phase cells without requirement of in vitro cell cycle progression into mitosis; furthermore, it is highly quantitative and can be performed rapidly on thousands of cells in a short time [1].

By means of simultaneous immunophenotyping and determination of DNA-content can be estimated without the necessity of previously applying special separation techniques (f.e. FACS-sorting; MACS-technology). The combination of both techniques is already of great benefit for the detection of minimal residual disease in acute leukemias. Sensitivity in finding MRDs by flow cytometry is additionally increased by "Continuous Gating" [4, 5, 7].

Summary

In summary, FACS analysis is highly applicable to the detection and classification of leukemias due to the techniques' advantages. The combination of immunophenotype supported measurement of cellular DNA-aneuploidy on single cell suspensions with new analysis software CG enables a new feasible tool to detect MRD, even when no aberrant marker combinations are expressed/known and no sufficient metaphases can be evaluated for cytogenetic analyses, and no chromosomal translocations are known to perform PCR-analysis.

The present study confirms that the combined usage of CG with flow cytometric immunophenotyping and DNA-ploidy studies is a suitable approach for MRD investigation in acute leukemia patients based on their applicability and sensitivity (up to 10^{-5}).

CG simplifies and standardizes immunological estimation of ploidy status by automatically evaluation.

Requirements for applying CG in MRD are the knowledge of relevant marker profile of leukemic blast cells as well as the availability of aneuploid DNA-index.

References

1. Barlogie B, Stass S, Dixon D, Keating M, Cork A, Trujillo JM, McCredie KB, Freireich EJ: DNA Aneuploidy in Adult Acute Leukemia. Cancer Genet Cytogenet 28:213-228 (1987)
2. Coustan-Smith E, Behm FG, Sanchez J, Boyett JM, Hancock ML: Immunological detection of minimal residual disease in children with acute lymphoblastic leukaemia. The Lancet 351:550-554 (1998)
3. Harbott J, Ritterbach J, Ludwig WD, Bartram CR, Reiter A and Lampert F: Clinical Significance of Cytogenetic Studies in Childhood Acute Lymphoblastic Leukemia: Experience of the BFM Trials. In: Recent Results in Cancer Research. Vol.131. Springer-Verlag Berlin.Heidelberg pp. 123-132 (1993).
4. Kleine HD, Zech I, Nowak R, Oelschlägel U, Kundt G, Freund M: Detection of residual aneuploid leukemic cells by „continuous gating". Cytometry 36(1):71-76 (1999)
5. Nowak R, Hietschold V, Koslowski R, Plat M: Die gleichzeitige Analyse von Zellmembranantigenen und des DNA-Gehaltes in Knochenmarkzellen - Potentielle Bedeutung für die Hämatologie. Z Klin Med 46:535-537 (1991)

6. Trueworthy R, Shuster, J, Look T, Crist W, Borowitz M, Carroll A, Frankel L, Harris M, Wagner H, Haggard M, Mosijczuk A, Steuber P, Land V: Ploidy of lymphoblasts is the strongest predictor of treatment outcome in B-progenitor cell acute lymphoblasic leukemia of childhood: A Pediatric Oncology Group study. J Clin Oncol 10:606 (1992)
7. Wehner S, Ebener U, Kornhuber B: Simultane Bestimmung des Immunphänotyps und DNA-Gehalts bei akut lymphoblastischen Leukämien im Kindesalter (FACS-Analyse). J Cancer Res Clin Oncol (1995); abstract
8. Wörmann B, Safford M, Konemann S, Büchner T, Hiddemann W, Terstappen LW: Detection of aberrant antigen expression in acute myeloid leukemia by multiparameter flow cytometry. Recent Results Cancer Res 131;185-196 (1993)

Cord Blood Transplantation

Pilot Study – Lymphocyte Subset Reconstitution after Cord Blood Transplantation

T. Niehues[1], A.H. Filipovich[2], K.W. Chan[3], M. Körbling[3], and U. Göbel[1]

Dept. of Pediatric Hematology and Oncology Heinrich-Heine-University of Düsseldorf[1], Childrens Hospital Cinncinatti USA[2], Division of Pediatrics, The University of Texas MD Anderson Cancer Center, Houston, USA[3]

Abstract

It has been hypothesized that an insufficient lymphocyte number and function may be generated after cord blood transplantation (CBT) due to the immaturity of lymphocytes transplanted with cord blood (CB). Absolute numbers of T, B, and NK cells were collected retrospectively from 29 children and one young adult transplanted with CB at three centers. Long term reconstitution data ≥ 360 days were available from 14 patients (mean observation period: 652±228 days). In the majority of children near normal B and NK cell numbers are reached quickly at 30–60 days after CBT. T cell recovery kinetics shows a slow increase during the first 12–16 months post transplant similar to data reported after T cell depleted BMT. However, in contrast to BMT there is no inversion of CD4/CD8 T cell ratios in the majority of children at any time point. In half of the individuals there is T (CD3) cell deficiency (≤ 5th percentile) at 360-480 days, but >480 days after CBT all children show normal T cell numbers (defined as >5th percentile). In conclusion, there appears to be a relatively fast B cell and slow CD8 cell recovery, which may be associated with less GvH in CBT. A prospective analysis of immune recovery and clinical course is needed to investigate which patients are at an increased risk for relapse or immunodeficiency after CBT.

Introduction

Cord blood (CB) can be used as a stem cell source for transplantation to treat hematological malignant disease, bone marrow failure syndromes, hemoglobinopathies, immunodeficiencies and inborn errors of metabolism [1–5]. The immaturity of immunological effector cells in CB has been associated with a relatively low incidence of GvH disease after cord blood transplantation (CBT) [6, 7]. CB stem cells are used as an alternative stem cell source in the situation where there is no allogeneic bone marrow donor with an acceptable number of HLA mismatches available.

Immune recovery and T cell reconstitution in particular is of central importance for the occurrence of relapse, GvH, and infectious complications after stem

---

This work was supported by the Elterninitiative der Kinderkrebsklinik e. V. Düsseldorf

cell transplantation. The current model of T cell reconstitution after conventional BMT [8, 9] describes two pathways. First, there is a thymus-dependent pathway that resembles ontogeny and takes at least 2–3 months after T cell depleted BMT until T cells can be detected in peripheral blood: transplanted bone marrow (BM) $CD34^+$ stem cells differentiate to lymphoid progenitors that enter the thymus. This pathway depends on thymic function which decreases with age [10]. It is largely unknown to what extent $CD34^+$ CB stem cells differ qualitatively from $CD34^+$ BM stem cells in their capacity to generate lymphoid progenitors [11]. Second, there is a thymus-independent generation of T cells, which involves expansion of mature donor T cells present in the graft (peripheral expansion). This pathway is thought to be faster and less influenced by age. However, with respect to the thymus-independent pathway, quality and quantity of donor lymphocytes transplanted with BM and CB clearly differ: CB lymphocytes have repeatedly been characterized as immature and therefore a less efficient expansion of donor CB T cells in the thymus-independent pathway may be expected.

Although infectious complications are documented to be a major cause of death after CBT [3, 4] there are few data on the immune recovery after CBT. Prompted by two cases with evidence for severe immunodeficiency after CBT – one overwhelming fatal septicemia and one case of long term T lymphopenia at one of our institutions (HHU Düsseldorf) – we addressed the following questions to centers actively performing CBT: What is the time course of lymphocyte recovery after CBT? Is there long term reconstitution of normal lymphocyte numbers?

Material and Methods

Patient and graft characteristics

Data from 30 patients of three institutions (Childrens Hospital Cinncinatti, USA, n=14, Division of Pediatrics, The University of Texas MD Anderson Cancer Center, Houston, USA, n=13, Dept. of Pediatric Hematology and Oncology Heinrich-Heine-University of Düsseldorf, n=3) were included. Inclusion criteria were transplantation with cord blood as stem cell source and availability of lymphocyte subset counts at any given time point after CBT. Patient data were excluded if immunocompetent cells had been transferred post transplantation. Administration of cytokines in vivo or ex vivo was not a regarded as an exclusion criterion. Patient and graft characteristics are given in Table 1. Cord blood transplants were provided by cord blood banks in New York (n=16), Düsseldorf, Germany (n=4), St. Louis, USA (n=4), Barcelona, Spain (n=4), Louvain, Belgium (n=1) and New Jersey, USA (n=1). Cord blood transplants were collected, processed and thawed following published procedures [12, 13]. The most common conditioning regimens used were TBI, fludarabine, melphalan (n=8), ATG, CTX, busulfan, VP16 (n=7), thiotepa, busulfan, cyclophosphamide (n=5) and ATG, TBI, CTX (n=5). The following regimens were used for GvH prophylaxis: CSA and prednisone (n=14), FK506 and MTX (n=12), CSA and MTX (n=1) and FK 506 or CSA alone (n=3).

Table 1. Patient and graft characteristics in 30 patients

Patient and graft characteristics	Total study group
Age	median: 5,0 years ±4,5 SD (7 monts–21 years)
< 5 years	16
>5 years (5–10 years, 11–21 years)	14 (12, 2)
Diagnosis	
ALL	10
AML	4
MDS	3
CML Large cell lymphoma	1
Fanconi´s anemia	4
Wiskott Aldrich Syndrome	3
Hemophagocytic lymphohistiocytosis	2
CMV Status	
IgG positive	14
IgG negative	14
Not available	2
Graft	
$CD34^+$ cells x 10^6/kg body weight of recipient*	median 0,27±0,2 SD (0,01 - 0,75)
available	23
not available	7
NC x 10^7/kg body weight of recipient*	median: 4,2±4,2 SD (0,9–17,5)
Available	30
Not available	–
Donor	
Related	2
Unrelated	28
HLA matching	
>1/6 mismatch§	8
≤1/6 mismatch (Identical)	22 (3)
Conditioning regimen	
TBI	13
No TBI	17
Serotherapy	16
No Serotherapy	14
GvH prophylaxis	
MTX	13
No MTX	17
Prednisone	14
No Prednisone	16

* after thawing; § Mismatches were determined by serologic and/or high resolution molecular typing for HLA-A and B, and by molecular typing for DRB1

Table 1. Continued

Patient and graft characteristics	Total study group
Acute GvH	
≤ grade I (None, grade I)	19 (16, 3)
> grade I (grade II, III, IV)	11 (4, 5, 2)
Hematopoietic engraftment	
Neutrophils**	median 24d ± 9 SD
Available	29
Not available	1
Platelets#	median 60d ± 36 SD
Available	22
Not available	8
Events	
Relapse, alive	1
Death	8
relapse	4
infection	3
graft failure	1

** absolute neutrophil count >500/ml on 3 consecutive days; # platelet count >20000/ml on 7 consecutive days

Determination of lymphocyte subsets and CD34+ cells in the graft

In each institution analyses were performed by laboratories specialized in immunophenotyping blood samples of children before and after stem cell transplantation. $CD34^{+}$ cells in the graft and lymphocyte subpopulations in peripheral blood after CBT were analyzed by flow cytometry. with monoclonal antibodies for classical T (anti-CD3, CD4 and CD8), B (anti-CD19), and NK cell antigens (anti-CD56, CD16). Absolute numbers were calculated using the percentages of CD3, CD4, CD8, CD19, and CD56/CD16 staining and the lymphocyte count of the same sample. CD4/CD8 ratios represented the absolute number of CD4 cells divided by the number of CD8 cells at a given time point. As normal values in childhood vary considerably with age absolute numbers of CD3, CD4, CD8, B- and NK cells were transformed into percentages of age specific normal values, which were taken from two studies on Pediatric reference values for blood lymphocytes [14, 15] (*age adjusted percentages*). In addition absolute values for lymphocyte subsets were plotted into 5th and 50th percentiles [15].

Analysis of Kinetics

The mean observation period was 367±233 days SEM after CBT (range 40–1040 days). For the kinetic study data were grouped by the following time intervals: 0-29 (n=7), 30-59 (n=13), 60-89 (n=6), 90-119 (n=17), 120-239 (n=19), 240-359 (n=8), 360-480 (n=12) and >480 days (n=10) after CBT. At these time points the numbers of analyzed patients vary as some patients have not yet reached later time points or died later. If more than 1 value was available during these intervals, mean values were used.

Statistical analysis

The mean percentage of lymphocyte reconstitution between CD4 and CD8 cell reconstitution at >480 days was compared using the paired, one-tailed Student t-test. P-values $\leq$0,05 were considered as statistically significant.

Results

B and NK cell reconstitution

B and NK cells engrafted fast in the majority of individuals (Fig. 1): An age-adjusted percentage of more than 50% B cells was reached by the majority (9/16) children at day 90–119 with a mean age related percentage of 118%±105. NK cell recovery was even faster: After 30–59 days, the majority of patients (8/11) had already engrafted normal NK cell numbers above the 5th percentile. B and NK cell reconstitution was stable long term: At the time points 240–359, 360–480 and >480 days none of the children analyzed had B and NK cell numbers below the 5th percentile.

T cell reconstitution

The kinetics for CD3, CD4 and CD8 cells showed a slow increase (Fig. 1): At the first three time points after CBT (0–89 days) mean age-adjusted percentages of T (CD3) cell numbers were below 20 %, approached near normal age-adjusted percentages between 23–52% at 90-480 days and reached 77%±38 after >480 days. 6/12 individuals were either on or below the 5th percentile for normal CD3 cell numbers at 360–480 days (Fig. 2, left panel). Interestingly an increase occurred in all individuals after 480 days (Fig. 2, right panel) except in one individual who was left with CD3, CD4 and CD8 cell numbers below the 5th percentile (see discussion).

While CD4 cells showed a recovery similar to total T cells the reconstitution of CD8 cells was characterized by a less efficient reconstitution after >480 days: Compared to CD4 cell reconstitution (81%±40), the mean age-related percentage of CD8 cell reconstitution was significantly lower (57%±27, $p=0.01$). There was one additional individual left with CD8 cell numbers below the 5th percentile at >480 days. Inversion of CD4/CD8 ratios was observed only in single individuals and mean CD4/CD8 ratios were $\geq$2,0 at all time points (data not shown).

Discussion

Lymphocyte recovery after CBT has systematically been reported in few patients so far [16–19]. There are no lymphocyte recovery data reported beyond 1 year

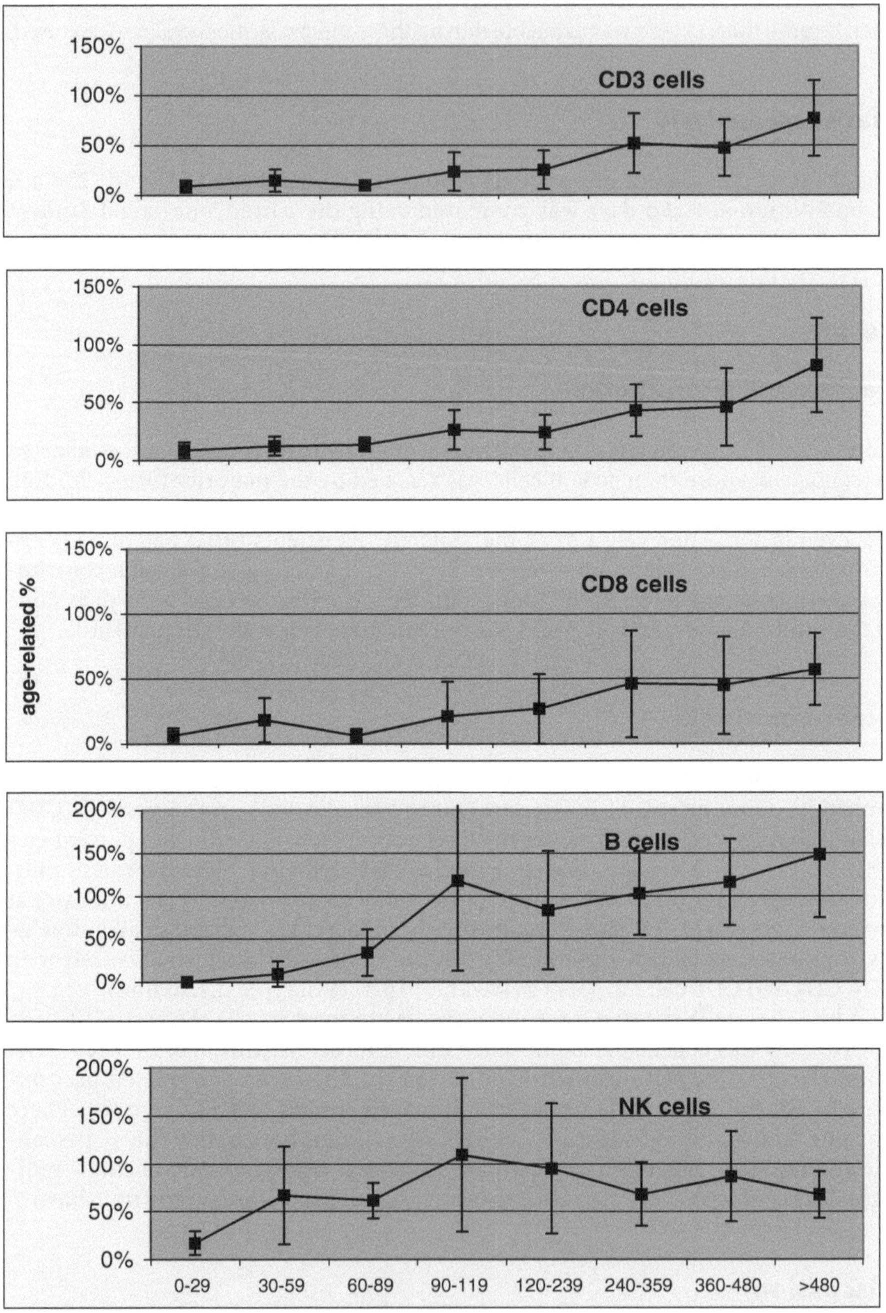

Fig. 1. Lymphocyte subset reconstitution kinetics after CBT. The x-axis represents different time intervals after CBT , values on the y-axis represent the mean age-related percentages ± SEM at each time point.

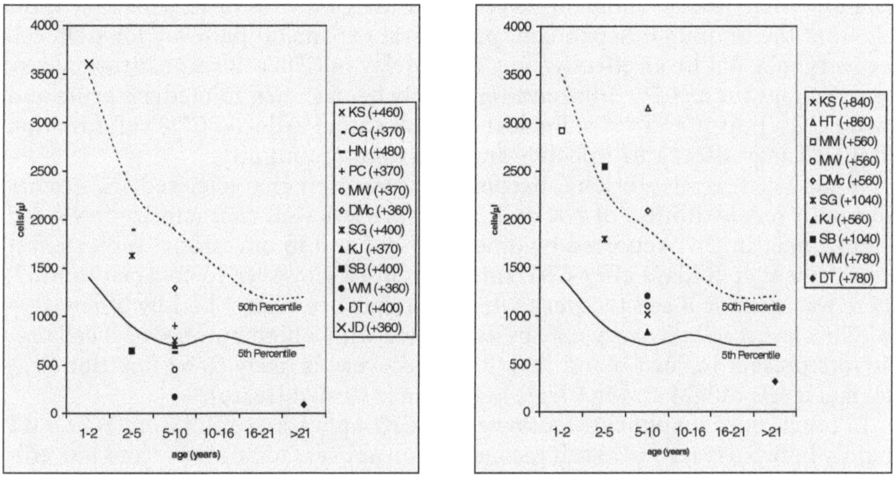

Fig. 2. Long term T cell reconstitution after CBT. The x-axis represents age at CBT expressed as different age intervals in years. Values on the y-axis show absolute number of CD3 cells/ml at 360-480 days (left panel) and >480 days (right panel) after CBT. Each symbol represents the number of CD3 cells of an individual patient (patient initials, day after CBT) and was plotted into 5th and 50th percentiles (calculated from reference 15).

after CBT. In this analysis, long term lymphocyte reconstitution after CBT is presented, based on a mean observation period of one year.

Most data on immune reconstitution after BMT in children are on T cell depleted (TCD) grafts. Immune recovery was reported to be complete within one year in earlier, smaller studies [20–22]. TCD and non-depleted BMT did not differ in long term lymphocyte recovery (22). The analysis of Kook on immune reconstitution after TCD-BMT in 102 children reported normalization (defined as >5th percentile) of CD3 cells within 18–36 months [23]. At the latest time point (18–24 months) in the analysis of 42 children by Small et al. there were also several children with T cell counts well below 1000/ml (Percentiles not given) [24]. In CBT we find that within 16-36 months all patients except one (see below) were above the 5th percentile, which is very similar to the large studies on TCD BMT by Kook and Small.

Long term T cell deficiency 16 months after CBT was observed only in one patient. This patient was the oldest patient (21 years) in the study group and received the lowest number of graft CD34$^+$cells/kg (0,01 x 10^6) and graft NC cells/kg (0,4 x 10^7). A multivariate analysis in a larger cohort is needed in order to identify independent risk factors influencing lymphocyte recovery and outcome (e.g. age, number of graft CD34$^+$ cells, graft NC cells/kg etc.).

What are the differences in lymphocyte recovery between CBT and BMT? Faster recovery of CD8 as compared to CD4 cells has been repeatedly observed in BMT and this has been attributed to peripheral expansion of mature CD8 cells transplanted with the graft. Even in TCD allogeneic BMT, reconstitution of CD8 cells is faster than that of CD4 cells [23, 24]. In CBT, however, our data as well as data by others [18, 19] show no inversion of the CD4:CD8 ratio. This may indicate that the thymus-independent, peripheral expansion pathway for CD8 cell recovery may not be as effective in CBT. A delay in CD8 cell reconstitution may be advantageous as CD8 cells have repeatedly been shown to mediate acute and chronic GvH. At present it is unclear to what extent reduced CD8 cell function after CBT may affect anti-infective and anti-tumor immunity.

While T cell reconstitution is becoming increasingly characterized, the mechanisms for reconstitution of NK and B cells are less well characterized. NK cell engraftment in CBT reported by others [16–19] and in our cohort indicate fast engraftment at 90 days after CBT, similar to BMT. However, in contrast to BMT, there was a faster B cell recovery, which also has been described by others [17–19]. This fast B cell recovery may be associated with a high number of B cell precursors present in cord blood [25]. B cell recovery is likely to be functional, as normal levels of IgM and IgA have been demonstrated [18, 19].

In conclusion, lymphocyte recovery after CBT appears to differ from TCD BMT mainly in two aspects: CD8 cell reconstitution appears to be slower and less efficient while engraftment of normal B cell numbers appears faster. This may result in an earlier availability of humoral immunity and less acute and chronic GvH in CBT compared to BMT. Persistence of normal numbers of lymphocyte subsets for years to come after CBT remains to be investigated. These preliminary findings may form the basis for a prospective analysis in a larger cohort (with a BMT control group) including determination of T cells in the CB transplant, testing of lymphocyte origin with donor/recipient specific markers, determination of naive and memory subsets, standardized immunological functional testing, and systematic recording of infectious complications and relapse after CBT.

Acknowledgements. We would like to thank E. Gluckman, V. Rocha and the EUROCORD group for discussion of the data, F. Locatelli, P. Wernet and G. Kögler for critical reading of the manuscript and S. Özbek for help in the preparation of the manuscript.

References

1. Wagner JE, Rosenthal J, Sweetman R, Shu XO, Davies SM, Ramsay NK, McGlave PB, Sender L, Cairo MS (1996) Successful transplantation of HLA-matched and HLA-mismatched umbilical cord blood from unrelated donors: analysis of engraftment and acute graft-versus-host disease. Blood 88: 795-802.
2. Kurtzberg J, Laughlin M, Graham MLSmith C, Olson JF, Halperin EC, Ciocci, Carrier C, Stevens CE, Rubinstein P (1996) Placental blood as a source of hematopoietic stem cells for transplantation into unrelated recipients. N Engl J Med 335: 157-166.
3. Gluckman E, Rocha V, Boyer-Chammard A Locatelli F, Arcese W, Pasquini R, Ortega J, Souillet G, Ferreira E, Laporte JP, Fernandez M, Chastang C (1997) Outcome of cord-blood transplantation from related and unrelated donors. Eurocord Transplant Group and the European Blood and Marrow Transplantation Group. N Engl J Med 337: 373-381.
4. Rubinstein P, Carrier C, Scaradavou A Kurtzberg J, Adamson J, Migliaccio AR, Berkowitz RL, Cabbad M, Dobrila NL, Taylor PE, Rosenfield RE, Stevens CE (1998) Outcomes among 562 recipients of placental-blood transplants from unrelated donors. N Engl J Med 339: 1565-1577.

5. Locatelli F, Rocha V, Chastang C, Arcese W, Michel G, Abecasis M, Messina C, Ortega J, Badell-Serra I, Plouvier E, Souillet G, Jouet JP, Pasquini R, Ferreira E, Garnier F, Gluckman E (1999) Factors associated with outcome after cord blood transplantation in children with acute leukemia. Eurocord-Cord Blood Transplant Group. Blood 93: 3662-3671.
6. Madrigal JA, Cohen SB, Gluckman E, Charron DJ (1997) Does cord blood transplantation result inlower graft-versus-host disease? It takes more than two to tango. Hum Immunol 56: 1-5.
7. Rocha V, Wagner JE Jr, Sobocinski KA, Klein JP, Zhang MJ, Horowitz MM, Gluckman E (2000) Graft-versus-host disease in children who have received a cord-blood or bone marrow transplant from an HLA-identical sibling. Eurocord and International Bone Marrow Transplant Registry Working Committee on Alternative Donor and Stem Cell Sources. N Engl J Med 342: 1846-1854.
8. Parkman R, Weinberg KI (1997) Immunological reconstitution following bone marrow transplantation. Immunol Rev 157: 73-78.
9. Mackall CL, Gress RE (1997) Pathways of T-cell regeneration in mice and humans: implications for bone marrow transplantation and immunotherapy. Immunol Rev 157: 61-72.
10. Mackall CL, Fleisher TA, Brown MR, Andrich MP, Chen CC, Feuerstein IM, Horowitz ME, Magrath IT, Shad AT, Steinberg SM, Wexler LH, Gress RE (1995) Age, thymopoiesis, and CD4+ T-lymphocyte regeneration after intensive chemotherapy. N Engl J Med 332: 143-149.
11. Noort WA, Willemze R, Falkenburg JH (1998). Comparison of repopulating ability of hematopoietic progenitor cells isolated from human umbilical cord blood or bone marrow cells in NOD/SCID mice. Bone Marrow Transplant 22 (Suppl. 1): S58-60.
12. Rubinstein P, Dobrila L, Rosenfield RE Adamson JW, Migliaccio G, Migliaccio AR, Taylor PE, Stevens CE (1995) Processing and cryopreservation of placental/umbilical cord blood for unrelated bone marrow reconstitution. Proc Natl Acad Sci U S A 92: 10119-10122.
13. Kögler G, Callejas J, Hakenberg P, Enczmann J, Adams O, Daubener W, Krempe C, Göbel U, Somville T, Wernet P (1996) Hematopoietic transplant potential of unrelated cord blood: critical issues. J Hematother 5: 105-116.
14. Erkeller-Yuksel FM, Deneys V, Yuksel B Hannet I, Hulstaert F, Hamilton C, Mackinnon H, Stokes LT, Munhyeshuli V, Vanlangendonck F (1992) Age-related changes in human blood lymphocyte subpopulations. J Pediatr Feb 120: 216-222.
15. Comans-Bitter WM, de Groot R, van den Beemd R Neijens HJ, Hop WC, Groeneveld K, Hooijkaas H, van Dongen JJ (1997) Immunophenotyping of blood lymphocytes in childhood. Reference values for lymphocyte subpopulations. J Pediatr 130: 388-393.
16. Knutsen AP, Wall DA. Kinetics of T-cell development of umbilical cord blood transplantation in severe T-cell immunodeficiency disorders (1999) J Allergy Clin Immunol 103: 823-832.
17. Locatelli F, Maccario R, Comoli P, Bertolini F, Giorgiani G, Montagna D, Bonetti F, De Stefano P, Rondini G, Sirchia G, Severi F (1996) Hematopoietic and immune recovery after transplantation of cord blood progenitor cells in children. Bone Marrow Transplant 18: 1095-1101.
18. Abu-Ghosh A, Goldman S, Slone V van de Ven C, Suen Y, Murphy L, Sender L, Cairo M (1999) Immunological reconstitution and correlation of circulating serum inflammatory mediators/cytokines with the incidence of acute graft-versus-host disease during the first 100 days following unrelated umbilical cord blood transplantation. Bone Marrow Transplant 24: 535-544.
19. Giraud P, Thuret I, Reviron D, Chambost H, Brunet C, Novakovitch G, Farnarier C, Michel G (2000) Immune reconstitution and outcome after unrelated cord blood transplantation: a single paediatric institution experience. Bone Marrow Transplant 25: 53-57.
20. Daley JP, Rozans MK, Smith BR, Burakoff SJ, Rappeport JM, Miller RA (1987) Retarded recovery of functional T cell frequencies in T cell-depleted bone marrow transplant recipients. Blood 70: 960-964.
21. Cowan MJ, McHugh T, Smith W, Wara D, Matthay K, Ablin A, Casavant C, Stites D (1987) Lymphocyte reconstitution in children receiving soybean agglutinin T-depleted bone marrow transplants. Transplant Proc 19: 2744.
22. Foot AB, Potter MN, Donaldson C, Cornish JM, Wallington TB, Oakhill A, Pamphilon DH (1993). Immune reconstitution after BMT in children. Bone Marrow Transplant 11: 7-13.
23. Kook H, Goldman F, Padley D Giller R, Rumelhart S, Holida M, Lee N, Peters C, Comito M, Huling, D, Trigg M (1996) Reconstruction of the immune system after unrelated or partially

matched T-cell-depleted bone marrow transplantation in children: immunophenotypic analysis and factors affecting the speed of recovery. Blood 88: 1089-1097.
24. Small TN, Papadopoulos EB, Boulad F Black P, Castro-Malaspina H, Childs BH, Collins N, Gillio A, George D, Jakubowski A, Heller G, Fazzari M, Kernan N, MacKinnon S, Szabolcs P, Young JW, O'Reilly RJ (1999) Comparison of immune reconstitution after unrelated and related T-cell-depleted bone marrow transplantation: effect of patient age and donor leukocyte infusions. Blood 93: 467-480.
25. Hannet I, Erkeller-Yuksel F, Lydyard P Deneys V, DeBruyere M (1992) Developmental and maturational changes in human blood lymphocyte subpopulations. Immunol Today 13: 215-218

Altered Growth Characteristics of Cord Blood after in vivo Exposure of the Mother to Chemotherapy

T. Fietz[1], R. Arnold[2], G. Massenkeil[2], H. Radtke[3], B. Reufi[1], E. Thiel[1], and W.U. Knauf[1]

[1]Dept. of Hematology, Oncology and Transfusion Medicine, Benjamin Franklin Hospital, Free University; [2]Dept. of Hematology and Oncology, [3]Dept. of Transfusion Medicine, Charité Hospital, Humboldt University, Berlin

Introduction

The biology of human umbilical cord blood cells is of growing interest regarding stem cell transplantation, since banked cord blood units might in the future represent the stem cell source of choice for certain patients lacking a suitable related or unrelated donor.

The content of $CD34^+$ progenitor cells in fetal blood decreases towards the end of pregnancy. Progenitor cells of term as well as of preterm neonates do have extensive proliferative capacities [1]. The influence of maternal malignant hematologic disease with or without chemotherapy on the development of fetal hematopoiesis is unknown.

Growth characteristics of cord blood cells from 2 newborns were studied. Both mothers were diagnosed with acute myeloid leukemia (AML) during pregnancy and in one case treated with one course of standard chemotherapy prior to cesarian section. Cord blood cells from 7 term newborns with healthy mothers were used as controls.

Material and Methods

Cord blood A (CB A)

Mother diagnosed with AML in the 31th week of gestation. No chemotherapy, cesarian section in gestational week 32.

Cord blood B (CB B)

Mother diagnosed with AML in the 26th week of gestation. Chemotherapy with thioguanin, ara C and doxorubicin (TAD 9) was given for remission induction. Cesarian section was performed in partial remission in week 30.

Controls

Cord blood cells from 7 term neonates from healthy mothers were used as controls.

All cord blood samples were obtained by puncture of the umbilical vein immediately after delivery and frozen in 5% DMSO. Prior to analysis cells were thawed according to the Rubinstein protocol and mononuclear cells (MNC) were isolated on Ficoll. Cultures were initiated in 24 well plates at a concentration of $1x10^6$ c/ml. Refeeding and reseeding at the initial cell concentration were on day 7, culture medium was IMDM containing SCF, flt-3 L, IL-3, IL-6, EPO and G-CSF. Methylcellulose assays were performed to assess colony (CFU-GM) growth, flow cytometry was applied to determine $CD34^+CD45^+$ cell content.

Results

Viability after thawing was 84% for CB A, 84% for CB B and mean 91% for control MNCs. The content of $CD34^+CD45^+$ progenitor cells was 2.7% in CB B, 1.64% in CB A and 1.56% for controls (this difference was not unexpected, since the content of $CD34^+$ progenitors in cord blood is high during fetal life and decreases towards birth). After short term culture the controls showed an increase in progenitor cells to 2.58% on day 7 with a decrease towards day 14. CB A – no chemo-

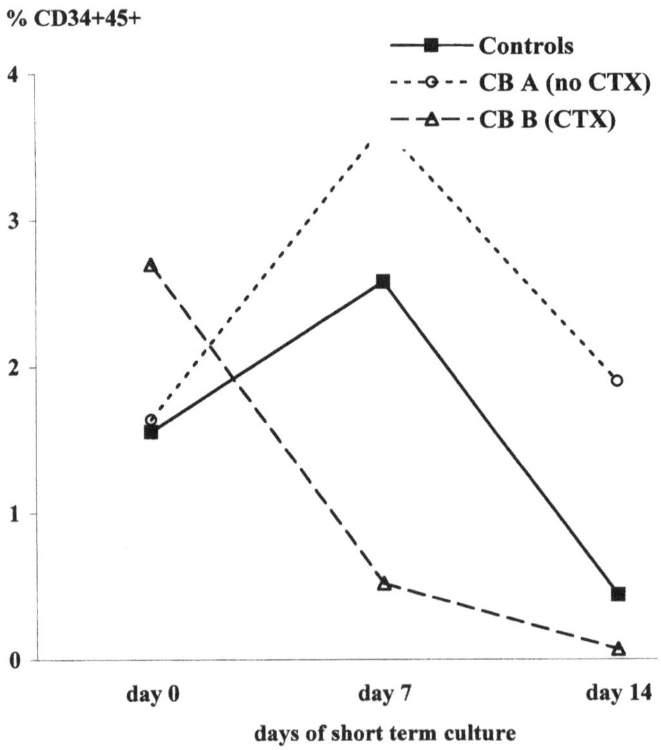

Fig. 1. % CD34 positive cells from human umbilical cord blood

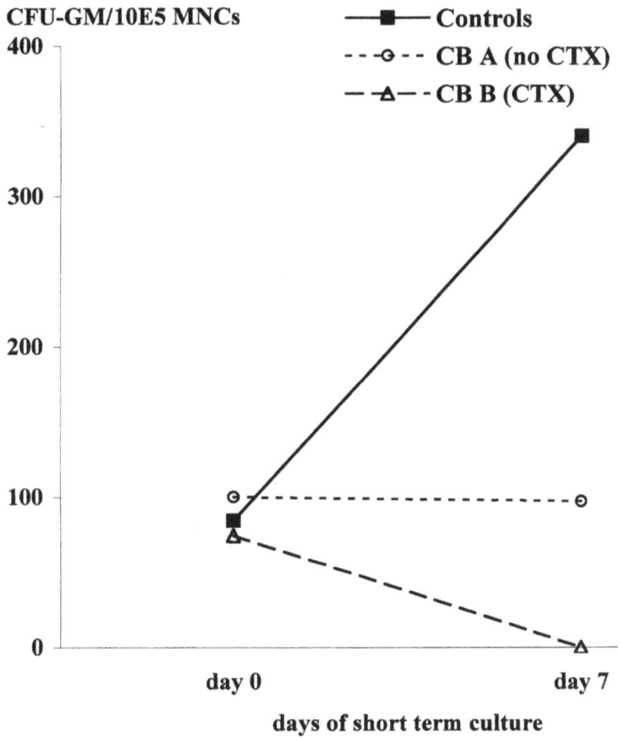

Fig. 2. CFU-GM from human cord blood per 10E5 seeded cells

therapy – showed the same proliferative pattern as the controls in contrast to CB B – harvested after TAD 9 chemotherapy – which showed a decrease to 0.52% on day 7 with less than 0.1% $CD34^+$ cells on day 14 (Fig. 1). On day 0 the frequency of CFU-GM was similar in all three groups. However, on day 7 CB A did not expand the number of colonies, and CB B showed no colonies at all (controls: 4 fold expansion) (Fig. 2).

The cloning efficiency (CFU-GM/$CD34^+$ cells) increased for controls from mean 5.4 on day 0 to 13.2% on day 7. CB A showed a decrease from 6.1 to 2.7% and CB B from 2.7 to 0%.

Discussion

The unexpected reduction in colony forming potential after short term culture (which cannot be seen in preterm cord blood obtained without maternal hematologic disease[1]) indicates a reduced growth potential of cord blood after in vivo exposure to maternal leukemia. Also the increased CD34 content on day 0 with a

[1] Wyrsch A et al. *Exp Hematol*, 1999: 1338-1345

reduced proliferation of CD 34^{+} cells for CB B compared to CB A during culture (Fig. 1) points towards an additional differentiation stimulating or toxic effect of chemotherapy.

Although conclusions must be drawn with caution due to the singularity of our samples, these data indicate that cord blood mononuclear cells in neonates with maternal leukemia show a normal CD34 content, viability and colony growth on day 0. After short term culture, however, the reduced proliferative potential becomes overt. Pre partum exposure to chemotherapy seems to further enhance this effect.

Mismatched Donor Transplantation

Bone Marrow Transplantation from Mismatched Unrelated Donors

A. R. Zander, T. Zabelina, C. Löliger, W. Krüger, T. Eiermann, H. Renges, M. Dürken, F. v. Finckenstein, H. Kabisch, R. Erttmann, and N. Kröger

Univ-Klinikum Hamburg-Eppendorf, Klinik und Poliklinik für Innere Medizin, Einr. für Knochenmarktransplantation, Martinistr. 52, D-20246 Hamburg, Germany

Introduction

Bone marrow transplantation is an accepted treatment for several haematological diseases like acute and chronic leukaemias, severe aplastic anaemia as well as inborn errors of metabolism and immune deficiency syndromes. Suitable family donors can be found in less than 30 percent of the cases. International registries for matched unrelated donors include world-wide more than seven million volunteers [2, 4, 11]. The probability to find a suitable HLA-A, -B, -DR-matched donor for a Caucasian recipient is about 70 percent. Matched unrelated donor transplants have been reported to have a higher incidence of transplant related mortality, specifically of acute and chronic graft-versus-host disease [5, 9, 13, 14, 15]. We explored Anti-Thymocyte-Globulin (Fresenius) as a part of a five-fold GvHD prevention programme [3, 6, 7, 8, 10, 12, 16]. Anti-Thymocyte-Globulin given prior to transplant has been shown to modify graft-versus-host disease in recipients of marrow from unrelated donors. Metronidazol, an antibiotic with high effectiveness against anaerobic bacteria, has been shown in a randomised study to reduce the incidence of gastrointestinal acute GvHD. HLA-mismatched allogeneic donor transplantation carries even the worst prognosis in matched unrelated donor transplants with a higher incidence of acute and chronic graft-versus-host disease and transplant related mortality. We therefore explored this GvHD prevention programme in HLA-matched and -mismatched unrelated donor transplants [16].

Materials and Methods

Patient Population

One hundred twenty eight consecutive recipients of unrelated donor stem cell transplantation treated between March 1994 and December 1999 at the University Hospital Hamburg-Eppendorf; 21 patients received an HLA-mismatched marrow, 107 an HLA-matched marrow. The median follow-up is 412 days for the mismatched and 905 days for the matched recipients. The median age was 30 years (range, 1–58 years) for the mismatched and 31 years (range, 1–56 years) for the HLA-matched patients. The following diagnoses (HLA-mismatched/HLA-matched) were transplanted: AML (1/18), ALL (6/19), CML (9/47), HLH (haemophagocytic lymphohistiocytosis) (2/7), other (3/16).

HLA-Mismatch, HLA-Typing and Donor Matching

HLA-A and -B antigens were typed by serologic methods [2, 16]. HLA-DRB1 and HLA-DQB1 alleles were typed by sequence-specific oligonucleotide probes [2, 6]. Donors were required to match the recipient for the serological defined HLA-A and -B antigens as well as HLA-DRB1 alleles and DQB1 alleles. In all patients the pretransplantation lymphocyte cross match with patient sera and donor cells was performed. There were 21 mismatches (HLA-A: 3, HLA-B: 1, HLA-B and -C: 4, HLA-B and DQB1: 3, DRB1: 6, DRB1 and DQB1: 4).

Stem Cell Source

109 recipients received bone marrow (mismatched: 19, matched: 90), 19 PBSC (mismatched: 2, matched: 17). The median cell dose of $CD34^+$ cells was 3.6 x 10^6 per kilogram body weight for the HLA-mismatched (range, 0,7–15,8) and 4.58 for the HLA-matched (range, 0,6–30,7). The CMV-status of the patients and donors was: Negative/negative (mismatched: 8, mismatched: 49), negative/positive (mismatched: 5, matched: 16), positive/negative (mismatched: 5, matched: 28), positive/positive (mismatched: 3, matched: 14).

Transplant-Preparative Regimens

The conditioning consisted of either total body irradiation/Cyclophosphamide plus/minus VP-16 or busulfan/cyclophosphamide plus/minus VP-16. There was an equal distribution of conditioning regimens [16].

GvHD Prophylaxis and Treatment

The GvHD prophylaxis consisted of Ciclosporine A (3 mg/kg body weight) and was given from day –1 with several reductions for six months post transplantation. The dose of Ciclosporine A was adjusted to Ciclosporine A levels, tapered from day 84 and discontinued at day 180. Methotrexate (10 mg/m^2) was given at day 1, 3 and 6 post transplantation. Anti-Thymocyte-Globulin (Fresenius, Bad Homburg, Germany) was given in 101 patients at a dose of 30 mg/kg over 12 hours on day -3, -2, -1 and in 18 patients at a dose of 30 mg/kg over 12 hours on day -1. Immunglobulin was given on day 1, 7, 14, 21, 28. 120 patients received additionally Metronidazol (Clont, Bayer, Leverkusen, Germany) at a dose of 400 mg i. v. given three times a day from conditioning until discharge from the unit. Standard criteria were used for the diagnosis of acute and chronic graft-versus-host disease [13]. Acute GvHD was treated with high dose steroids, and extensive chronic GvHD with Ciclosporine A and steroids. Chronic GvHD was evaluated in patients who survived at least 80 days with sustained engraftment.

Supportive Care

All patients were nursed in single rooms with hepa-filtered air. Antibiotic prophylaxis consisted of Ofloxacin or Ciprofloxacin, and antifungal prophylaxis of Fluconazol, and – in case of prior mycotic infection – of Amphotericin. Aciclovir was given as Herpes prophylaxis from day 1 until day 180. Pneumocystis carinii prophylaxis consisted of either Trimethoprim/Sulfamethoxazol or monthly inhalation with Pentamidin. All blood products were radiated before infusion and only blood products from CMV-negative donors were given. Weekly monitoring of blood and urine for CMV-antigen by PCR and short term culture was carried out. In case of repeated positivity an antiviral therapy with Ganciclovir was initiated.

Our patients received haematopoietic growth factors (G-CSF, 5 µg/kg) intravenously beginning on day 1 and continued until absolute granulocyte count was > 1.0 /nl for three consecutive days. Prostaglandin E1 (Prostavasin, Schwarz-Pharma, Mannheim, Germany) at a dose of 500 µg was given daily as continuous infusion for patients with hepatotoxicity upon a rise of total bilirubine above 2.0.

Statistical Methods

Statistical analysis was performed by using WIN-STAT software (Kalmia Co., Inc., Cambridge, MA, USA). Survival curves for disease free survival and overall survival were estimated by the Kaplan-Meier method.

Results

Engraftment and Graft Failure

Two graft failures occurred, 1 in the mismatched and 1 in the matched group. A leukocyte engraftment of > 1.0 /nl was seen on day 17 (range, 11–24) in the mismatched and on day 16 (range, 11–45) in the matched group. Platelets of > 20 /nl were seen on day 25 in the mismatched and on day 24 in the matched group.

GvHD

The incidence of acute GvHD II-IV was identical in both groups (34 percent), III in 4 patients (5 percent) in the mismatched and 17 (16 percent) in the matched group (details as per Table 1). Chronic GvHD was seen in 2/17 patients in the mismatched group for limited chronic GvHD and 11/74 (14 percent) in the matched group. Extensive chronic GvHD occurred in 3/17 (18 percent) in the mismatched and in 13/77 (17 percent) in the matched group (details as per Table 2).

Table 1. Unrelated Donor Transplantation acute GvHD

Grade	mismatched	matched
I	6 (29 %)	10 (9 %)
II	6 (29 %)	20 (18 %)
III	1 (5 %)	12 (11 %)
IV	0	5 (5 %)
II–IV	7 (34 %)	37 (34 %)
III + IV	1 (5 %)	17 (16 %)

Table 2. Unrelated Donor Transplantation chronic GvHD

	mismatched (n = 17)	matched (n = 77)
limited	2 (12 %)	11 (14 %)
extensive	3 (18 %)	13 (17 %)

Table 3. Unrelated Donor Transplantation Causes of Death

	mismatched	matched
Relapse	3 (14 %)	11 (10 %)
Regimen-related toxicity	1 (5 %)	6 (6 %)
acute GvHD	0	7 (6 %)
Fungal infection	3 (14 %)	7 (6 %)
CMV infection	1 (5 %)	4 (4 %)
graft failure	1 (5 %)	1 (1 %)
other	0	5 (5 %)
TRM	n = 6 (29 %)	n = 30 (28 %)

Cause of Death

Both groups are listed in Table 3. The transplant related mortality was identical in both groups (29 vs. 28 percent).

Side Effects of ATG

Mainly fever, chills, flush and one case of anaphylactic reaction with bronchospasm and hypertension, responding to administration of cortico-steroids were noted. Three patients developed serum sickness, successfully treated with cortico-steroids.

Overall and Disease-free Survival

The outcome of the 21 mismatched unrelated donors is shown in detail in Table 4. The disease free survival of both groups (matched and mismatched) was identi-

Table 4. Mismatched Unrelated Donor

Patient	Graft-failure	aGvHD	cGvHD	Survival	Cause of Death
1	no	2	0	> 2783	
2	no	0	NE	44	toxicity
3	no	1	extensive	> 1748	
4	no	1	0	100	fungal infection
5	no	2	extensive	> 1341	
6	no	1	0	1033	relapse
7	no	2	NE	64	CMV-infection
8	no	3	limited	300	relapse
9	no	2	0	> 732	
10	no	2	0	286	relapse
11	no	0	NE	21	fungal infection
12	no	2	0	> 469	
13	no	0	limited	> 454	
14	no	0	0	> 369	
15	no	0	extensive	171	fungal infection
16	no	1	limited	> 237	
17	no	1	0	> 186	
18	no	1	0	> 158	
19	no	0	0	> 136	
20	no	0	0	> 83	
21	yes	0	NE	51	graft failure

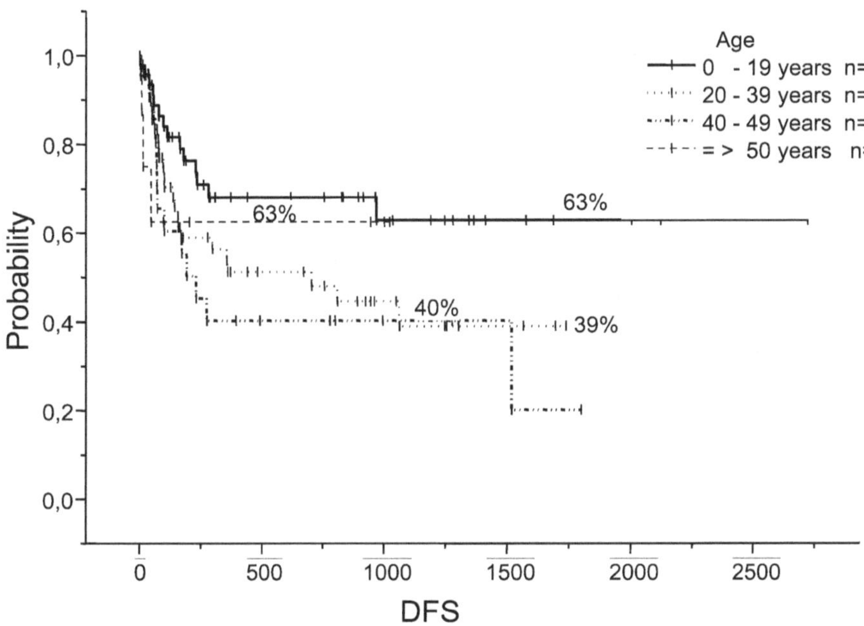

Fig. 1. Disease-free survival times by age groups

cal (about 45 percent at 3 years). Breaking down the disease free survival by age, a small advantage for the young group < 20 years of age is seen. Interestingly enough, the small group of 8 patients > 50 years of age shows similar results (Fig. 1).

Discussion

With the use of Anti-Thymocyte-Globulin (ATG) in the conditioning regimen we observed no difference in the outcome of mismatched and matched unrelated donor transplant recipients. The transplant related mortality was 29 and 28 percent respectively. The incidence of clinical relevant acute GvHD (II–IV) was 34 percent in both groups. Graft failure was low (1 case in each group). The haemopoietic recovery was fast with leukocyte engraftment in 16 days. One case of lymphoproliferative disorder was observed at autopsy in a patient who died of acute GvHD.

Our data compare favourably with reports of unrelated donor transplant from the literature [1, 9, 13, 14, 15]. Sullivan reported in HLA-A, -B, -DRB1 matched donor recipient a graft failure rate of 3 percent, with one antigen mismatched graft failure of 5 percent, acute GvHD (II–V) of 78 percent and with one antigen mismatch of 94 percent, acute GvHD (III-IV) of 36 percent in the matched group, 51 percent with 1 antigen mismatch, extensive chronic GvHD of 61 percent in the matched group, 74 percent in the mismatched group.

The reduction of the incidence of acute and chronic GvHD by administration of ATG (Fresenius) has been documented by several groups [6, 7, 8, 10, 12, 16]. ATG (Fresenius) is produced from rabbits which are immunised with a JURKAT cell line, a cell line resembling activated T-lymphocytes [3]. Therefore it might be that ATG (Fresenius) suppresses the immune system without simultaneously depriving it completely from defence mechanisms against infections and malignancies. Serum from patients treated with ATG were shown to suppress the PHA response of normal peripheral blood mononuclear cells [3]. ELISA based measurements of rabbit IgG is detectable beyond day 22 post ATG-administration. The effect of ATG as part of the pretransplant conditioning is likely to lead to an *in vivo* T-cell effect on donor marrow which is less radical than a T-cell depletion.

ATG as part of the preparative regimen in matched unrelated stem cell transplantation reduces the risk of severe acute and chronic GvHD without an obvious increase of relapse or severe infections. Further studies are necessary to optimise the dose for unrelated donor transplantation.

References

1. Anasetti C, Beatty PG, Storb R, Martin PJ, Mori M, Sanders JE (1990) Effect of HLA incompatibility on graft versus host disease, relapse, and survival after marrow transplantation for patients with leukemia and lymphoma. Hum Immunol 29:79
2. Beatty PG, Clift RA, Mickelson EM, Nisperos B, Flournoy N, Martin PJ, Sanders JE, Stewart P, Buckner CD, Storb R, Thomas D, Hansen JA (1985) Marrow transplantation from related donors other than HLA-identical siblings. N Engl J Med 313:765

3. Eiermann TH, Lambrecht P, Zander AR (1999) Monitoring anti-thymocyte globulin (ATG) in bone marrow recipients. Bone Marrow Transplant 23:779
4. Goldman JM, Apperley JF, Jones L, Marcus R, Goolden AWG, Batchelor R, Hale G, Waldmann H, Reid CD, Hows J, Gordon-Smith E, Catovsky D, Galton DAG (1986) Bone marrow transplantation for patients with chronic myeloid leukemia. N Engl J Med 314:202
5. Hansen JA, Gooley TA, Martin PJ, Appelbaum F, Chauncey TR, Clift RA (1998) Bone marrow transplants from unrelated donors for patients with chronic myeloid leukemia. N Engl J Med 338:962
6. Holler E, Ledderose G, Knabe H, Muth A, Günther C, Wilmanns W, Kolb HJ (1998) ATG Serotherapy during pretransplant conditioning in unrelated donor BMT: Dose dependent modulation of GvHD. Bone Marrow Transplant 27 (Suppl 1): 105 (Abstr)
7. Horstmann M, Stockschläder M, Krüger W, Hoffknecht M, Betker R, Kabisch H, Zander A (1995) Cyclophosphamide/antithymocyte globulin conditioning of patients with severe aplastic anemia for marrow transplantation from HLA-matched siblings: preliminary results. Ann Hematol 71:77
8. Hows J, Downie T, Gore S, Brookes S, Howard M, Bradley B, on behalf of centres participating in the IMUST Study (1997) Pretransplant serotherapy reduces GvHD without increasing relapse after unrelated donor (UD) BMT. Bone Marrow Transplant 19 (Suppl 1)
9. Kernan NA, Bartsch G, Ash RC, Beatty PG, Champlin R, Filipovich A, Gajewski J, Hansen JA, Henslee-Downey PJ, McCullough J, McGlave P, Perkins HA, Phillips GL, Sanders J, Stroncek D, Thomas ED, Blume KG (1993) Analysis of 462 transplantations from unrelated donors facilitated by the national marrow donor program. N Engl J Med 328:593
10. Kolb HJ, Holler E, Knabe H, Ledderose G, Mittermueller J, Schleuning M, Mayer F, Goldmann SF, Fischer M, Lorenz T, Hill W, Schuh R (1995) Conditioning treatment with Antithymocyte Globulin (ATG) modifies Graft-vs-Host Disease in recipients of marrow from unrelated donors. Blood 86: (Suppl 1): 952a
11. Krivit W, Shapiro E, Hoogerbrugge PM, Moser HW (1992) State of art review. Bone marrow transplantation in treatment for storage diseases. Bone Marrow Transplant (suppl 1): 10:87
12. Kröger N, Zabelina T, Krüger W, Renges H, Rüssmann B, Dürken M, Stockschläder M, Erttmann R, Kabisch H, Zander AR (1998) Anti Human T-lymphocyte globulin (ATG) as part of conditioning regimen in unrelated bone marrow transplantation of patients with CML in chronic or accelerated phase. Blood 92 (Suppl 1): 578
13. McGlave P, Bartsch G, Anasetti C, Ash R, Beatty P, Gajewski J, Kernan NA (1993) Unrelated donor marrow transplantation for chronic myelogenous leukemia: initial experience of the National Marrow Donor Program. Blood 81:543
14. Nademanee A, Schmidt GM, Parker P, Dagis AC, Stein A, Snyder DS, O'Donnell M, Smith EP, Stepan DE, Molina A, Wong KK, Margolin K, Somlo G, Littrell B, Woo D, Sniecinski I, Niland JC, Forman SJ (1995) The outcome of matched unrelated donor bone marrow transplantation in patients with hematologic malignancies using molecular typing for donor selection and graft versus host disease prophylaxis regimen of cyclosporine, methotrexate, and prednisone. Blood 86:1228
15. Szydlo R, Goldman JM, Klein JP, Gale RP, Ash RC, Bach FH, Bradley BA, Casper JT, Flomenberg N, Gajewski JL, Gluckman E, Henslee-Downey PJ, Hows JM, Jacobsen N, Kolb HJ, Lowenberg B, Masaoka T, Rowlings PA, Sondel PM, van Bekkum DW, van Rood JJ, Vowels MR, Zhang MJ, Horowitz MM (1997) Results for allogeneic bone marrow transplants for leukemia using donors other than HLA-identical siblings. J Clin Oncol 14:1767
16. Zander AR, Zabelina T, Kröger N, Renges H, Krüger W, Löliger C, Dürken M, Stockschläder M, de Wit M, Wacker-Backhaus G, Bielack S, Jaburg N, Rüssmann B, Erttmann R, Kabisch H (1999) Use of a five-agent GvHD prevention regimen in recipients of unrelated donor marrow. Bone Marrow Transplant 23:889

Immune Reconstitution after Haploidentical Stem Cell Transplantation

P.G. Schlegel, C. Leiler, T. Croner, P. Lang, M. Schumm, R. Handgretinger, K. Schilbach, P. Bader, J. Greil, D. Niethammer, T. Klingebiel, and M. Eyrich

University Children's Hospital, D-72076 Tuebingen and D-97080 Würzburg

With increasing efficacy and safety of the procedure in recent years, the transplantation of hematopoietic stem cells has become an important therapeutic modality for patients with a variety of malignant and nonmalignant diseases. However, the scarcity of available HLA-identical donors necessitates the search for alternative donors in many cases. Haploidentical donors offer the advantages of a high availability and motivation to donate several times if necessary. Limitations such as GvHD and resistance to engraftment across HLA-barriers have been successfully overcome by the introduction of T-cell depletion, transplantation of megadoses of stem cells and immunological conditioning regimens [1-3]. Although immune reconstitution is one of the prime factors determining the outcome of a T cell depleted, HLA-mismatched transplant, little data are known about the pattern of immune reconstitution in this particular transplant setting so far. At the University Children's Hospital in Tübingen, we are transplanting highly purified $CD34^+$ hematopoietic stem cells, isolated from the peripheral blood of a G-CSF mobilized parental donor. A purity of 98–99% CD34 positivity is achieved by several steps of positive selection using a MACS-device following immunomagnetic labeling [2]. 17 high-risk patients (ALL 8, AML 5, CML 3, NHL 1) with malignant diseases lacking a conventional HLA-matched donor have been included in our pilot study in which we prospectively analysed the patterns of immune reconstitution by phenotypic and functional analysis at monthly intervals after transplantation. T-cell receptor (TCR) repertoire complexity was monitored using the RT-PCR *Spectratyping* approach measuring the size distribution of the CDR3-regions every three months [4]. All patients received megadoses of $CD34^+$ cells (median 21×10^6 / kg BW) which had been rigorously T-cell depleted (median 10×10^3 $CD3^+$ cells/kg BW). The GvHD-prophylaxis consisted only of T-cell depletion, no posttransplant immunosuppression was given. None of our patients showed significant acute GvHD ($\geq$ II°). However, one patient developed severe intestinal GvHD after repeated T-cell addbacks in an attempt to convert an increasing mixed chimerism. This patient died of multiorgan failure subsequently. Eight patients succumbed to relapse of the underlying malignant disease after a median of 125 days. One patient developed severe autoimmune hemolytic anemia and required profound immunosuppression to control the anemia. He died subsequently of an invasive aspergillosis. So far, this was the only case of an autoimmune disease in our series of haploidentical transplants. Only one patient developed a fatal infectious complication (disseminated varicella infection). Six patients are alive and well after a median of 1130 days.

The non-specific cellular elements of immunity (granulocytes) are the first to reconstitute after transplant. Granulocyte recovery (neutrophil count > 500/µl after stimulation with G-CSF) occured after a median of 10 days. Thereafter, the NK-cell compartment reconstituted rapidly and reached a median of 348/µl CD16/56$^+$ cells on day 30. NK-cells were the predominant lymphoid cells in the early phase after transplant, making up to 74% of the total lymphoid count on day 30. As a consequence, peripheral mononuclear cells (PMNC) on day 30 proliferated only in response to IL-2, but did not show any response to other mitogens such as anti-CD3, PHA or to SEA. The percentage of NK-cells returned to 26% of lymphoid cells on day 100.

Elements of specific, cellular immunity recovered subsequently. T-cells reached a median of >100/µl CD3$^+$ T-cells as early as 67 days (median). As in conventional allogeneic bone marow or autologous stem cell transplantats, CD8$^+$ T-cells were observed to reconstitute more rapidly than the CD4$^+$ fraction, resulting in an inverted CD4/CD8 ratio. The progressive increase in T-cell number was paralleled by an increase in the proliferative capacities of PMNCs. Proliferation assays on day 100 showed an increased mitogenic response to PHA, PMA and ionomycin, IL-2, anti-CD3 and SEA. This represented a marked increase as compared to proliferation assays on day 30. Although proliferation did increase further during the following months, normal levels were not reached even after 12 months post transplant.

In order to characterize T-cell subsets more in detail, further phenotypic analysis was carried out. T-cell reconstitution could be divided into two waves, that were not detectable when considering only CD3$^+$ T-cell numbers. The early reconstituting T-cells showed predominantly a phenotype of activated, mature T-cells expressing CD45RO, HLA-DR and the adhesion molecules CD11a and CD29 (Fig. 1). T-cell repertoire analysis by RT-PCR *Spectratyping* in the early stages of regeneration revealed a markedly skewed repertoire, suggesting that the early

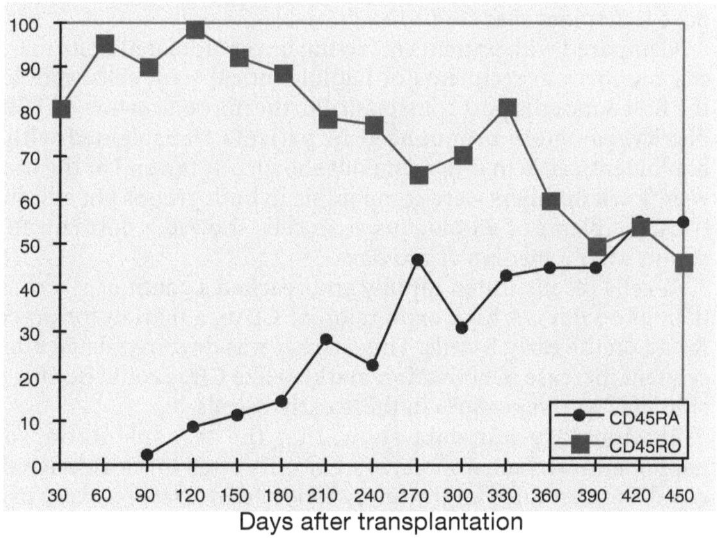

Fig. 1. Regeneration of CD45RA$^+$ naive versus CD45RO$^+$ primed CD4$^+$ T-helper cells after haploidentical stem cell transplantation in children (n=17)

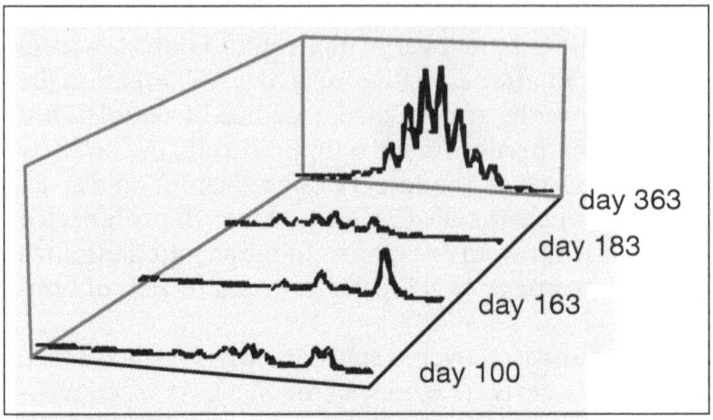

Fig. 2. Development of the peripheral T-cell repertoire during the first year post-transplant. Exemplary reconstitution of the Vβ6.2 family in a patient with ALL

appearing T-cells are derived from a limited number of oligoclonally expanded, mature T-cells. The origin of these early T-cells remains to be determined. Although they could be identified as donor-type T-cells by PCR analysis of VNTR-regions, it remains to be elucidated, if they are derived from the expansion of graft-contaminating mature T-cells or if they reflect de novo T-cells, that have rapidly matured in the host environment.

Levels of unprimed, naive $CD45RA^+$ T-cells were found to be very low in the first 6 months following transplant, with the depression being more profound in the $CD4^+$ subset. After 6 months however, the $CD45RA^+$ population increased accompanied by an increase in the expression of the costimulatory molecule CD28 and L-selectin (Fig. 1). This reflects the maturation of new T cells derived from the hematopoietic stem cell via the thymus, or in some instances also via an extrathymic pathway [5]. Together with the increase in $CD45RA^+$ T cells the repertoire complexity as demonstrated by spectratyping normalized and was indistinguishable from normal subjects in most Vβ-families by the end of the first post-transplant year (Fig. 2).

Compared with patients receiving unmanipulated bone marrow, peripheral T cell numbers in recipients of haploidentical stem cells were lower only during the first 6 months post transplant. Furthermore, skewing of TCR-repertoire complexity was more pronounced in patients transplanted with T-cell depleted, haploidentical stem cells (data not shown). At the end of the first post-transplant year, T cell numbers were comparable in both groups but still subnormal. In contrast, recipients of autologous stem cells showed a normalization of their T cell counts after a median of 250 days.

B-cells reconstituted rapidly and reached a count of > 100 cells/μl after a median of 69 days. A high expression of CD10, a marker for precursor B-cells was found on the early B-cells. This marker was downregulated afterwards, and subsequent increase in activation markers like CD23 could be observed. The expression of CD40 was > 80% in these early B-cells.

In summary our data show, that the transplantation of megadoses of haploidentical, hematopoietic stem cells after myeloablative therapy results in rapid and sustained engraftment followed by a fast recovery of the NK-cell compartment around day 30. T- and B-cells start to reconstitute as early as day 70.

The surprisingly low incidence of infectious complications in our pediatric patients indicates, that the early appearing NK-cell compartment together with the limited T-cell repertoire seems to be capable of controlling infections in the majority of cases. Therefore, a haploidentical transplant should be considered in all pediatric patients with malignant diseases, who are in remission at time of transplant and lack a conventional HLA-matched donor. Studies investigating clinical outcome and immune reconstitution of haploidentical transplantations in patients with nonmalignant diseases are currently in progress.

The rate of early relapses in our high risk patient cohort remains a challenge and underlines the need for posttransplant immunotherapy. The presented insights into the kinetics of immune reconstitution will help us to design novel strategies, directed at augmenting the anti-tumor effect of the graft without putting the patient at risk for GvHD.

References

1. Reisner Y, Martelli MF: Transplantation tolerance induced by „mega dose" CD34+ cell transplants. Exp Hematol 28:119-27, 2000
2. Handgretinger R, Schumm M, Lang P, Greil J, Reiter A, Bader P, Niethammer D, Klingebiel T: Transplantation of megadoses of purified haploidentical stem cells. Ann N Y Acad Sci 872:351-61; discussion 361-2, 1999
3. Schlegel P, Eyrich M, Bader P, Handgretinger R, Lang P, Niethammer D, Klingebiel T: OKT-3 based reconditioning regimen for early graft failure in HLA-non-identical stem cell transplants. Br J Haematol 111:668-673, 2000
4. Gorski J, Yassai M, Zhu X, Kissela B, Kissella B [corrected to Kissela B, Keever C, Flomenberg N: Circulating T cell repertoire complexity in normal individuals and bone marrow recipients analyzed by CDR3 size spectratyping. Correlation with immune status. J Immunol 152:5109-19, 1994
5. Mackall CL, Gress RE: Pathways of T-cell regeneration in mice and humans: implications for bone marrow transplantation and immunotherapy. Immunol Rev 157:61-72, 1997

Clinical Transplantation – Hematologic Malignancies

Autografting and Allografting for Chronic Lymphocytic Leukemia: Is there a Rationale?

P. DREGER

Second Department of Medicine, University of Kiel, Germany

Allogeneic and autologous stem cell transplantation (SCT) are increasingly considered for treatment of patients with chronic lymphocytic leukemia (CLL). In order to assess the potential therapeutic value of SCT for CLL, the present article reviews the most important clinical studies in this field, thereby attempting to answer the following crucial questions for both allo- and auto-SCT:

1. Is SCT a curative treatment?
2. Does SCT improve the dismal prognosis of poor-risk CLL?
3. Do risk factors exist which are useful for defining prognostic groups in terms of feasibility and post transplant outcome?

Autologous stem cell transplantation

To date, only four studies on autologous SCT for CLL are available which comprise sufficiently large patient numbers with informative analyses of prognostic factors to allow an approach to these three critical issues: The recent update of the CLL database of the European Group for Blood and Marrow Transplantation (EBMT) [3], the International Project on CLL Transplants [8], the 2nd interim analysis of the CLL3 study of the German CLL Study Group (to be published), and the series from Kiel [4].

Is auto-SCT a curative treatment?

As summarized in Table 1, all of these four studies are characterized by a low treatment-related mortality (TRM) on the one hand and the lack of a plateau in the event- or relapse-free survival curves on the other hand. The fact that patients continue to relapse up to 5 years post transplant does at least not support the hypothesis that autografting can be curative in certain subsets of patients with CLL.

Another argument against the curative potential of auto-SCT comes from results of the molecular follow-up of the patients from the Kiel series: Allele-specific PCR amplification of the complementary determining region 3 of the IgH gene (ASO CDR3 PCR) detected residual disease in at least two follow-up samples

---

Supported by the José Carreras Leukämie-Stiftung (DJCLS-R16)

Table 1. Autologous SCT in CLL

Trial	EBMT [3]	Int. Project [8]	Kiel [4]	GCLLSG
Trial type	registry data, retrospective	registry data, retrospective	single center prospective	single center prospective
n	370	107	77	105
TRM	10%	7%	4%	5%
2y-EFS	na	69%	87%	na
4y-EFS	na	37%	69%	na
2y-OS	82%	83%	94%	88%*
4y-OS	69%	65%	94%	na
plateau	no	no	no	no

TRM = treatment-related mortality; 2y-EFS = event-free survival 2 years post SCT; 2y-OS = overall survival 2 years post SCT; * survival of all patients included 2 years after start of treatment (intent-to-transplant analysis)

in 28 of 35 cases (80%) with specific CDR3 primers available, although more than half of the patients with a positive ASO PCR had no evidence of disease by consensus primer PCR, flow cytometry, or clinical assessment. Molecular persistence or recurrence of CLL post transplant was not correlated with Binet stage. This implies that complete disease eradication was not possible by this intensive approach in the vast majority of patients even though the Kiel protocol included highly effective tools for in-vivo and ex-vivo CLL cell depletion and focused on individuals with early (though poor-risk) disease. Taken together, there is limited hope that CLL can be cured by standard myeloablative therapy with reinfusion of ex-vivo B-cell depleted autografts alone.

Does auto-SCT improve the prognosis of patients with CLL?

A reliable evaluation of the impact of SCT on the prognosis of CLL requires prospectively randomized studies comparing autografting with conventional palliative treatment. As such studies are completely lacking to date, the possible prognostic benefit of SCT can only be roughly extrapolated from the results of the published single-arm series. These studies, however, usually suffer from patient heterogeneity and selection bias, and, thus, can hardly be compared with the generally accepted results of conventional therapy. Having these limitations in mind, the Barcelona group plotted the overall survival of the advanced-stage patients from the International Project against the overall survival of conventionally-treated but otherwise similar patients from their own database, and found a significant prognostic advantage for auto-SCT (Jordi Esteve, personal communication). In the Kiel series, we analyzed the 19 patients in whom autografting was attempted as part of a second-line strategy. In these 19 individuals, freedom from

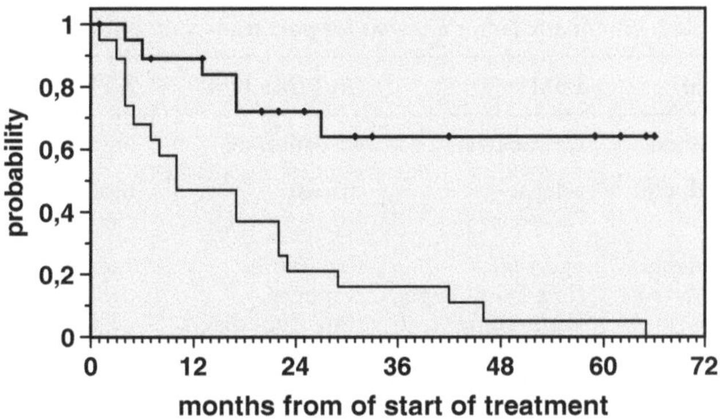

Fig. 1. Freedom from treatment failure (FFTF) in the patients who underwent salvage SCT. Thin line: FFTF after the last conventional regimen prior to SCT attempt. Bold line: FFTF after start of high-dose protocol (by intention-to-treat).

treatment failure (FFTF) post mobilization (= SCT attempt) was compared to FFTF after the last conventional regimen prior to mobilization. It became apparent that FFTF after SCT attempt was much longer than after the last standard chemotherapy (median FFTF 10 months vs. not reached, p=0.0002; Fig. 1), implying that SCT allows more efficient tumor control than conventional treatment. Taken together, although the results of the published trials are promising, data illustrating a clear-cut therapeutic benefit of autografting in CLL are still very sparse, and the results of the ongoing prospective studies have to be awaited.

Are there prognostic factors predicting the outcome after autologous SCT?

Prognostic factor analyses are important to identify subgroups of patients who are most likely to benefit from SCT, and to define the optimum timing of SCT. Possible explanatory variables predicting for the success of autografting can be divided into three groups:

1. Course-related risk factors are those which develop as the disease continues (e.g. stage, time from diagnosis, intensity of pretreatment, timing of transplant). Their prognostic impact may be bypassed by early transplant.
2. Biological risk factors are determined by genuine biological features of the tumor clone and cannot necessarily be eliminated by early timing of transplant (e.g. age, sex, lymphocyte count, lymphocyte doubling time, cytogenetics, mutational status).
3. Technical risk factors are related to the transplant procedure itself and, thus, can be influenced (e.g. source of stem cells, purging, high-dose regimen, remission status at transplant).

Prognostic factor analyses are available for all four studies mentioned. Their results are listed in Table 2 and can be summarized as follows: As far as analyzed, biological risk factors, such as lymphocyte count and adverse cytogenetics, are associated with an inferior post transplant outcome. Among the technical risk factors, insufficient remission at SCT and possibly the use of high-dose regimens

Table 2. Prognostic factor analysis for post transplant outcome in autologous SCT in CLL

Trial	EBMT	Int. Project	Kiel	GCLLSG
Method	Cox analysis	Cox analysis	log rank test	log rank test
Endpoint	relapse incidence	disease-free survival	molecular clonality	molecular clonality
Variables analyzed	age, sex, time from diagn., fludarabine treatment, status at SCT, purging, TBI	fludarabine response, time from diagn., pretreatment, status at SCT, purging, TBI	age, sex, time from diagn., pretreatment, lymphocyte count, Binet stage	caryotype, time from diagn., pretreatment, lymphocyte count, Binet stage, status at SCT
Favorable variables	CR at SCT, <36 mos. from diagn., TBI yes	CR at SCT	lymphocytes <50G/l	CR at SCT, caryotype other than del 11q-

TBI = total body irradiation; CR = complete remission

not containing total body irradiation (TBI) might have an adverse influence, whereas course-related factors, such as stage and time from diagnosis, appear to be less important.

Another issue is the question of pretransplant failure, i.e. which patients scheduled for transplant cannot undergo autografting do to lack of a suitable graft or a sufficient response. This question has been addressed in the prospective Kiel and GCLLSG trials. In both series, about one fifth of all patients considered for transplant experienced pretransplant failure. A history of Binet stage C disease was the predominant factor predicting for poor pretransplant outcome, as illustrated by a failure probability of 36% and 58%, respectively, in the Kiel and CLL3 studies.

Taking into account their preliminary character, these analyses support the requirement of a sufficient remission status at SCT as well as the use of TBI. Furthermore, they suggest that randomized trials on SCT might be best performed in a salvage setting, since the results of conventional second-line treatment in CLL are poor, whereas the outcome after autografting is encouraging and does not appear to be very much different between patients with early and advanced disease, respectively. Thus, the possible benefits of SCT will emerge easier and faster if studied as second-line treatment. Whether this, on the other side, questions the justification of further trials on early transplant remains highly debatable: Almost every patient with poor-risk features will progress to a symptomatic stage and, ultimately, fulfill the criteria for SCT. Delaying high-dose therapy until advanced stage or need for salvage treatment, however, implies that many patients will never receive an autograft due to mobilization failure and resistant disease.

Allogeneic stem cell transplantation

Allogeneic SCT is a treatment approach which is fundamentally different from autologous transplantation in particular in the context of indolent diseases such as CLL. Whereas efficacy (and complications) of autografting rely exclusively on the cytotoxic therapy administered, the crucial anti-leukemic principle of allotransplantation appears to be the immune-mediated anti-host activities conferred with the graft (GVL effects). Accordingly, autologous SCT adds nothing else than intensity (and perhaps a radiotherapeutic component) to conventional treatment. For this reason, the toxicity of autotransplantation is nowadays only slightly higher than that of intensive conventional chemotherapeutic regimens, but its capacity for complete eradication of resistant CLL clones seems to be limited, too. On the other hand, allogeneic transplantation introduces the entirely different modality of cellular immune therapy, which appears to be responsible for its superior anti-leukemic activity as well as for its considerably higher toxicity.

Is allo-SCT a curative treatment?

Three larger series on allogeneic SCT for CLL have been published and are summarized in Table 3 [5,7,9]. All three studies are characterized by a high TRM on the one hand and a very low relapse incidence on the other hand: The survival curves appear to approach a plateau in the long term, suggesting that allotransplantation may have curative potential in this disease. The superior tumor control provided by allografting in comparison to autografting suggests a pronounced susceptibility of CLL to GVL effects.

Another line of evidence for the presence of GVL activity and, thus, curative potential of allografting in CLL comes from the documented efficacy of donor lymphocyte infusions and the fact that CLL cells persisting after dose-reduced conditioning for allogeneic SCT disappear with the onset of chronic graft-versus-host disease [1].

Does allo-SCT improve the prognosis of patients with CLL?

In spite of the low relapse rate, the survival after allo-SCT is significantly lower than after autologous SCT at least during the first 4 years. The reason for this is the high toxicity associated with allografting for this particular indication. Even in well experienced centers, the TRM of allogeneic SCT in patients with CLL is reported to be up to 50% (Table 3). The causes of these detrimental results are not completely clear, but patient age, selection of poor risk patients with advanced disease and extensive pretreatment, and the CLL-associated incompetence of the immune system may all contribute to the high TRM observed. The recent development of conditioning regimens with reduced intensity may help to improve the tolerability of allo-SCT in CLL without affecting its GVL activities [2,4].

In conclusion, at the present time allo-SCT in CLL should be restricted to symptomatic patients with very high-risk disease, such as those with unfavorable cy-

Table 3. Allogeneic SCT in CLL

Trial	EBMT [7]	Omaha [9]	MD Anderson [5]
Trial type	registry data, retrospective	single center retrospective	single center retrospective
n	134	23	15
TRM	40%	30%	27%
4y-OS	54%	62%	57%
plateau	yes	yes	yes

TRM = treatment-related mortality; 2y-EFS = event-free survival 2 years post SCT; 2y-OS = overall survival 2 years post SCT; * survival of all patients included 2 years after start of treatment (intent-to-transplant analysis)

togenetics, early relapse after purine analogues, or failure of autografting. In these subgroups, the considerable risk of TRM should be more than outweighed by the prognostic improvement due to the effective disease control provided by allogeneic SCT.

Are there prognostic factors predicting the outcome after allogeneic SCT?

Conclusive prognostic factor analyses for identifying subgroups of patients who are most likely to benefit from allogeneic SCT for CLL are not available to date.

Conclusions and perspectives

Autologous and allogeneic stem cell transplantation appear to be fundamentally different treatment modalities for patients with CLL. The efficacy of auto-SCT relies exclusively on the cytotoxic therapy administered. With appropriate supportive care, it is safe and can induce long-lasting clinical and molecular remissions. Feasibility of autologous SCT appears to be best early during the course of the disease, but there is only limited hope that autotransplantation can cure the disease even in this favorable subgroup. Nevertheless, the results of the published series suggest that auto-SCT is capable of improving the prognosis of CLL with defined poor-risk features. Favorable conditions for successful autografting are less advanced disease, a sufficient remission status at SCT and use of a TBI-containing high-dose regimen. Since post transplant outcome does not appear to be very much different between patients with first-line and salvage SCT, respectively, randomized trials on auto-SCT might be best performed in a salvage setting, where the results of conventional second-line treatment in CLL are poor, and, thus, the possible benefits of SCT will emerge easier and faster. Such a trial has been started recently as a combined effort of the EBMT and the GCLLSG (CLL3R trial of the GCLLSG). Given the excellent feasibility of auto-SCT in early (but not in advanced) stages, further refinement of the procedure towards cure by implementing additional modalities, such as monoclonal antibodies, should focus on early patients. Along this line the GCLLSG CLL3C trial has been designed. The objective of this recently launched phase-II study is to investigate the safety and feasibility of the addition of CAMPATH-1H to the high-dose regimen for autologous SCT in patients with poor-risk CLL (Fig. 2).

The crucial anti-leukemic principle of allotransplantation in CLL consists in the immune-mediated GVL effects conferred with the graft. The GVL activity should be responsible for the better disease control observed. Thus, allografting seems to be a curative treatment for at least a subset of poor-risk patients. However, as long as allo-SCT in CLL is still associated with an excessively high TRM, only selected patients with advanced poor-risk disease and low probability of successful auto-SCT should be considered for allografting. The development of conditioning regimens with reduced intensity may allow to extend the indications of allogeneic SCT for CLL in the near future. To this end, the GCLLSG runs the EBMT-approved CLL3X trial, which studies fludarabine-based conditioning regimens in patients with very-high-risk CLL (Fig. 2).

Taken together, we believe that autologous transplantation is preferable for patients with early or sensitive disease. Selected patients with advanced poor-risk disease and low probability of successful auto-SCT should be considered for allografting. However, it must be kept in mind that both autologous and allogeneic stem cell transplantation are still experimental procedures which should not be performed outside of approved clinical trials.

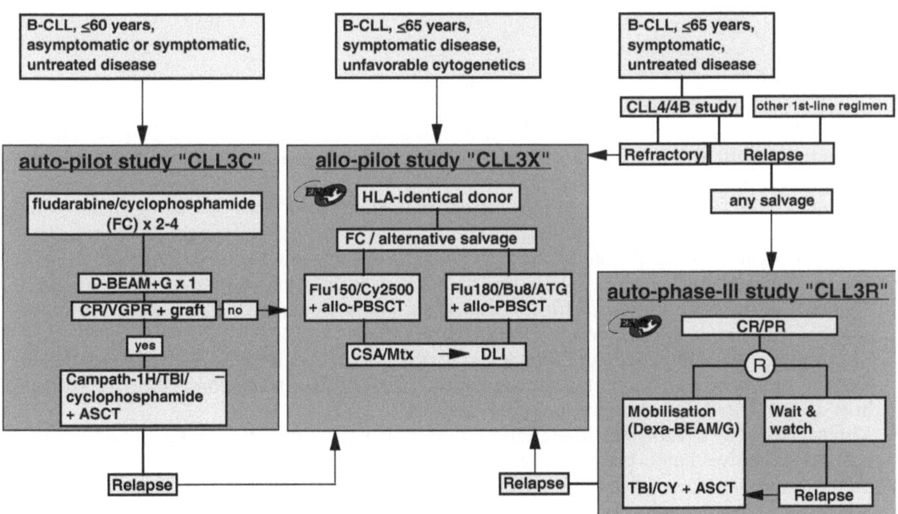

Fig. 2. Current GCLLSG transplant studies

Summary

Allogeneic and autologous stem cell transplantation (SCT) are increasingly considered for treatment of patients with chronic lymphocytic leukemia (CLL). In order to assess the potential therapeutic value of SCT for CLL, the present article aims at answering the following crucial questions:

1. Is SCT a curative treatment?
2. Does SCT improve the dismal prognosis of poor-risk CLL?
3. Do risk factors exist which are useful for defining prognostic groups in terms of feasibility and post transplant outcome?

The efficacy of auto-SCT relies exclusively on the cytotoxic therapy administered. To date, there is only limited hope that autotransplantation can cure the disease even in this favorable subgroup. Nevertheless, the results of the published series suggest that auto-SCT is capable of improving the prognosis of CLL with defined poor-risk features. Favorable conditions for successful autografting are less advanced disease, a sufficient remission status at SCT and use of a TBI-containing high-dose regimen. The crucial anti-leukemic principle of allo-SCT consists in the immune-mediated GVL effects conferred with the graft. The GVL activity should be responsible for the fact allografting seems to be a curative treatment for at least a subset of poor-risk patients. However, as long as allo-SCT in CLL is still associated with an excessively high treatment-related mortality, only selected patients with advanced poor-risk disease should be considered for allografting. The development of conditioning regimens with reduced intensity may allow to extend the indications of allogeneic SCT for CLL in the near future.

References

1. Dreger, P., et al.: „Reduced-intensity allogeneic stem cell transplantation as salvage treatment for patients with indolent lymphoma after failure of autologous SCT." Bone Marrow Transplant 26(2000):1361-1362.
2. Dreger, P., et al.: „Allogeneic stem cell transplantation for poor-risk CLL using fludarabine/cyclophosphamide (FC) conditioning." Bone Marrow Transplant 27(2001):S37(Abstract)
3. Dreger, P., et al.: „Prognostic factors for survival after autologous stem cell transplantation for chronic lymphocytic leukemia (CLL): the EBMT experience." Blood 96(2000a):482a(Abstract)
4. Dreger, P., et al.: „Feasibility and efficacy of early autologous stem cell transplantation for poor-risk CLL." Blood 96 Suppl.1(2000b):483a(Abstract)
5. Khouri, I., et al.: „Allogeneic blood or marrow transplantation for chronic lymphocytic leukaemia: timing of transplantation and potential effect of fludarabine on acute graft-versus-host disease." Br J Haematol 97(1997):466-473.
6. Khouri, I.F., et al.: „Transplant-lite: induction of graft-versus-malignancy using fludarabine-based nonablative chemotherapy and allogeneic blood progenitor-cell transplantation as treatment for lymphoid malignancies." J.Clin.Oncol. 16(1998):2817-2824.
7. Michallet, M., et al.: „Allotransplants and autotransplants in CLL." Bone Marrow Transplant 23 Suppl.1(1999):S53(Abstract)
8. Montserrat, E., et al.: „Autologous stem cell transplantation for CLL: analysis of the impact on overall survival in 107 patients from The International Project for CLL/transplants." Blood 94 Suppl.1(1999):397a
9. Pavletic, Z.S., et al.: „Outcome of allogeneic stem cell transplantation for B cell chronic lymphocytic leukemia." Bone Marrow Transplant 25(2000):717-722.

Results of Stem Cell Transplantation in Children with CML in Comparison with Treatment with Cytostatics alone or with Interferon alfa. Report of the Polish Children's Leukemia/Lymphoma Study Group

A. Chybicka[1], K. Kalwak[1], J. Boguslawska-Jaworska[1], A. Balcerska[3], W. Balwierz[4], M. Cwiklinska[4], A. Hicke[7], M. Kaczmarek-Kanold[6], P. Kolecki[6], J. Kowalczyk[5], A. Krauze[7], M. Matysiak[7], A. Ploszynska[3], R. Rokicka-Milewska[7], D. Sonta-Jakimczyk[8], B. Sikorska-Fic[7], H. Wisniewska-Slusarz[5], M. Wysocki[2], and J. Wachowiak[6]

Departments of Children's Hematology/Oncology in Wroclaw[1], Bydgoszcz[2], Gdansk[3], Kraków[4], Lublin[5], Poznan[6], Warsaw[7] and Zabrze[8], Poland

Introduction

Philadelphia positive chronic myeloid leukemia (CML Ph+) is a malignant clonal hematological disease of pluripotent stem cell representing 2–5% of all childhood leukemias [2]. The incidence of CML increases with age and is 1 per 100 000 at the age of 20 [2]. The male to female ratio is 1.8:1 [1]. CML in children remains one of the major problems, because of its progressive clinical course, unless cured by bone marrow transplantation (BMT). Conventional chemotherapy with the use of hydroxyurea (HU) or busulfan (BUS) relieves clinical symptoms and controls the leucocytosis in chronic phase of the disease, but hardly influences overall survival [2]. Interferon alfa (IFN) can lead to very adequate control of leucocytosis and in spite of its possible negative effect on BMT outcome, IFN seems to be an alternative option for those, who do not have a suitable donor for BMT. Moreover, a minority of patients can achieve a major cytogenetic response or elimination of the Philadelphia chromosome or the bcr/abl fusion product. At present, the only known potentially curative therapy is stem cell transplantation (SCT) from either HLA-matched related or unrelated donor [3]. This form of therapy is limited by the availability of a suitable donor [3, 11]. Children can have an 80% or greater chance of long-term survival with a matched related or unrelated donor, provided they are transplanted early in the disease course [4].

The aim of the study was a retrospective analysis of treatment results in children with CML obtained from data of the Polish Children's Leukemia/Lymphoma Study Group.

Material and methods

A total number of 102 children with CML from 9 pediatric centers in Poland: 58 boys and 44 girls aged 1–17 years (median 9.4 years old) treated in the period

1975–1999 were included in the retrospective study. Forty-eight of 102 (47.1%) children were treated with cytostatic drugs without IFN: HU, BUS or etoposide (VP-16) and 6-mercaptopurine (6-MP). Fifty-four of 102 (52.9%) patients were treated with IFN after cytoreductive pretreatment (HU). IFN therapy was started between 2 weeks and 36 months from the disease onset. Either IntronA (Schering Plough), Berofor (Behring), Roferon (Hofmann La Roche) or Wellferon (Wellcome) were used in the dosis of 3×10^6 U every second day s.c. Two patients received IFN in the increasing dosis everyday [8]. The maximum tolerated dosis was 5×10^6 U/m^2 s.c. When the acceleration phase occurred, the children were treated either with IFN in the dosis as above plus HU 40 mg/m^2/d or idarubicin (IDA) and cytosine arabinoside (Ara-C) [8]. Treatment with HU + IFN was continued until leucocyte count decreased under 10G/l, which allowed to use IFN alone. Median observation time was 53 months.

In case blast crisis occurred, children were treated acc. to AML-BFM 83 or ALL-BFM 86, 90, 93 and ALL-BFM REZ 96 protocols.

Thirty of 102 (52.9%) patients underwent stem cell transplantation (SCT): 24 – matched related donor allogeneic BMT, 2 – matched unrelated donor allogeneic BMT, 1 – partially matched related donor T-cell depleted allogeneic peripheral blood progenitor cell transplantation (PBPCT), 1 – syngeneic allogeneic BMT and 2 – autologous PBPCT. Disease status at BMT was as follows: 1st chronic phase – n = 21, 2nd chronic phase – n = 8, accelerated phase – n = 1 (the latter patient underwent haploidentical T-cell depleted PBPCT).

Results

Time of BUS or HU administration ranged from 3 to 24 months, whereas IFN was given from 2 to 52 months with median 26 months. We observed 2 cytogenetic remissions in 2 children treated with IFN. After 3-37 months from the disease onset blast crisis occurred in 40 of 102 children (39.2%), including 15 of 54 patients (27.8%) treated with IFN and 25 of 48 children (52.1%) treated with cytostatics. The blast crisis was of lymphoblastic type (ALL) in 7 (17.5%) children and of myeloblastic type (AML) in remaining 33 (82.5%) patients.

Overall survival analysis revealed 46 of 102 (45.1%) children remaining alive: 5 of 35 (14.3%) children treated with cytostatics alone, 22 of 37 (59.5%) children treated with IFN and 19 of 30 (63.3%) patients treated with SCT.

Among SCT survivors there are 10 of 17 (58.8%) children treated with IFN prior to SCT and 9 of 13 (69.2%) patients treated with cytostatics alone prior to SCT. In the cohort of transplanted patients 11 of 30 (36.7%) died: 3 due to disease recurrence and 8 because of transplant related complications (Graft versus Host Disease, cytomegalovirus (CMV) infection, graft rejection).

Probability of 5-year survival is 0.51 in the group treated with SCT (median follow-up 58 months); 0.43 in the group treated with IFN alfa (median follow-up 53 months) and 0.23 in the group treated with cytostatics (median follow-up 31 months).

Discussion

Our data confirm, that allogeneic SCT is the treatment of choice in pediatric CML. IFN could be successfully applied as an alternative treatment to control the leucocytosis for those, who do not have a suitable donor for allogeneic SCT. Median follow-up is however shorter in this group. The percentage of cytogenetic remissions during IFN therapy (2 of 54; 3.7%) is much lower than in the cohort of adults, which might be due to more aggressive course of CML in children [2, 9, 10].

The retrospective analysis demonstrates, that the main reason of treatment failure is still insufficient amount of SCT (29.4%), due to lack of suitable related or unrelated bone marrow donor availability.

Every effort should be made to transplant children with CML within a year from diagnosis, because the duration of disease before transplantation was identified as a predictor of survival [4].

IFN administration before allogeneic SCT leads to the anti-IFN antibodies generation, bone marrow stroma changes, enhanced production of inflammatory cytokines and acc. to some authors to increased frequency and severity of acute Graft versus Host Disease (aGvHD) in patients receiving IFN just before SCT [6, 7]. We observed trend towards a better outcome post SCT in children, who were not treated with IFN prior to SCT. However, these data require confirmation in studies on larger groups of patients. It seems to be justified to stop IFN at least 90 days prior to planned SCT. Current recommendations accept HU as the only therapy before SCT in case, there is a great chance to find a suitable donor for transplantation. Clear candidates for early transplantation should not be pretreated with IFN [5].

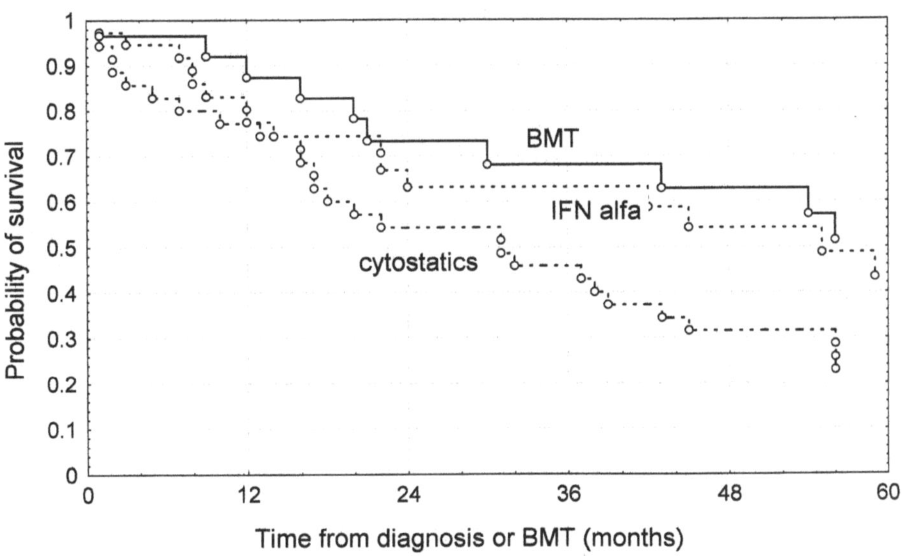

Fig. 1. Probability of survival in children with CML treated with BMT, IFN or cytostaticcs

The main reason of clinical failure in patients with CML in Poland remains still insufficient access to matched unrelated donor SCT. The situation is going to be improved by the year 2000.

Summary

Philadelphia positive chronic myeloid leukemia (CML Ph^+) in children remains one of the major problems, because of its progressive clinical course, unless cured by allogeneic bone marrow transplantation (BMT). In spite of its possible negative effect on BMT outcome, Interferon-alfa (IFN alfa) seems to be an alternative option for those, who do not have a suitable donor for allogeneic BMT.

Retrospective analysis of 102 children with CML from 9 pediatric centers in Poland has been performed. A total number of 102 children: 58 boys and 44 girls aged 1–17 years (median 9.4 years old) with CML treated in the period 1975-1999 were included in the study. Forty-eight of 102 (47.1%) children were treated with cytostatic drugs without IFN alfa: busulfan, hydroxyurea, 6-mercaptopurin or etoposide (VP-16). Fifty-four of 102 (52.9%) patients were treated with interferon alfa (IFN alfa) after cytoreductive pretreatment. Thirty of 102 (29.4%) pts underwent stem cell transplantation (SCT): 24 – matched related donor alloBMT, 2 – matched unrelated donor alloBMT, 1 – partially matched related donor T-cell depleted alloPBPCT, 1 – syngeneic alloBMT and 2 – autologous PBPCT. Disease status at BMT was as follows: 1st chronic phase – n = 21, 2nd chronic phase – n = 8, accelerated phase – n = 1.

Overall survival analysis revealed 46 of 102 (45.1%) children remaining alive: 5/35 (14.3%) children treated with cytostatics alone, 22/37 (59.5%) children treated with IFN alfa and 19/30 (63.3%) children treated with SCT. Among SCT survivors there are 10/17 (58.8%) children treated with IFN alfa prior to SCT and 9/13 (69.2%) children treated with cytostatics alone prior to SCT. Probability of 5-year survival is 0.51 in the group treated with SCT (median follow-up 58 months); 0.43 in the group treated with IFN alfa (median follow-up 53 months) and 0.23 in the group treated with cytostatics (median follow-up 31 months).

Our data show, that BMT is the treatment of choice in pediatric CML. IFN alfa could be successfully applied as an alternative treatment for those, who do not have a suitable donor for allogeneic BMT. Trend towards a better outcome post BMT in children, who were not treated with IFN alfa prior to BMT requires studies on larger groups of patients. However, it seems to be justified to stop IFN alfa therapy at least 3 months before BMT. The main reason of clinical failure in patients with CML in Poland remains still insufficient access to MUD-BMT.

References

1. Chybicka A, Kalwak K (1999) Chronic Myelogenous Leukemia (CML) in children. International Intensive Course of Oncology ERASMUS 1999. Recent advances in the knowledge of cancer. 450-64
2. Emanuel PD (1999) Myelodysplasia and myeloproliferative disorders in childhood. An update. Br J Hematol 105: 852-863

3. Goldman JM et al. (1986) Bone marrow transplantation for patients with chronic myeloid leukemia. N Engl J Med 314: 202-207
4. Hansen et al. (1998) Bone marrow transplants from unrelated donors for patients with chronic myeloid leukemia. N Engl J Med 338: 962-968
5. Hehlmann R et al. (1999) Interferon-alpha before allogeneic bone marrow transplantation in chronic myelogenous leukemia does not affect outcome adversely, provided it is discontinued at least 90 days before the procedure. Blood 94(11): 3668-77
6. Morton AJ et al. (1998) Association between pretransplant interferon-alpha and outcome after unrelated donor marrow transplantation for chronic myelogenous leukemia in chronic phase. Blood 92(2): 394-401
7. Prummer O et al. (1996) Antibodies to interferon-alpha: a novel type of autoantibody occurring after allogeneic bone marrow transplantation. Bone Marrow Transplant 17: 617-623
8. Suttorp M (1995) CML-Päd 95 Protokoll
9. Talpaz M et al. (1986) Hematologic remission and cytogenetic improvement induced by recombinant human interferon alpha in chronic myelogenous leukemia. N Engl J Med 314: 1065-1069
10. Talpaz M et al. (1993) Interferon alfa in the therapy of CML. Interferons and cytokines 23: 6-9
11. Thomas ED et al. (1986) Marrow transplantation for the treatment of chronic myelogenous leukemia. Ann Int Med 104: 155-163

Comparison of Allogeneic Matched Related Stem Cell Transplantation in 1st CR with Chemotherapy alone in Children with High-Risk AML

D. Reinhardt[1], M. Zimmermann[1], J. Ritter[1], Ch. Bender-Götze[2], and U. Creutzig[1]

[1]Pediatric Hematology/Oncology University of Muenster
[2]Childrens Hospital, University of Munich

Introduction

Intensive treatment modalities have continuously improved survival and cure of children with acute myeloid leukemia (Hurwitz et al., 1995; Mitus et al., 1995; Stevens et al., 1998; Vormoor et al., 1996). Allogeneic stem cell transplantation (SCT) after a bone marrow ablative conditioning regimen in first remission (CR) seemed to effect a favorable outcome in adults (Frassoni et al., 1996; Gale et al., 1996; Gorin et al., 1996; Proctor et al., 1995; Reiffers et al., 1996). However, a benefit of allogeneic SCT could not be proven in all studies (Klingebiel et al., 1996; Zittoun et al., 1995). The discussion about the indication of allogeneic SCT in 1st CR in children is much more controversial. Whereas the Children Cancer Study Group (CCG) (Sanders, 1997; Woods et al., 1996; Woods et al., 2001), the French Society of Pediatric Hematology and Immunology (SHIP) (Michel et al., 1996), the Italian study group (Amadori et al., 1993) and some single center studies (Matsuyama et al., 2000; Uderzo et al., 2000) recommended SCT without any limitation for AML in 1st CR, other groups demonstrated a significant advantage in risk-defined groups (Ortega et al., 1996; Ortega and Olive, 1998). By contrast, other study groups have not supported a general benefit of all children with AML and restricted their recommendation to patients with recurring or refractory AML, secondary AML, special chromosomal aberrations (monosomy 7) and proven myelodysplastic syndromes (Ladenstein et al., 1997; Vormoor et al., 1996). The theoretical efficacy of SCT was based on both, the intensification by a bone marrow ablative conditioning regimen and the postulated graft versus leukemia effect. In some studies this was supported by a reduced risk of relapse following allogeneic SCT compared to chemotherapy only. However, prognosis was frequently hampered by increased toxicity and treatment related mortality. Indeed, evidence of benefit from randomized controlled studies is lacking. (Dini et al., 1996; Ladenstein et al., 1997). The restriction of allogeneic SCT to children without favourable cytogenetics [t(8;21); t(15;17); inv(16)] is widely accepted (Dini et al., 1996; Ladenstein et al., 1997; Ortega and Olive, 1998; Pui, 1995). We herein compare the effect of matched related SCT with chemotherapy alone in children with AML in first remission.

Table 1. Characteristics of the AML-BFM 93 study patients. Data of the total group 471, standard risk and high risk group

	Patients AML BFM 93	SR patients	HR patients	p-value SR vs HR
Total (n)	471	161	310	
Gender male (%)	54	50	56	0.24 (chi)
Age, median, range (years)	7.6 (0–18)	9.5 (0–17)	6.6 (0–18)	0.001 (u-test)
Leukocytes, median, range (/µl)	18 150 (300–520,000)	19 000 (400–520 000)	17 980 (300–500 000)	0.8 (u-test)
Hepatomegaly > 5 cm	13%	7%	17%	0.004 (chi)
Splenomegaly > 5 cm	11%	7%	12%	0.10 (chi)
Blasts day 15 > 5%	25%	8%	35%	< 0.0001 (chi)
Follow-up in CCR (median, range, years)	3.9 (1–7)	3.9 (1–7)	4.0 (1–7)	0.6 (chi)

Patients and Methods

From January 1993 to June 1998, 471 patients were enrolled in study AML-BFM 93. Follow-up was as of December 2000. The diagnosis was confirmed by centralized review of a panel of hematologists. Cytogenetic analyses were performed at the laboratory of the Children's Hospital of Giessen (J. Harbott). Patients characteristics are summarized in Table 1.

In the AML-BFM 93 study, the standard risk (SR) group was defined by morphology (AML M1/M2 with Auer rods, AML M3, AML M4eo) or cytogenetics t(8;21); t(15;17); inv(16)) and response with less than 5% blasts at day 15 (not required for M3) (Creutzig et al., 1999). In children of the SR group allogeneic SCT was reserved for the 2nd CR. All other children of the high risk group (HR) were eligible for allogeneic SCT in 1st CR if a HLA-identical donor was available. According to risk definition, there were 161 SR and 310 HR patients (Table 1). Two hundred forty-three children of the high risk group achieved remission. Sixteen children had autologous (n=6), haploid (n=3) or matched unrelated SCT (n=7) and were excluded. Two hundred twenty seven were eligible for analyses. HR patients who received MR-SCT (n=28, including 1 syngenic), were compared with non-SCT HR patients (n=199).

In addition Cox regression analysis was performed.

Statistics

Univariate analysis was conducted by the Wilcoxon test for quantitative variables and Fisher´s exact test for qualitative variables. When frequencies were sufficiently large χ^2-statistic was used. Since estimated disease-free survival (DFS)

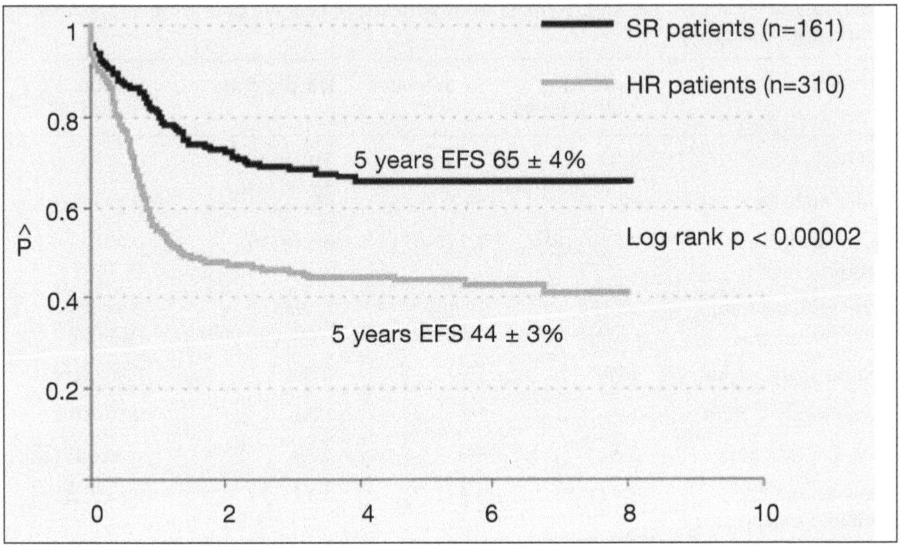

Fig. 1. AML-BFM-93 study: Estimated probability for event-free survival (EFS) of SR and HR-patients

of the SCT patients might be biased results were compared by Cox regression with SCT as time dependent variable.

Results

Overall outcome

In study AML-BFM 93, 387 of 471 (82%) patients achieved remission. The estimated probabilities for 5-year overall survival, event-free survival (EFS) and disease-free survival (DFS) were 60%±3%, 51%±2% and 62%±3%, respectively (Creutzig et al., 2001). Results of SR patients were favorable with an estimated 5-year survival of 74%±4%, EFS of 65%+4%, disease free survival of 73%±4%. HR patients had an estimated overall survival of 52%±3%, EFS 44%±3%, DFS 54%±3%, respectively (Fig. 1).

Chemotherapy versus allogeneic SCT

Children treated with chemotherapy alone or matched related SCT did not differ significantly regarding gender, median age, leukocyte count, clinical features or response (Table 2). Estimated 5-year DFS was 54%±4% for chemotherapy compared to 64%±9% in children with SCT (Mantel-Bayr p=0.31) (Fig. 2).

5-year overall survival was 65%±3% (CHT) versus 68%±9% (SCT; p=0.41 Fig. 3).

The Cox regression analysis revealed for MR-SCT a risk ratio (RR) of 0.56, 95% confidence interval 0.34-1.39, p=0.37.

Table 2. Characteristics and comparison of high risk group patients with and without SCT

	Total HR CR Patients	HR No SCT	HR with MR SCT	p-value
Total (n)	226*	199	28	
Gender male (%)	54	55	57	0.9 (chi)
Age, median, range (years)	5.2 (0–17)	4.9 (0.1–16.5)	10.1 (0.3–16.1)	0.2 (u-test)
Leukocytes, median, range (/µl)	16 985 (300–500,000)	16 000 (300–500,000)	26 050 (1200–394,000)	0.7 (u-Test)
Hepatomegaly > 5 cm	17%	16%	18%	0.7 (chi)
Splenomegaly > 5 cm	12%	13%	12%	0.9 (chi)
Blasts day 15 > 5%	35	32	36	0.7 (chi)
Follow-up in CCR (median, range, years)	3.8 (1–7)	3.9 (1–7)	3.7 (1–7)	

*Overall 243 children of the HR group achieved first remission. Sixteen patients were excluded because they received autologous, haplo-identical or matched unrelated SCT (Table III).

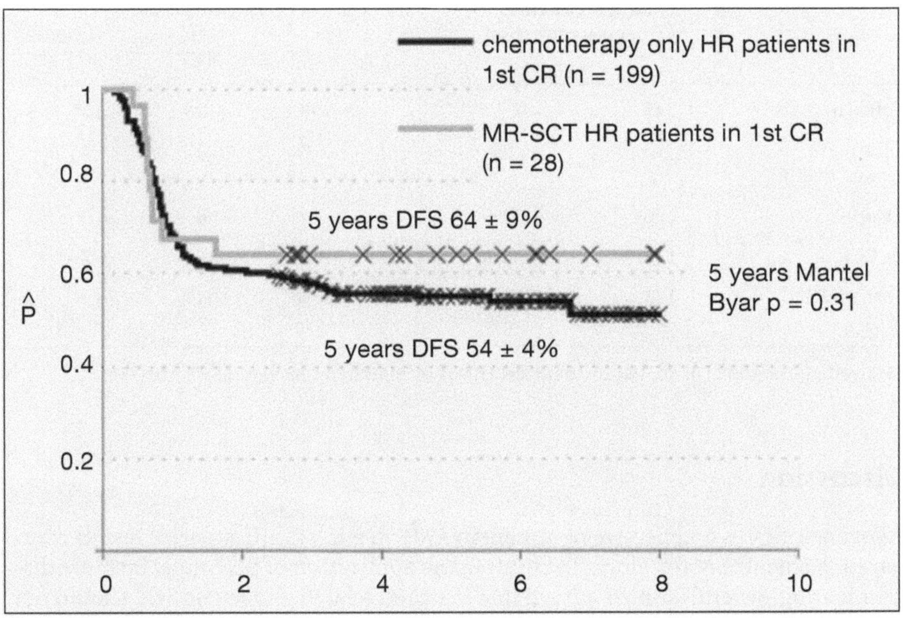

Fig. 2. Estimated probability for disease-free survival (DFS) in children either with SCT in 1st CR or chemotherapy alone.

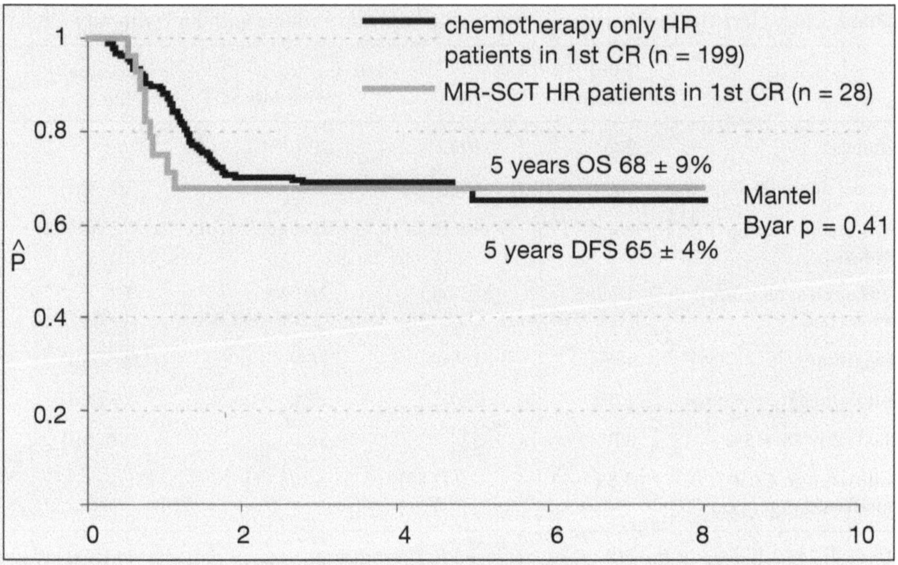

Fig. 3. Estimated probability for overall survival (OS) in children either with SCT in 1st CR or chemotherapy alone.

Table 3. Treatment and outcome of the high risk group patients in remission

	Total HR Patients achieving remission		SCT in 1st CR no	MR SCT	Other SCT
Total (n)	243		198	28	16*
Treatment related death	13	5%	8	2	3
Relapse	96	39%	82	8	6
In CCR	134	55%	108	18	7
5-yr. pDFS (SE)	143	55% 3%	57% (4%)	64% (9%)	47 (12%)

received autologous (n=6), haplo-identical (n=3) or matched unrelated SCT (n=7)

Discussion

Allogeneic SCT is an effective treatment in AML in adults with superior results compared to chemotherapy alone. In children the application of SCT must be more discriminating. Several authors agreed that matched related allogeneic SCT should not be recommended in children with favorable prognostics factors like t(15;17), t(8;21) or inv(16) (Creutzig et al., 2001; Gibson et al., 2000; Ladenstein et al., 1997).

However, other study groups postulated a general indication of allogeneic SCT in children AML (Sanders, 1997; Woods et al., 1996), but all of these studies were characterized by a low efficacy of chemotherapy (Amadori et al., 1993; Sanders, 1997; Woods et al., 1996). The remission rate reported from the CCG 2891 study was 70% with a standard timing and 75% with an intensive timing treatment strategy. Event-free survival was 42±7% and 27±6%, respectively (Woods et al., 1996; Woods et al., 2001). The Italian AIEOP/LAM 8204 study revealed a remission rate of 79% and a DFS of only 31% (Amadori et al., 1993). The French LAME 89/91 study showed a DFS of 48%±10% in the chemotherapy group. These results are low compared to the results of the MRC 10/12 (Gibson et al., 2000; Stevens et al., 1998) or AML-BFM 93 studies (Creutzig et al., 2001). Remission rates in the latter studies with a more intensive induction treatment, consolidation and re-intensification ranged between 82% and 86%, the 5-years event-free survival was 48%±3% (MRC10) and 51%±3% (AML-BFM 93). 5 years DFS in the AML-BFM-93 study was 62 ±3%, mainly achieved by chemotherapy alone. As demonstrated, matched related allogeneic SCT revealed no significant advantages even in high risk patients in first remission (Fig. 2 and 3). Similar results were presented by the MRC10 (Stevens et al., 1998) and MRC12 studies (Gibson et al., 2000).

The best results in the treatment of AML with an overall survival of more than 80% were reported in single center studies (Matsuyama et al., 2000; Ortega et al., 1996; Uderzo et al., 2000). Interestingly, these studies revealed similar outcomes with allogeneic and autologous SCT suggesting a minor influence of the graft versus leukemia effect but a major influence of supportive care and experience in AML therapy. Overall, an intensive chemotherapy combined with sufficient supportive care provided similar rate of cure and survival as allogeneic SCT in first remission, probably with less severe late effects. Whereas in adults severe late side effects of SCT were comparable to those of chemotherapy (Lowsky et al., 1994), children suffered more often from academic difficulties and growth impairment. In addition, SCT compared to CHT alone was associated with lower weight and the development of growth hormone deficiency, hypothyroidism, hypogonadism including infertility, chronic graft-versus-host disease and cataracts (Leung et al., 2000; Afify et al., 2000; Alter et al., 1996; Huma et al., 1995; Leahey et al., 1999).

Considering late adverse effects associated with SCT a risk factor analysis is warranted to identify patients in whom allogeneic SCT in 1st CR is mandatory.

Summary

The indication for allogeneic matched related stem cell transplantation (SCT) in children with high risk acute myeloid leukemia in 1st complete remission is still controversial. In the AML-BFM 93 study 471 children were enrolled between 1993 and 1998. According to morphology, cytogenetic and response[1] 161 children were

[1] Standard risk = AML M1/M2 with Auer rods or t(8;21), AML M4eo or inv(16) and less than 5% blasts at day 15, AML FAB M3 with t(15;17) regardless of their blast count on day 15 high risk = all other

defined as standard risk patients and 310 as high risk patients. All children were treated intensively (according treatment protocol) with 2-3 intensive chemotherapy blocks and 6weeks consolidation. Complete remission was achieved in total by 387 children (82%), 243 of the high risk group (78%). If a matched related (MR) donor was available, SCT was recommended after consolidation. Twenty-eight patients received matched related SCT (1 syngen), 199 children had chemotherapy only (CHT) and 16 patients were transplanted allogeneic unrelated (n=7), autologous (n=6) or haplo-identical (n=3). The three groups did not differ regarding gender, median leukocyte count, hemoglobin concentration, clinical features or response. Four of the 7 children receiving an allogeneic unrelated, 3 of 6 patients with autologous and 1 of 3 with haplo-identical SCT were in first or second continuous remission. Estimated 5-year DFS was 54%±4% for patients with CHT compared to 64%±9% in children with MR-SCT (Mantel-Bayr p=0.31). 5-year overall survival was 65%±4% (CHT) versus 68%±9% (MR-SCT; p=0.64). The Cox regression analysis revealed a risk ratio of 0.56, 95% confidence interval 0.23-1.34.

In conclusion there was no significant advantage of MR-SCT in HR-patients with AML in 1st remission. Considering adverse late effects associated with SCT a risk factor analysis is warranted to identify patients in whom allogeneic SCT in 1st remission is mandatory.

References

Afify Z, Shaw PJ, Clavano-Harding A, Cowell CT (2000), Growth and endocrine function in children with acute myeloid leukaemia after bone marrow transplantation using busulfan/cyclophosphamide. *Bone Marrow Transplant* 25:1087-1092

Alter CA, Thornton PS, Willi SM, Bunin N, Moshang T, Jr. (1996), Growth in children after bone marrow transplantation for acute myelogenous leukemia as compared to acute lymphocytic leukemia. *J Pediatr Endocrinol Metab* 9:51-57

Amadori S, Testi AM, Arico M, Comelli A, Giuliano M, Madon E, Masera G, Rondelli R, Zanesco L, Mandelli F (1993), Prospective comparative study of bone marrow transplantation and postremission chemotherapy for childhood acute myelogenous leukemia. The Associazione Italiana Ematologia ed Oncologia Pediatrica Cooperative Group. *J Clin Oncol* 11:1046-1054

Creutzig U, Ritter J, Zimmermann M, Hermann J, Gadner H, Blütters-Sawatzki D, Niemeyer CM, Schwabe D, Selle B, Boos J, Kühl J, Feldges A (2001) Idarubicin improves blast cell clearance during indiction therapy in children with AML: results of the study AML-BFM 93. Leukemia in press.

Creutzig U, Zimmermann M, Ritter J, Henze G, Graf N, Löffler H, Schellong G (1999), Definition of a standard-risk group in children with AML. *Br J Haematol* 104:630-639

Dini G, Cornish JM, Gadner H, Souillet G, Vossen JM, Paolucci P, Manfredini L, Miano M, Niethammer D (1996), Bone marrow transplant indications for childhood leukemias: achieving a consensus. The EBMT Pediatric Diseases Working Party. *Bone Marrow Transplant* 18 Suppl 2:4-7

Dinndorf P, Bunin N (1995), Bone marrow transplantation for children with acute myelogenous leukemia. *J Pediatr Hematol Oncol* 17:211-224

Frassoni F, Labopin M, Gluckman E, Prentice HG, Vernant JP, Zwaan F, Granena A, Gahrton G, De Witte T, Gratwohl A, Reiffers J, Gorin NC (1996), Results of allogeneic bone marrow transplantation for acute leukemia have improved in Europe with time—a report of the acute leukemia working party of the European group for blood and marrow transplantation (EBMT). *Bone Marrow Transplant* 17:13-18

Gale RP, Buchner T, Zhang MJ, Heinecke A, Champlin RE, Dicke KA, Gluckman E, Good RA, Gratwohl A, Herzig RH, Keating A, Klein JP, Marmont AM, Prentice HG, Rowlings PA, Sobocinski KA, Speck B, Weiner RS, Horowitz MM (1996), HLA-identical sibling bone marrow transplants vs chemotherapy for acute myelogenous leukemia in first remission. *Leukemia* 10:1687-1691

Gibson BE, Webb D, Wheatley K (2000), Does transplant in first remission CR have a role in paediatric AML? A review of the MRC AML10&AML12 trials. *Blood* 96:2248

Gorin NC, Labopin M, Fouillard L, Meloni G, Frassoni F, Iriondo A, Brunet MS, Goldstone AH, Harousseau JL, Reiffers J, Esperou-Bourdeau H, Gluckman E (1996), Retrospective evaluation of autologous bone marrow transplantation vs allogeneic bone marrow transplantation from an HLA identical related donor in acute myelocytic leukemia. A study of the European Cooperative Group for Blood and Marrow Transplantation (EBMT). *Bone Marrow Transplant* 18:111-117

Huma Z, Boulad F, Black P, Heller G, Sklar C (1995), Growth in children after bone marrow transplantation for acute leukemia. *Blood* 86:819-824

Hurwitz CA, Mounce KG, Grier HE (1995), Treatment of patients with acute myelogenous leukemia: review of clinical trials of the past decade. *J Pediatr Hematol Oncol* 17:185-197

Klingebiel T, Pession A, Paolucci P, Rondelli R (1996), Autologous versus allogeneic BMT in AML: the European experience. Report of the EBMT—Pediatric Diseases Working Party. *Bone Marrow Transplant* 18 Suppl 2:49-52

Ladenstein R, Peters C, Gadner H (1997), The present role of bone marrow and stem cell transplantation in the therapy of children with acute leukemia. *Ann N Y Acad Sci* 824:38-64

Leahey AM, Teunissen H, Friedman DL, Moshang T, Lange BJ, Meadows AT (1999), Late effects of chemotherapy compared to bone marrow transplantation in the treatment of pediatric acute myeloid leukemia and myelodysplasia. *Med Pediatr Oncol* 32:163-169

Leung W, Hudson MM, Strickland DK, Phipps S, Srivastava DK, Ribeiro RC, Rubnitz JE, Sandlund JT, Kun LE, Bowman LC, Razzouk BI, Mathew P, Shearer P, Evans WE, Pui CH (2000), Late effects of treatment in survivors of childhood acute myeloid leukemia. *J Clin Oncol* 18:3273-3279

Lowsky R, Lipton J, Fyles G, Minden M, Meharchand J, Tejpar I, Atkins H, Sutcliffe S, Messner H (1994), Secondary malignancies after bone marrow transplantation in adults. *J Clin Oncol* 12:2187-2192

Matsuyama T, Horibe K, Kato K, Kojima SS (2000), Bone marrow transplantation for children with acute myelogenous leukaemia in the first complete remission. *Eur J Cancer* 36:368-375

Michel G, Leverger G, Leblanc T, Nelken B, Baruchel A, Landman-Parker J, Thuret I, Bergeron C, Bordigoni P, Esperou-Bourdeau H, Perel Y, Vannier JP, Schaison G (1996), Allogeneic bone marrow transplantation vs aggressive post-remission chemotherapy for children with acute myeloid leukemia in first complete remission. A prospective study from the French Society of Pediatric Hematology and Immunology (SHIP). *Bone Marrow Transplant* 17:191-196

Mitus AJ, Miller KB, Schenkein DP, Ryan HF, Parsons SK, Wheeler C, Antin JH (1995), Improved survival for patients with acute myelogenous leukemia. *J Clin Oncol* 13:560-569

Ortega JJ, Olive T (1998), Haematopoietic progenitor cell transplant in acute leukaemias in children: indications, results and controversies. *Bone Marrow Transplant* 21 Suppl 2:S11-S16

Ortega JJ, Olive T, Diaz dH, Coll MT, Bastida P, Massuet L (1996), Allogeneic and autologous bone marrow transplantation in AML in first remission. The Spanish experience. *Bone Marrow Transplant* 18 Suppl 2:53-58

Proctor SJ, Taylor PR, Stark A, Carey PJ, Bown N, Hamilton PJ, Reid MM (1995), Evaluation of the impact of allogenic transplant in first remission on an unselected population of patients with acute myeloid leukaemia aged 15-55 years. The Northern Regional Haematology Group *Leukemia* 9:1246-1251

Pui CH (1995), Childhood leukemias—current status and future perspective. *Chung Hua Min Kuo Hsiao Erh Ko I Hsueh Hui Tsa Chih* 36:322-327

Reiffers J, Stoppa AM, Attal M, Michallet M, Marit G, Blaise D, Huguet F, Corront B, Cony-Makhoul P, Gastaut JA, Laurent G, Molina L, Broustet A, Maraninchi D, Pris J, Hollard D, Faberes C (1996), Allogeneic vs autologous stem cell transplantation vs chemotherapy in patients with acute myeloid leukemia in first remission: the BGMT 87 study. *Leukemia* 10:1874-1882

Sanders JE (1997), Bone marrow transplantation for pediatric malignancies. *Pediatr Clin North Am* 44:1005-1020

Stevens RF, Hann IM, Wheatley K, Gray RG (1998), Marked improvements in outcome with chemotherapy alone in paediatric acute myeloid leukemia: results of the United Kingdom Medical Research Council's 10th AML trial. MRC Childhood Leukaemia Working Party. *Br J Haematol* 101:130-140

Uderzo C, Biagi E, Rovelli A, Balduzzi A, Schiro R, Longoni D, Arrigo C, Nicolini B, Placa L, Da Prada A, Mascaretti L, Giltri G, Galimberti S, Valsecchi MG, Locasciulli A, Masera G (2000), Bone marrow transplantation for childhood hematological disorders: a global pediatric approach in a twelve year single center experience. *Pediatr Med Chir* 21:157-163

Vormoor J, Boos J, Stahnke K, Jürgens H, Ritter J, Creutzig U (1996), Therapy of childhood acute myelogenous leukemias. *Ann Hematol* 73:11-24

Woods WG, Kobrinsky N, Buckley JD, Lee JW, Sanders J, Neudorf S, Gold S, Barnard DR, DeSwarte J, Dusenbery K, Kalousek D, Arthur DC, Lange BJ (1996), Timed-sequential induction therapy improves postremission outcome in acute myeloid leukemia: a report from the Children's Cancer Group. *Blood* 87:4979-4989

Woods WG, Neudorf S, Gold S, Sanders J, Buckley JD, Barnard DR, Dusenbery K, DeSwarte J, Arthur DC, Lange BJ, Kobrinsky NL (2001), A comparison of allogeneic bone marrow transplantation, autologous bone marrow transplantation, and aggressive chemotherapy in children with acute myeloid leukemia in remission: a report from the Children's cancer group. *Blood* 97:56-62

Zittoun RA, Mandelli F, Willemze R, De Witte T, Labar B, Resegotti L, Leoni F, Damasio E, Visani G, Papa G (1995), Autologous or allogeneic bone marrow transplantation compared with intensive chemotherapy in acute myelogenous leukemia. European Organization for Research and Treatment of Cancer (EORTC) and the Gruppo Italiano Malattie Ematologiche Maligne dell'Adulto (GIMEMA) Leukemia Cooperative Groups. *N Engl J Med* 332:217-223

Stem Cell Transplantation in Acute Myeloid Leukemia after Conditioning with Busulfan, Cyclophosphamide and Different Dosages of Etoposide (VP-16)

N. Kröger, T. Zabelina, S. Sonnenberg, W. Krüger, H. Renges, N. Stute, F. Finkenstein, U. Mayer, K. Holstein, W. Fiedler, H. Colberg[2], R. Sonnen[2], R. Kuse[2], D. Braumann[3], B. Metzner[4], F. del Valle[4], R. Erttmann, H. Kabisch, and A. R. Zander

Bone Marrow Transplantation, University Hospital Hamburg-Eppendorf, Germany and [2]A.K. St. Georg, Hamburg, [3]A.K. Altona, Hamburg, [4]Städtische Kliniken, Oldenburg, Germany

Abstract

To evaluate the efficacy and toxicity of two different etoposide dosages (30 or 45 mg/kg) in combination with busulfan/cyclophosphamide as conditioning regimen followed by stem cell transplantation in patients with acute myeloid leukemia (AML).

90 patients with AML received either 30 mg/kg (n=60) or 45 mg/kg (n=30) etoposide in combination with busulfan (16 mg/kg) and cyclophosphamide (120 mg/kg). Stem cell source was allogeneic related bone marrow (BM) (n= 53), allogeneic unrelated BM (n=5), allogeneic unrelated PBSC (n=2), syngeneic BM (n=2), autologous BM purged (n=9) or unpurged (n=9), autologous PBSC (n=10). 56 patients (63%) were in 1.CR, 26/90 (29%) were >1.CR and 8/90 (8%) were transplanted in relapse. Main toxicity in both groups were mucositis and hepatotoxicity. 45 mg/kg etoposide resulted in a greater hepatic toxicity (p =0.03) and a higher incidence of VOD (23 vs 12%, p=0.04). The treatment-related mortality was 17% in the 30 mg/kg group and 33% in the 45 mg/kg group and mainly due to infections, intestinal pneumonia and GvHD. Hematological recovery of leukocyte 1/nl was comparable in both groups (17 vs 16 days). After a median follow-up of 16 months 18% in the 30 mg/kg group and 26% in the 45 mg/kg group relapsed. In patients with allogeneic related bone marrow transplantation in first CR no relapse was observed after a median follow-up of 3 years. For all patients the 3-years estimated disease-free survival was 62% in the 30 mg/kg group and 40% in the 45 mg/kg group (p=0.03). For patients in 1.CR and allogeneic related stem cell-transplantation the 3 years disease-free survival was 80% and 66%, respectively (p=0.4). We conclude that etoposide, busulfan and cyclophosphamide is a highly active regimen in bone marrow transplantation of patients with AML with a low relapse rate. Conditioning with 30mg/kg etoposide resulted in less toxicity and a better overall survival due to a lower transplant related mortality than 45 mg/kg.

Introduction

Intensive chemotherapy for acute myeloid leukemia achieves approximately 65–80% complete remission, but only 20-30% of patients will maintain durable remission with standard consolidation therapies [1–3]. The use of allogeneic or autologous bone marrow transplantation increases the rate of long-term survivors, however a substantial number of patients will relapse of their disease despite allogeneic or autologous stem cell transplantation [4–6]. The most common preparartive regimen in acute myeloid leukemia is busulfan and cyclophosphamide or TBI plus cyclophosphamide [7, 8]. It has been already shown that an intensified preparative regimen can lower the relapse rate in allogeneic as well as in autologous transplantation [5, 9, 31]. We incorporated etoposide in escalating doses (30 and 45 mg/kg) to a conditioning regimen consisting of busulfan (16 mg/kg) plus cyclophosphamide (120 mg/kg) to investigate the efficacy and toxcitity of this new preparative regimen in patients with acute myeloid leukemia undergoing autologous or allogeneic stem cell transplantation [10, 28–30]. Etoposide has been administrated in doses up to 60 mg/kg, which represents a 10 fold increase over the conventional dosage. The dose-limiting factor of high-dose etoposide is stomatitis. Other side effects are hepatic and pulmonary toxicity, particulary in extensively pretreated patients [11–14].

Patients and Methods

Between 1991 and 1998, 90 patients were enrolled in the protocol. The median age was 32 years (range: 1–64); The median follow-up was 16 months (range 1 to 94). The patient characteristics are listed in Table 1. The conditioning protocol consisted of 16 mg/kg busulfan administered orally in four divided doses daily for four days, Cyclophoshamide 60 mg/kg was given intravenously over 1 hour for two days and etoposide 30 mg/kg (n=60) or 45 mg/kg (n=30) was administered intravenously undiluted over 6 hours. The transplant protocol was approved by the local ethic commission and all patients gave written informed consent.

GvHD Prophylaxis

GvHD prophylaxis consisted in allogeneic transplantation of cyclosporin A (3 mg/kg) started on day -1 until day 180. Patients received 10 or 15 mg/kg methotrexate on day 1 and 10 mg/kg on day 3 and 6. Acute GvHD was diagnosed and graded according to the Glucksberg criteria [15]. Since 1995 all patients addionally received metronidazole as GvHD prophylaxis. In unrelated transplantation further GvHD prophylaxis contained anti-thymocycte globulin (90 mg/kg) as part of the conditioning regimen, metronidazole and IgM enriched immunoglobulins as described previously [16].

Table 1. Patient characteristics

	VP-16: 30mg/kg	VP-16:45 mg/kg
Number	60 (66%)	30 (33%)
Allogeneic related	32 (53%)	21(70%)
Allogeneic unrelated	2 (3%)	5 (17%)
Syngeneic	2 (3%)	0
Autologous BMT	8 (13%)	1 (3%)
Autologous BMT purged	6 (10%)	3 (10%)
Autologous PBSCT	10 (17%)	0
Gender: m:f	32:28	10:20
Age (range)	33,5(14-59)	31,5(1-64)
FAB-Classification		
M0	1	0
M1	12	9
M2	15	7
M3	0	1
M4	21	9
M5	6	4
M6	5	0
1. CR	39 (65%)	17 (57%)
2. CR	17 (28%)	8 (26%)
3. CR	1 (2%)	1 (3%)
1. Relapse	0 (0%)	2 (7%)
2. Relapse	2 (3%)	2 (7%)
1. PR	1 (2%)	1 (3%)

Regimen-Related Toxicity

Regimen-related toxicity was graded using the Bearman score [17]. Skin toxicity was described as mild in case of erythema or as more severe in case of desquamation.

Results

Transplant-related –toxicity and GvHD

The main toxicity in both VP-16 groups was mucositis grade II and hepatotoxicity.

Treatment with 45mg/kg VP-16 resulted in a higher incidence of grade I/II liver toxicity than with 30 mg/kg (67% vs 43%, p=0.03). The incidence of VOD was also higher in the 45mg than in the 30mg/kg group (23% vs 12% , p=0.04). The treatment related mortality was 16% in the 30mg- group and 26% in the 45 mg/kg-group (p=0.1) and mainly due to Infection (fungal, sepsis, CMV). Skin toxicity was mild in both groups (18 and 26%). GvHD grade I/I and III/IV was higher in the 45 mg group (30 vs 18% and 13 vs 5%; p=0.2).

Table 2. Toxicities according the VP-16 dose

Organ-toxicity	Grade	VP 16 30 mg/kg (n=60)	VP-16 45mg/kg (n=30)	p-value
Cardiac	I/II	3%	3%	n.s.
Bladder	I/II	5%	1%	n.s.
Renal	I/II	68%	57%	n.s.
	III	2%	0%	n.s.
Lung	I/II	8%	13%	n.s.
	III	8%	16%	n.s.
	IV	5%	3%	n.s.
Liver	I/II	43%	67%	0.03
	IV	2%	0%	n.s.
ZNS	I-IV	0%	0%	n.s.
GI-tract	I/II	34%	43%	n.s.
Stomatitis	I/II	94%	96%	n.s.
	III/IV	3%	3%	n.s.
Skin	I-III	18%	26%	n.s.
Veno-occlusive disease	I-III	12%	23%	0.04

Hematopoietic engraftment

The median days to leucocyte engraftment >1/nl was 17 days (range 9-39) in the 30 mg/kg group and 16 days (range 12-47) in the 45 mg/kg group. In the 45 mg-group platelet engraftment was observed after a median of 21 days (range 13-158) and in the 30 mg/kg group after a median of 22 days (range 22-365).

Response, relapse and survival

After a median follow-up of 16 months 11 patients (18%) of the 30mg/kg group and 8 patients (26%) of the 45 mg/kg group relapsed. The overall relapse-rate was 20% and occured mostly after autologous transplantation (40%) or allogeneic transplantation beyond first complete remission (27%). In patients with allogeneic related transplantation in first CR no relapse was observed after a median follow-up of 3 years in both groups. Only 1 patient developed MDS 4 years post transplantation but with 100% donor cells. The 3 vears estimated disease-free survival for all patients was 62% in the 30mg/kg group and 40% in the 45mg/kg group (p=0.03) (Fig. 1). The 3-years estimated overall survival was 63% in the 30mg/kg group and 41% in the 45 mg/kg group (p=0.06) (Fig. 2). For the homogenous group of patients transplanted in first CR with HLA-identical sibling the estimated 3-years overall and disease-free survival was 80% in the 30 mg/kg group and 66% in the 45 mg/kg group (p=0.4) (Fig. 3).

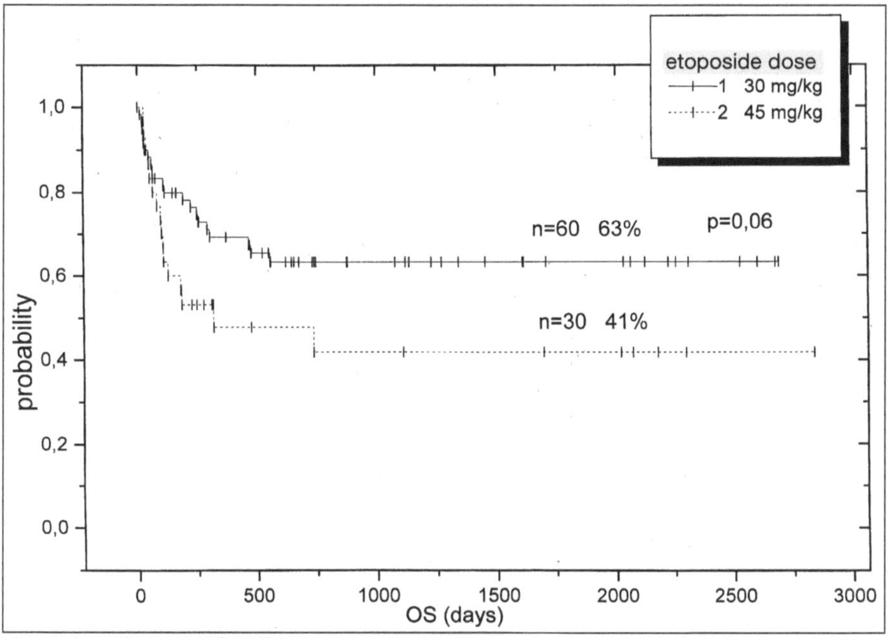

Fig. 1. Overall survival for all patients

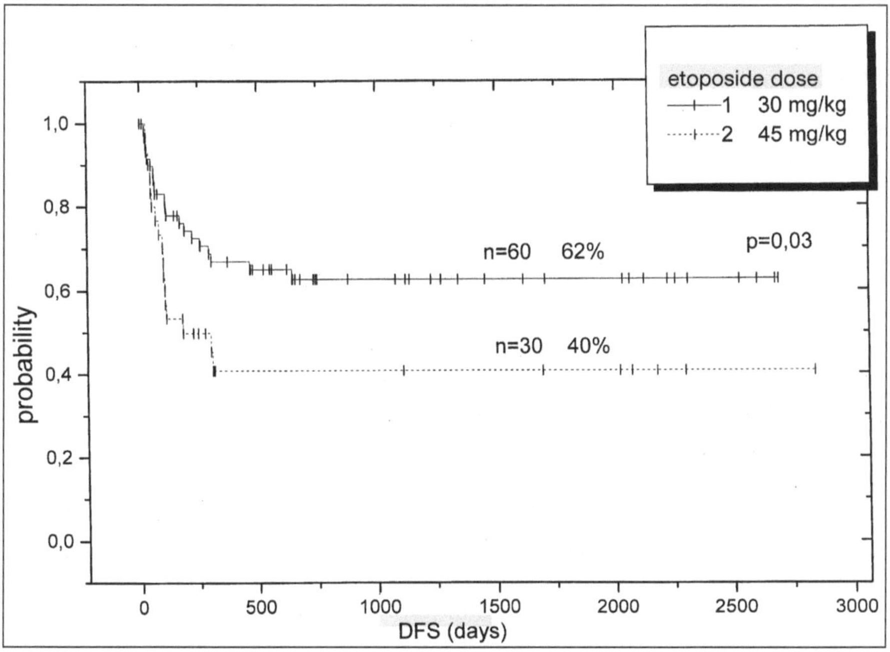

Fig. 2. Disease-free survival of all patients

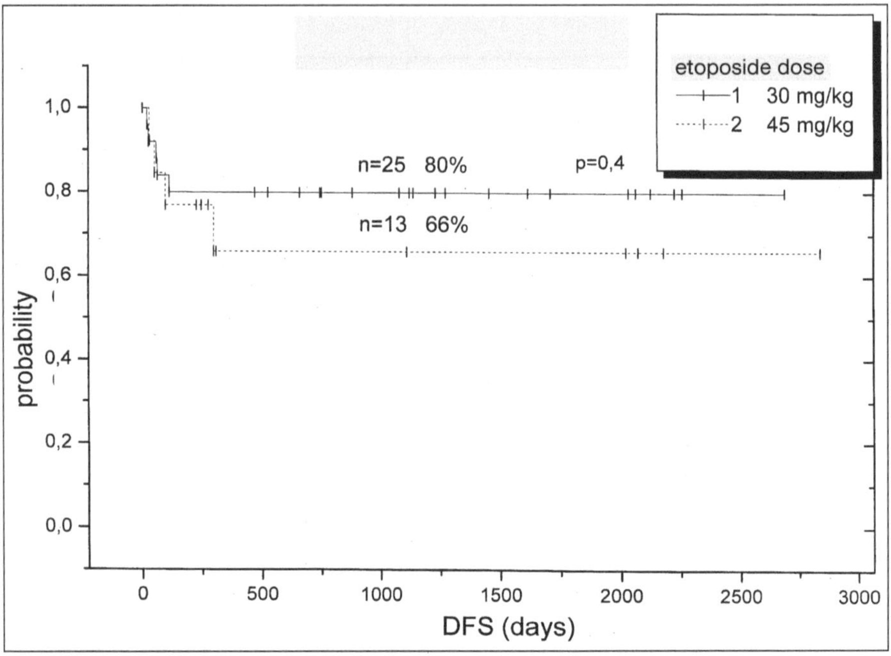

Fig. 3. Disease-free survival of patients transplanted in 1. CR with HLA-identical sibling

Discussion

The combination busulfan plus cyclophosphamide (Bu/Cy) has been widely used in patients with hematological malignancies. Initially studies using busulfan (16 mg/kg) and cyclophosphamide (200 mg/kg) provided an effective alternative to TBI plus cyclophosphamide in treatment of AML [19]. Modification of this regimen by lowering the cyclophosphamide dose to 120 mg/kg appears to be equally effective and less toxic [20] Recently, a follow-up of a french study comparing busulfan/cyclophosphamide (120 mg/kg) with TBI/cyclophosphamide in allogeneic transplantation in patients with 1.CR in AML showed a lower relapse-rate (28% vs 38%) and a longer disease-free survival (58% vs 48%) for patients treated with TBI/Cyclophosphamide. Furthermore, the Bu/Cy regimen resulted in a higher incidence of liver toxicity and GvHD [21]. A retrospective study of the European Cooperative Group for Blood and Marrow Transplantion (EBMT) compared TBI/Cy with Bu/Cy for allogeneic and autologous stem cell transplantation in AML and ALL.Relapse, survival and disease-free survival did not differ between the regimens, but VOD was more common in the Bu/Cy group [33]. A recent meta-analysis compared five randomized trials of Bu/Cy versus TBI containing regimens in allogeneic stem cell transplantation. Survival and disease-free survival were better in the TBI group but the differences did not reach statistical significance. There was a significantly higher incidence of VOD with the Bu/Cy regimen [32]. However, both arms had a substantial relapse-rate. In several studies the high efficacy of high-dose etoposide in advanced hematological malignancies has been confirmed [11–13]. In combination with TBI, high dose etoposide followed by allogeneic stem cell transplantation resulted in a disease-free survival of 43% and a relapse-rate of 32% in patients with advanced leukemia [25, 26]. In a comparison study of AML beyond first CR, Bu/Cy showed an advantage without significance in terms of survival, but the TBI/Cy regimen resulted in less VOD and GvHD [34].

The feasibility and toxicity of high-dose busulfan, cyclophosphamide and etoposide has been mainly evaluated in allogeneic bone marrow transplantation of high risk patients and guilded a high treatment-related mortality, mainly due to GVHD, aspergillosis and failure to engraftment [23, 24]. A study with Bu/Cy/etoposide (40 mg/kg) was conducted by Crilley et al. [25] in 84 patients with hematologic malignancy and autologous or allogeneic bone marrow transplantation. Mucositis and skin symptoms were noted as frequent extramedullary toxicity. Toxic death because of VOD or pulmonary hemorrhage occured in 8% of the patients.

The critical issue of etoposide in high-dose chemotherapy is the dose. Several studies observed a dose-response effect of etoposide in terms of extramedullary toxicity, with a maximum tolerated dose of 60–70 mg/kg [11–13, 27]. Escalating dose of etoposide (30 to 40 mg/kg) were added to busulfan and cyclophosphamide in 11 patients undergoing allogeneic or autologous transplant. The authors conclude that the regimen could be administered with tolerable toxicity, but expressed concern over skin and hepatic toxicity [13]. Toxicity of the liver and mucositis was the main toxicity in our study. Liver toxicity and veno-occlusive disease was more frequent in the 45 mg/kg group, however the only fatal case of VOD occured in the 30 mg/kg group. The treatment related mortality for all patient was 20% and 23% for allogeneic transplantation in 1.CR., mainly due to fungal and viral infection, intestinal pneumonia, liver toxicity or GvHD. The treatment related mortality was higher for patients treated with 45mg/kg etoposide than for those patients treated with 30 mg/kg (30 vs 20%). Fatal intestinal pneumonia with pulmonary hemorrhage was observed in 4 cases (three at 30mg/kg and one at 45 mg/kg) within 100 days after tranplantation, which might be due to high-dose etoposide [14]. However, several other factors like busulfan can cause intestinal pneumonia or pulmonary hemorrhage.

High-dose etoposide in combination with busulfan followed by autologous transplantation has been used in patients with acute non-lymphoblastic leukemia with a disease-free survival of 57% and a relapse-rate of only 28% [5]. The relapse–rate of all patients in our study with busulfan, cyclophosphamide and etoposide was only 20% and for patients transplanted with HLA-identical sibling in first remission no relapse was observed after a median follow-up of three years, indicating the high efficacy of this regimen [22]. Most relapse occured after autologous stem cell transplantation, especially in advanced disease (40%). We observed no difference in relapse rate between 30 mg/kg and 45 mg/kg etoposide, suggesting that a the lower dose of etoposide might be sufficient to prevent relapse.

In conclusion, etoposide in dose of 30 or 45 mg/kg in combination with busulfan and cyclophosphamide is a highly active preparative regimen in AML with a low relapse rate and tolerable toxicity, especially for patients in 1. CR with HLA-identical sibling undergoing allogeneic stem cell transplantation. Toxicity profile is in favour to 30 mg/kg etoposide. Furthermore, 30 mg /kg etoposide leads to a better overall survial than 45 mg/kg due to a lower transplanted related mortality without an increase of the relapse-rate.

References

1. Weinstein HJ, Mayer RJ, Rosenthal DS, Coral FS, Camitta BM, Gelber RD. Chemotherapy for acute myelogenous leukemia in children and adults: VAPA update. Blood 62:315, 1983.
2. Cassileth PA, Lynch E, Hines JD, et al. Varying intensity of postremission therapy in acute myeloid leukemia. Blood 1992; 79:1924-1930.
3. Büchner T, Urbanitz D, Hiddemann W, et al. Intensified induction and consolidation with or without maintenance chemotherapy for acute myeloid leukemia. J Clin Oncol 1985;3:1583-1589.
4. Appelbaum FR. Allogeneic hematopoietic stem cell transplantation for acute leukemia. Semin Oncol 1997,24:114-123.
5. Linker CA, Ries CA, Damon LE, Rugo HS, Wolf JL. Autologous bone marrow transplantation for acute myeloid leukemia using busulfan plus etoposide as a preparative regimen. Blood 1993;81:311-318.
6. Gorin NC, Najman A, Duhamel G. Autologous bone marrow transplantation in acute myeloid leukemia. Lancet 1977;1:1050.
7. Tutschka PJ. Copelan EA,. Klein JA, et al. Bone marrow transplantation for leukemia following a new busulfan and cyclophosphamide regimen. Blood 1987; 70:1382-1388.
8. Körbling M, Hunstein W, Fliedner TM ,et al. Disease-free survival after autologous bone marrow transplantation in patients with acute myelogenous leukemia. Blood 1989;74:1898-1904.
9. Clift RA, Buckner CD, Appelbaum FR, Bryant E, Bearman SI, Petersen FB, Fisher LD, Anasetti C, Beatty P, Bensinger WI, Doney K, Hill RS, McDonald GB, Martin P, Meyers J, Sanders J, Singer J, Stewart P, Sullivan KM, Witherspoon R, Storb R, Hansen JA, Thomas ED. Allogeneic marrow transplantation in patients with acute myeloid leukemia in first remission: A randomized trial of two irradiation regimens. Blood 1990;76:1867.
10. Henwood JN, Brodgen RN. Etoposide: a review of its pharmacodynamic and pharmacokinetic properties, and therapeutic potential in combination chemotherapy of cancer. Drugs 1990;39:438-490.
11. Stadtmauer, E,A, Casselith PA, Gale RP, et al. Etoposide in leukemia, lymphoma and bone marrow transplantation. Leuk.Res. 1989;13:639-650.
12. Wolff SN, McKay CM, Hande KR, et al. High-dose VP16-213 and autologous bone marrow transplantation for refractory malignancies- aphase I study. J Clin Oncol 1983;1:701-705.
13. Spitzer TR, Cottler-Fox M, Torrisi J, et al. Escalating doses of etoposide with cyclophosphamide and fractionated TBI or busulfan conditioning for BMT. Bone Marrow Transplantation 1989;4:559-565.
14. Crilley P, Topolsky D, Styler MJ, Bernstein E, Resnik K, Mullaney R, Bulova S, Brodsky I, Marks DI. Extramedullary toxicity of a conditioning regimen containing busulfan, cyclophosphamide and etoposide in 84 patients undergoing autologous and allogeneic bone marrow transplantation. Bone Marrow Transplantation 1995;15:361-365.
15. Glucksberg H, Storb R, Fefer A, et al. Clinical manifestations of graft vs host disease in human recipients of marrow from HLA-matched sibling donors.. Transplantation 1974;18:295.
16. Zander AR, Zabelina T, Kröger N, Renges H, Krüger W, Löliger C, Dürken M, Stockschläder M, de Wit M, Wacker-Backhaus G, Bielack S, Jaburg N, Rüssmann B, Erttmann, Kabisch H. Use of a five-agent GvHD prevention regimen in recipients of unrelated donor marrow. Bone Marrow Transplantation 1999; 23:889-893.
17. Bearman SI, Appelbaum FR, Buckner CD, et al. Regimen related toxicity in patients undergoing bone marrow transplantation. J Clin Oncol 1988;6:1562-68.
18. Kaplan E, Meier P. Non-parametric estimation from incomplete observations. J Am Stat Assoc 1958;53:457-81.

19. Santos GW, Tutschka Pj, Brookmeyer et al. Marrow transplantation for acute non-lymphomic leukemia after treatment with busulfan and cyclophosphamide. N Engl J Med 1983, 309:1347-1353.
20. Tutschka PJ, Copelan EA, Klein, JA et al.: Bone marrow transplantatiom for leukemia following new busulfan and cyclophosphamide regime. Blood 1987, 70:1382-88.
21. Blaise D, Maraninchi D, Michallet M, Reiffers J, Deverdie A, Jouet JP, Milpied N, Attal M, Ifrah N, Kuentz M, Dauriac C, Bordigoni P, Gratecos N, Guilhot F, Guyotat D, Gluckmann E. BuCy(120) versus TBI/Cy to prepare allo-BMT for CR1 AML: a follow-up of a study from GEGMO. Bone Marrow Transplant 1999;23 (Suppl 1):228.
22. Zander AR, Berger C, Kröger N, Stockschläder M, Krüger W, Horstmann M, Grimm J, Zeller W, Kabisch H, Erttmann, Schönrock P, Kuse R, Braumann D, IlligerHJ, Fiedler W, de Wit M, Hossfeld DK, Weh HJ: High-Dose Chemotherapy with Busulfan, Cyclophosphamide and VP 16 as Conditioning Regimen for Allogenic Bone Marrow Transplantation for Patients with Acute Myeloid Leukemia in First Complete Remission Clin Cancer Res 1997;3:2671-75.
23. Spitzer TR, Cottler-Fox M, Torrisi J, et al.: Escalating doses of etoposide with cyclophosphamide and fractionated total body irradiation or busulfan as conditioning for bone marrow transplantation. Bone Marrow Transplant 1989;4:559-565.
24. Vaughan WP, Dennison JD, Reed EC, et al. Improved results of allogenic bone marrow transplantation for advanced hematologic malignancy using busulfan, cyclophosphamide and etoposide as cytoreductive and immunosuppressive therapy. Bone Marrow Transplant 1991;8:489-495.
25. Blume KG, Forman SJ, O'Donnel MR, Doroshow JH, et al. Total body irradiation and high-dose etoposide : a new preparative regimen for bone marrow transplantation in patients with advanced hematological malignancies. Blood 1987;69:1015-1020.
26. Schmitz N, Gassmann W, Rister M, Johannson W, Suttorp M, Brix F, Holthuis JJM, Heit W, Hertenstein B, Schaub J, Löffler H. Fractionated total body irradiation and high-dose VP 16-213 followed by allogeneic bone marrow transplantation in advanced leukemias. Blood 1988;72:1567-1573.
27. Chao NJ, Stein AS, Longo GD, Negrin RS, Amylon MD, Wong RM, Forman SJ, Blume KG. Busulfan/etoposide-initial experience with a new preparatory regimen for autologous bone marrow transplantation in patients with AnLL. Blood 1993;81:319-323.
28. Mathe G, Schwarzenberg L, Pouillart P, Oldham R, Weiner R, Jasmin C, Rosenfeld C, Hayat M, Misset JL, Musset M, Schneider M, Amiel JL, de Vassal F. Two epidophyllotoxin derivates VM 26 and VP16-213 in the treatment of leukemias, hematosarcomas, and lymphomas. Cancer 1974;34:985.
29. Smith IE, Gerken ME, Clink HM, McElwain TJ. VP 16-213 in acute myelogenous leukemia. Postgrad Med J 1976;52:66.
30. van Echo DA, Wiernik PH, Aisner J. High-dose VP 16-213 for treatment of patients with previously treated acute leukemia. Cancer Clin trials 1980;3:325.
31. Zander AR, Culbert S, Jagannath S, Spitzer G, Keating M, Larry N, Cockerill K, Hester J, Horwitz L. Vellekoop L, Swan F, McCredie K, Dicke K. High-dose cyclophosphamide, BCNU, and VP-16 as a conditioning regimen for allogeneic bone marrow transplantation for patients with acute leukemia. Cancer 1987;59:1083-1086.
32. Hartmann AR, Williams SF, Dillon JJ. Survival, disease-free survival and adverse effects of conditioning for allogeneic bone marrow transplantation with busulfan/cyclophosphamide vs total body irradiation: a meta-analysis. Bone Marrow Transplantation 1998;22:439-443.
33. Ringden O, Labopin M, Tura S. A comparison of busulphan versus total body irradiation combined with cyclophosphamide as conditioning for autograft or allograft bone marrow transplantation in patients with acute leukemia. Brit J Haematol 1996;93:637-645.
34. Blume KG, Kopecky KJ, Henslee-Downey JP, et al. A prospective randomized comparison of total body irradiation-etoposide versus busulfan-cyclophosphamide as preparatory regimens for bone marrow transplantation in patients with leukemia who were not in first remission: a Southwest Oncology Group Study. Blood 1993;81:2187-2193.

The Occurrence of Acute Graft-Versus-Host Disease and Infectious Complications in Patients with Acute and Chronic Myeloid Leukemia who Underwent Allogeneic Peripheral Blood Stem Cell Transplantation

M. MACHACZKA[1], M. RUCINSKA[1], J. WILCZYNSKI[2], B. ZAWILINSKA[3], B. PLATKOWSKA-JAKUBAS[1], D. URACZ[4], and A.B. SKOTNICKI[1]

[1] Department of Hematology; [2] Department of Virology, Panstwowy Zaklad Higieny, ul. Chocimska 24, 00-791 Warszawa, Poland; [3] Department of Virology, Institute of Microbiology; [4] Molecular Biology Laboratory, Department of Clinical Biochemistry Collegium Medicum of the Jagiellonian University, ul. Kopernika 17, 31-501 Krakow, Poland

Introduction

Allogeneic hematopoietic cell transplantation (HCT) is a well established and widely accepted method of treatment for eligible patients with acute and chronic myeloid leukemia (AML and CML) [1]. Intensive clinical investigations are done world-wide to determine risk/benefit ratio of allogeneic transplants using peripheral blood stem cells (PBSCT) mobilized by growth factors (e.g. G-CSF, GM-CSF) compared with allogeneic bone marrow transplantation (BMT) [2]. Expectations of above trials include superior to marrow the tempo of engraftment (neutrophilis and platelets recovery) without significant increase of severity in acute graft-versus-host disease (GVHD), even with unmanipulated PBSCT containing many more T-cells than are present in a normal marrow graft [2–7]. Faster neutrophils and monocytes engraftment should also contribute to decreased frequency of bacterial and fungal complications in early post-transplant period.

Graft-versus-host disease is a consequence of donor T cells recognizing host antigens as foreign. GVHD has been divided into acute (aGVHD) and chronic phases [1]. Traditionally, aGVHD occurs within the first 100 days following allogeneic HCT. However, it is clear now that cases of aGVHD occur within 30-40 days posttransplant and chronic GVHD, defined both by clinical and histological criteria, can occur as early as 50 days of allogeneic HCT. Classicaly, affected by aGVHD organs are skin, liver and gut. The usual triad of aGVHD symptoms is dermatitis (rash), hepatitis (jaundice) and gastroenteritis (diarrhea, nausea/vomiting).

The aim of our study was to analyse the incidence and severity of aGVHD as well as a profile of infectious complications in patients diagnosed for AML and CML, who underwent unmanipulated G-CSF mobilized peripheral blood stem cells transplansplants from related matched and one antigen mismatched donors.

Patients and Methods

Seven patients with myeloid leukemia (4/7 AML in first complete remission; 3/7 CML in first chronic phase) underwent PBSCT. Median age of patients was 32 (range 17-48), and sex distribution was 4F/3M. Median time from diagnosis to transplantation was 8.6 months for AML patients and 9.0 months for CML patients.

Donor/recipient histocompatibility was typed using serological methods for a HLA class I and molecular methods (Sequence Specific Oligonucleotide Probes – SSOP) for a HLA class II. Additionally, mixed lymphocyte culture (MLC) was performed. 6/7 patients had completely matched donor and one patient had a one loci HLA-A mismatched donor. Donors were mobilized with rhG-CSF (daily dose range: 10-20 mg/kg of donor body weight) administered by subcutaneous injection for 5 days. Mean number of obtained CD34+ cells was 3.1 x 10^6/kg (range 2.28 to 4.31).

The preparative regimen consisted of oral busulfan 1 mg/kg body weight (b.w.) every 6 hours, total of 16 doses (days –7 to –4) and intravenous (i.v.) cyclophosphamide 120 mg/ kg b.w. in two divided doses (days –3 to –2).

All patients have received cyclosporin A (CSP) and methotrexate (MTX) for the prevention of GVHD. Initially, CSP 3 mg/kg b.w./day i.v. in two divided doses was started since day –1. After 4 days of treatment first CSP dose adjustment was done to keep CSP blood level between 150 to 450 ng/ml (target level). As soon as the patient begins eating, CSP was switched to oral form (x 2.5 of i.v. dose) with further control of CSP blood levels. MTX was administered in a dose of 15 mg/m^2 i.v. on day +1 and in a dose of 10 mg/m^2 i.v. on days +3, +6, +11. Two patients didn't receive 4th MTX dose because of development grade IV mucositis after 3rd MTX dose. Assessment of aGVHD was based on clinical, laboratory and histological criterias as described elsewhere. Routine day +28 and +80 evaluation was performed for each patient.

Fluconazole and acyclovir were administered routinely as a prophylaxis of fungal and herpes viruses infections, respectively. Trimethoprim/Sulfamethoxazole was used as prophylactic therapy against *Pneumocystis carinii* pneumonia. Routine blood cultures and cytomegalovirus (CMV) tests were performed on weekly basis. CMV infection was tested using different methods (pp65 antigenemia, polymerase chain reaction, shell vial culture). More microbiological tests were done if necessary, depending on clinical situation.

Results

All of the patients engrafted, reaching an absolute neutrophil count (ANC) > 0.5 x 10^9/L between day +11 to +17 (median +15) and platelet counts > 20 x 10^9/L between day +14 to +34 (median +23).

All transplanted patients have developed grade +1 skin aGVHD. Five of them had grade +1 liver aGVHD. One of patients had grade +1 and two of patients grade +3 gut aGVHD. Although only two patients developed overall grade III aGVHD and no resistance to first line treatment with intravenous methylprednisolon (2 mg/kg b.w./day) was observed (Table 1). None of patients has developed fungal complications. Symptomatic bacteriemia was documented for

Table 1. Patient's characteristic – selected parameters

UPN	Age	Sex	Diagnosis	Karnofsky performance score	Donor		Tempo of engraftment (day after transplantation with ANC > 0.5 x 10^9/L)	Acute graft-versus-host disease				Infectious complications		Patient status
					histocompatibility	sex		Grade Skin	Grade Liver	Grade Gut	Treatment initiated	CMV infection	other	
035	39	F	CML-CP	100	MRD	F	+17	+1	+1	0	no	yes	no	alive
044	41	M	CML-CP	80	MRD	M	+11	+1	+1	+3	yes	yes	CMV disease	died (+69)
046	18	F	CML-CP	100	MRD	M	+16	+1	+1	0	no	yes	Adenovirus disease	died (+95)
052	25	F	AML CR1	90	MRD	F	+14	+1	+1	0	no	yes	Adenovirus infection, *Enterococcus spp, E.coli*	alive
057	17	F	AML CR1	100	MRD	M	+17	+1	0	0	no	yes	*Enterococcus spp.*	alive
065	30	M	AML CR1	90	MRD	M	+15	+1	0	+1	no	yes	no	alive
075	38	M	AML CR1	90	one HLA-A misMRD	F	+15	+1	+1	+3	yes	yes	*Staphylococcus epidermidis*	alive

MRD- matched related donor

3 patients (*Staphylococcus epidermidis, Escherichia coli, Enterococcus spp.*). All of them have responded to targeted antibiotics treatment. Nevertheless, in all of presented patients despite of pre-transplant patient/donor CMV status, cytomegalovirus infection was diagnosed with further initiation of pre-emptive therapy with ganciclovir (GCV). One patient (UPN 044) has developed disseminated, treatment-resistant CMV disease (enteritis, hepatitis) and died on day +69 after transplant. Two patients developed adenovirus disease. The first one with multiorgan involvement (UPN 046) died on day +95. The second one developed urinary tract infection but recovered after treatment with a new, promising antiviral agent – intravenous cidofovir.

Discussion

The first successful allogeneic unmodified PBSCTs were performed in the early 1990s [8, 9]. The results of successive trials confirmed better tempo of granulocyte and platelet recovery after allogeneic PBSCT than seen with BMT [3-5]. The next trials, contrary to widespread expectations showed no significant increase in acute GVHD with the use of allogeneic PBSCT compare with allogeneic marrow [6, 7]. Finally, some recent studies suggest superior survival [10] and lower relapse rate [11] rather after allogeneic PBSCT than after marrow.

Our results of primary allogeneic PBSCTs from matched and one loci mismatched related donors in patients with acute and chronic myeloid leukemia showed development of aGVHD in all of analized patients. However an overall aGVHD grade was low (I-II) for the majority of patients. Our study confirm a lack of significant increase in high grade (III-IV) acute GVHD after allogeneic PBSCT. All of the patients achieved rapid post-transplant engraftment and didn't suffer from fungal and serious bacterial complications in early post transplant period (up to day +100). Nevertheless CMV infection occured in 100% patients (7/7) and adenovirus infection in 28% (2/7) of our patients. 28% of patients (2/7) developed disseminated, treatment-resistant viral diseases.

We conclude that allogeneic PBSCT for hematologic cancers seems to be an interesting alternative source of transplant in comparison with marrow. However, we suggest that the risk of infectious (particularly viral) complications after allogeneic PBSCT requires further investigations in control clinical trials.

Acknowledgements. This work was supported by educational grants of Collegium Medicum of the Jagiellonian University: BBN-Wl/313/KL/L and BBN-501/KL/L/406/L.

References

1. Deeg H-J, Klingemann H-G, Phillips GL, Van Zant G (1999) A guide to blood and marrow transplantation. Springer-Verlag, Berlin, Heidelberg, New York
2. Appelbaum FR (1999) Choosing the source of stem cells for allogeneic transplantation: no longer a peripheral issue. Blood 94:381-383

3. Schmitz N, Dreger P, Suttorp M, et al. (1995) Primary transplantation of allogeneic peripheral blood progenitor cells mobilized by filgrastim (granulocyte colony-stimulating factor). Blood 85:1666-1672
4. Korbling M, Przepiorka D, Huh YO, et al. (1995) Allogeneic blood stem cell transplantation for refractory leukemia and lymphoma: potential advantage of blood over marrow allogrefts. Blood 85:1659-1665
5. Bensinger WI, Weaver CH, Appelbaum FR, et al. (1995) Transplantation of allogeneic peripheral blood stem cells mobilized by recombinant human granulocyte colony-stimulating factor. Blood 85: 1655-1658
6. Bensinger WI, Clift R, Maritn P, et al. (1996) Allogeneic peripheral blood stem cell transplantation in patients with advanced hematologic malignancies: a retrospective comparison with marrow transplantation. Blood 88:2794-2800
7. Przepiorka D, Anderlini P, Ippoliti C, et al. (1997) Allogeneic blood stem cell transplantation in advanced hematologic cancers. Bone Marrow Transplant 19:455-460
8. Dreger P, Suttorp M, Haferlach T, et al. (1993) Allogeneic granulocyte colony-stimulating factor-mobilized peripheral blood progenitor cells for treatment of engraftment failure after bone marrow transplantation. Blood 81:1404-1407
9. Russell NH, Hunter A, Rogers S, et al. (1993) Peripheral blood stem cells as an alternative to marrow for allogeneic transplantation. Lancet 341:1482
10. Champlin R, Schmitz N, Horowitz M for the IBMTR and EBMT (1998) Allogeneic blood stem cell (BSC) vs. bone marrow transplantation (BMT); improved leukemia free survival in high risk but not in low risk patients. Blood 92 (suppl 1):657a
11. Elmaagacli AH, Beelen DW, Opalka B, et al. (1999) The risk of residual molecular and cytogenetic disease in patients with Philadelphia-chromosome positive first chronic phase chronic myelogenous leukemia is reduced after transplantation of allogeneic peripheral blood stem cells compared with bone marrow. Blood 94:384-389

Long-Term Survival after Stem Cell Transplant in Adult Acute Lymphoblastic Leukemia

X. THOMAS[1], C. DANAÏLA[1], N. RAUS[1], J. TRONCY[1], C. SEBBAN[1], V. LHÉRITIER[1], M. MICHALLET[1], and D. FIERE[1]

[1]Service d'Hématologie clinique, Hôpital Edouard Herriot, Lyon, France

Introduction

Over the past decade, great progress has been made in the treatment of adult acute lymphoblastic leukemia (ALL). Improvements in the quality and availability of broad-spectrum antibacterial antibiotics, antifungal agents, and platelet transfusions, as well as greater understanding of the optimal use of a variety of antineoplastic agents, have resulted in gradual improvements in CR rates and the identification of a significant fraction of patients achieving long-term disease free survival [6, 9, 11–13, 16, 17]. Stem cell transplantation (SCT) is one of the post-remission strategies for the eradication of residual disease in ALL. Long-term disease-free survival for patients with ALL after management with chemotherapy plus SCT is now widely accepted [7, 8, 20]. However, little data is still available on long-term survival beyond 3 years.

We, therefore, reviewed data on 111 ALL patients, admitted to our department from 1978 to 1999, who underwent SCT at least one time during the evolution of the disease. These findings should prove useful both in clinical practice and in the design of future studies. Although there are many publications that describe the outcome of clinical trials in ALL, few of them include the results of long-term follow-up beyond 3 years after study entry. Furthermore, this retrospective study might better reflect the outcome for a non-selected population of patients.

Patients and Methods

Patients

From 1978 to 1999, a total of 378 consecutive adult ALL patients have been referred to the Edouard Herriot Hospital (Lyon, France) for newly diagnosed ALL. Among those patients, 111 (29%) received SCT (allogeneic transplant or autologous transplant) at least one time during the evolution of the disease. Diagnosis of ALL was established on the basis of bone marrow aspirate. ALL were morphologically classified according to the French-American-British (FAB) criteria [1], completed by cytochemical and immunological analyses. Based on the pattern of reactivity, lymphoblasts were assigned as T (CD7+, CD5+ or CD2+), early pre-B (CD19+, HLA-DR+, CD10±, CD22±, CD7-, cIg-, sIg-), pre-B (cIg+), or B (sIg+) ALL subgroups [4]. Cytogenetic analysis was performed in 84 of the 111 patients (76%) on bone marrow and/or on peripheral blood cells before initiation of therapy, using short unstimulated cultures and RHG banding [5]. Molecular characterization of BCR/ABL, E2A-PBX1, HRX-AF4 rearrangements at diagnosis were routinely performed since 1992.

Treatment

Different successive protocols were active during the 21-year accrual period. Details of the specific protocols and the methods of analysis have been published previously. Induction chemotherapy consisted of an corticosteroid, vincristine, cyclophosphamide, anthracycline, ± bleomycin combination. According to our institution policy, all young ALL patients who achieved a CR and had an HLA-identical familial donor were scheduled to receive allogeneic bone marrow transplantation (BMT). The presence of an HLA-identical familial donor was ascertained by serologic typing of HLA-A, -B, -C, and -DR determinants. Histocompatibility within the HLA-D region was defined by mutual unresponsiveness in mixed lymphocyte culture. The conditioning regimen for allogeneic BMT consisted of cyclophosphamide 60 mg/Kg/day on 2 consecutive days and total body irradiation (TBI), either 10 Gy in a single fraction or 12 Gy in 6 fractions over 3 days, with lung shielding after 10 Gy. Prophylaxis of graft-versus-host disease (GVHD) following allogeneic BMT consisted of either cyclosporine A alone, at the initial dose of 5 mg/m^2/day intravenously (IV) from the day before BMT until 6 months after BMT, or cyclosporine A at the same dose in combination with methotrexate 10 mg/m^2 IV on days 1, 3, 6, and 11 after BMT, or cyclosporine A, at the initial dose of 3 mg/m^2/day IV from the day before BMT until 6 months after BMT, and methotrexate 15 mg/m^2 IV on day 1, and 10 mg/m^2 IV on days 3, 6, ± 11 after BMT.

In absence of sibling donor, or in older patients, post-remission therapy could consisted, since 1987, in autologous BMT or autologous SCT according to the protocol criteria in which patients were included in. The preparative regimen for autologous SCT combined cyclophosphamide and total body irradiation (TBI). Since 1994, conditioning regimen (autologous and allogeneic transplants) also comprised etoposide 50 mg/Kg on one day preceding cyclophosphamide and TBI administration in case of Ph+ ALL.

Since 1993, matched BMT from unrelated donors have been proposed, at time of relapse or in refractory ALL, in absence of HLA-identical sibling. Conditioning regimen included anti-lymphocyte globulins (ALG) at 5 mg/Kg/day for 4 days (from day -8 to day -5) combined with the regular combination of cyclophosphamide and TBI.

In case of second SCT, conditioning regimen included busulfan 4 mg/Kg/day for 4 days followed by cyclophosphamide 60 mg/Kg/day for 2 days.

Statistical analysis

CR was defined according to the CALGB criteria as less than 5% blasts in bone marrow aspirates with evidence of maturation of cell lines and restoration of peripheral blood counts [10]. Hematological relapse was considered when more than 5% blasts were seen in two bone marrow aspirates obtained at 15-day interval [10]. Survival data were updated as of November 1999. Overall survival (OS) was calculated from the date of diagnosis (or from the date of relapse when studying OS after a second line therapy) to the date of death (failure) or the date the patient was last known to be alive (censored). Kaplan-Meier curves were then generated based on the updated data and were compared for statistical significance by the log rank test [15]. Leukemia-free survival (LFS) duration was calculated from the date of first or second CR achievement to the date of relapse (failure), the date of death during intensification (failure), the date of other deaths in CR (censored), or the date last alive without evidence of relapse (censored). Long-term survivors (LTS) were defined as survival of 3 years or more after initial diagnosis. Specifically, patients who continued in LFS for at least 3 years were considered "cured" because relapse was extremely rare after that time point. Computations were performed using BMDP PC-90 statistical program (BMDP Statistical Software, Los Angeles, CA, USA).

Results

The entire cohort was composed of 111 patients (78 males and 33 females) with a median age of 25 years (range: 15–57 years). By FAB classification, 68% were L1, 29% L2, 3% L3. By immunophenotype, 37% of patients presented with T-lineage ALL, and 63% with B-lineage ALL. Regarding cytogenetic analysis, 19 of the 84 analyzed patients (23%) displayed a normal karyotype, 19 patients (23%) had Ph+ chromosome, 4 patients (5%) had t(4;11), and only 1 patient presented with t(1;19). Fifty-nine patients (group 1) (median age: 24 years; range: 15–50 years) were allografted in first CR (CR1), 16 patients (group 2) (median age: 33 years; range: 17–51 years) were autografted in CR1, 34 patients (group 3) (median age: 33 years; range: 16–57 years) were allografted in second CR (CR2) (13 patients) or with progressive disease (21 patients), and 10 patients (group 4) (median age: 22 years; range: 16–38 years) were autografted in CR2. In group 3, 8 patients received allogeneic BMT from an unrelated HLA-identical donor. Five patients, who received a first allogeneic BMT as consolidation therapy during the first line treatment, underwent another allogeneic BMT in second line therapy, and were included in both group 1 and group 3.

Figure 1 illustrates the overall survival of all 111 patients. When considering the entire cohort, the probability of survival at 3 years and at 5 years after diagnosis was 46% and 38% respectively (36% and 30%, 59% and 56% respectively for B- and T-cell lineage ALL). Overall survival of all patients grafted in CR1 (group 1 and group 2) is shown in Figure 2. Median survival durations were respectively of 119 months and 14 months after allogeneic transplant and autologous transplant in CR1 (Table 1). In group 1, the probability of survival 3 years and 5 years after allogeneic BMT was 50% and 46% for B-cell lineage ALL, and 76% for T-cell lineage ALL. Treatment-related mortality (TRM) occurred in 11 cases (19%), while relapse occurred in 16 cases (27%; median: 14 months; range: 3-31months). The probability of survival 3 years (as well as 5 years) in group 2

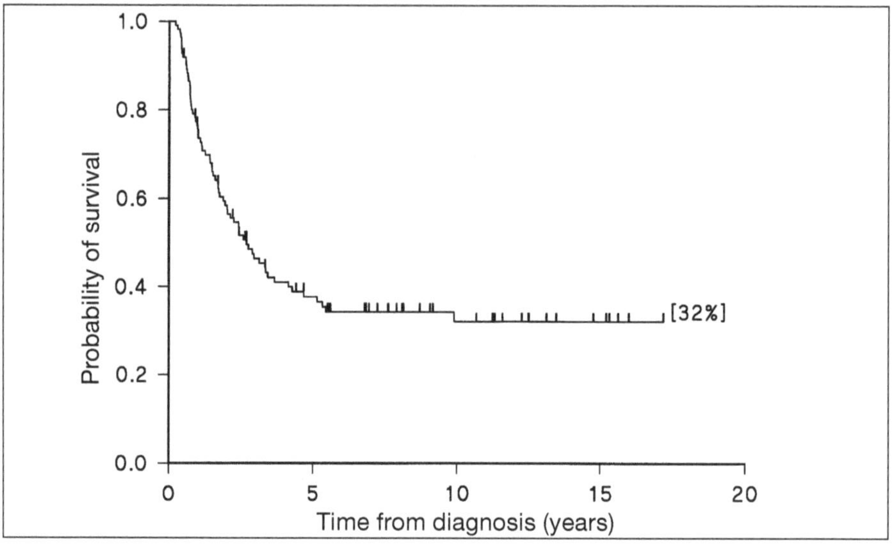

Fig. 1. Overall survival of the entire cohort (111 patients who underwent at least 1 stem cell transplant)

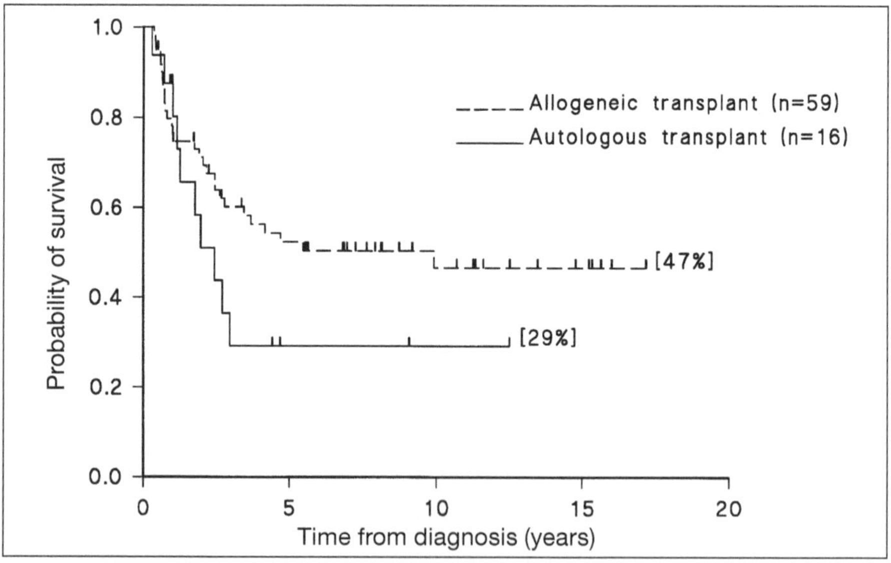

Fig. 2. Overall survival of patients grafted in CR1

was 28%, and 33% for B- and T-cell lineage ALL respectively. Relapse was the major reason for failure after autologous transplant in CR1. All 8 relapses (50%) had occurred by year 3. When considering patients grafted after a second line therapy, median survival was 8 months after allogeneic BMT with 8% of survival at 3 and 5 years. Among patients undergoing allogeneic BMT from an HLA-identical unrelated donor, 3 were still alive at time of analysis (2 of which in CR2, and 1 of which in relapse), and 5 patients died (2 relapses, and 3 toxic deaths) (Fig. 3). All 5 patients undergoing a second allogeneic BMT died (3 relapses, and 2 toxic deaths). Median survival after autologous SCT was 10 months without any long-term survivor (Table 1 and Fig. 3).

Of the 111 patients, 44 (40%) have survived for ≥ 3 years and could therefore be considered as long-term survivors (LTS). There were several categories of LTS. The largest group is composed of patients who remained in their first remission for 3 years (33 patients): 29 patients after allogeneic bone marrow transplanta-

Table 1. Long-term follow-up of transplanted patients

Status	Number of patients (months)	Median OS	3-year OS	5-year OS
Allogeneic transplant in CR1	59	119	60%	52%
Autologous transplant in CR1	16	14	29%	29%
Allogeneic transplant during second line therapy*	34**	8	8%	8%
Autologous transplant in CR2	10	10	0%	0%

* patients allografted in CR2 or in evolutive disease; ** including 8 allogeneic BMT from unrelated HLA-identical donor, and 5 second allogeneic BMT.

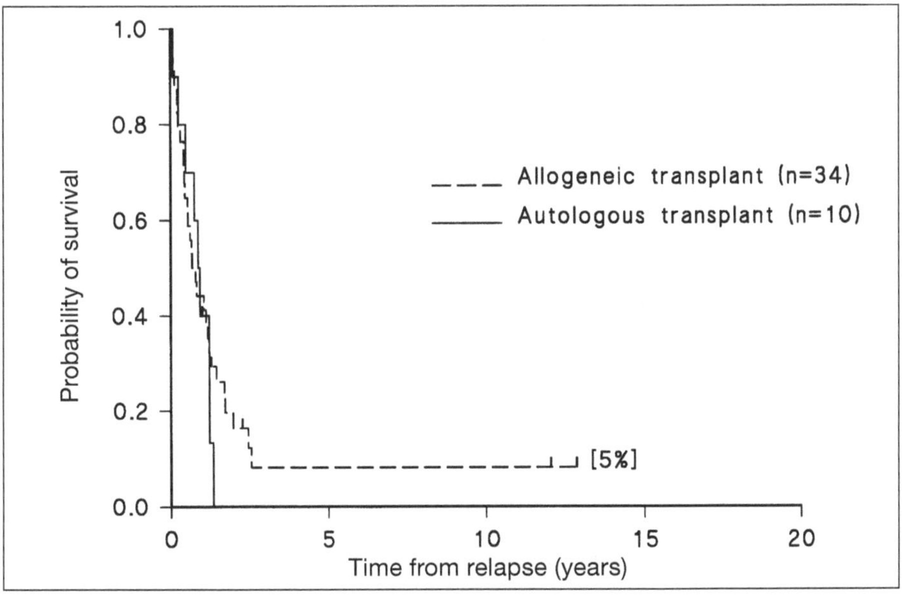

Fig. 3. Overall survival of patients grafted in second line Therapy

tion (BMT) (2 of which died while in CR1), and 4 patients after autologous SCT. The second group is composed of those whose remission was < 3 years in duration and who survived for ≥ 3 years (11 patients). In that group, 5 patients, undergoing allogeneic transplantation in second line of treatment, survived more than 3 years, 3 patients, receiving autologous transplant in second line of treatment, survived more than 3 years, and 3 patients, receiving one allogeneic BMT in first line therapy and another allogeneic BMT in second line of treatment, survived more than 3 years.

Because failure rates declined to relatively low levels after a first or later CR of more than 3 years duration, such patients comprised a „potentially cured" cohort. The criterion for entry into this cohort was fulfilled by 35 patients (33 patients in first CR, and 2 patients in further CR): 31 patients after allogeneic bone marrow transplantation (BMT), and 4 patients after autologous SCT. An additional 10 patients remain alive and in CR (5 in group 1, 2 in group 2, 2 in group 3, and 1 in group 4) at < 3 years and could become „potentially cured" (follow-up shorter than 3 years).

Discussion

Bone marrow transplantation is one of the post-remission strategies for the eradication of residual disease in ALL and can replace consolidation/maintenance treatment. Although the concept of cure of ALL is now widely accepted, few studies with prolonged follow-up have been reported. This study, which provides prolonged follow-up confirms that cure of ALL is not infrequent. Over the years, the proportion of patients who received an allogeneic BMT, autologous BMT or PSC transplantation increased in our department. The exact role of allogeneic BMT or autologous transplantation is better assessed by prospective studies with analyses based on the intention-to-treat principle. However, data about patients effectively grafted may be of interest both in clinical practice and in the design of future trials. Compared to randomized trials, this historical single center study on a large population of patients avoids selection biases and reflects more accurately the prognosis of adult ALL. Several groups have reported long term disease-free survivals in the region of 45 to 70% [2, 3, 14] after allogeneic BMT in CR1. Relapse rates after first remission BMT range between 10 to 20%. In second remission, the data from individual and multiple centers show a long term survival between 15 and 45% [3, 8, 21]. This high figure reflects the selection of poor risk patients for BMT. Better prognosis groups are children, patients with standard risk features or with slow disease.

In our series, the initial failure rate was higher for patients in second CR. However, in both cases (first and second CR) the failure rate fell to a relatively low level after 3 years in CR. Results of allogeneic BMT are better in good risk leukemia. This goes almost exclusively on the account of a lower risk of relapse. Relapse is the particular complication that confronts transplantation attempts in ALL. It occurs from any stage in the early post-transplant period up to about 3 years after BMT and may arise either in the bone marrow, extramedullary sites, or lymph nodes. With rare exceptions, relapse occurs in recipient cells that have failed to be eradicated by the transplant procedure. Ultimately, patients who relapse after BMT die of recurrent disease but, nevertheless, several long term survivors have been reported whom current remission exceeds the interval between the BMT and the relapse. The question of further BMT in these patients has not been completely resolved. Second BMT have a high relapse rate and a high incidence of BMT complications [19]. BMT in relapse for ALL was an endstage experimental procedure and the overall survival appears commensurate with the selection of a highly resistant disease group. It is therefore disappointing that there has been no improvement in the results for relapsed patients which still give a low overall survival rate and a high relapse rate.

Autologous graft started as an alternative approach for patients lacking a matched donor or over age limit for receiving allogeneic transplant. The survival rate for autologous BMT in CR1 is inferior to that for allogeneic BMT in CR1. In advanced stages, the results are again inferior to those of allogeneic BMT. Factors affecting the success of autologous transplant are the quality of remission as the optimal time to perform the graft, and the potential benefit of „in vivo" pre-transplant ablative therapy. However, autologous transplants in CR1 seems promising with survival rates of 29%. Autologous BMT is a readily available alternative and can be performed in patients up to 65 years old. The major disadvantage is the high relapse rate probably caused to some extent by the reinfusion of leukemic blasts, but more by the lack of GVL effects. Purging of the marrow graft may reduce the leukemia cell burden [18].

The observations from this study have several significant clinical implications. First, the data reflect the degree to which ALL treatment remains unsuccessful. Only approximately 31% of patients entered the potentially cured cohort. Second, the results suggest a time (3 years) at which it becomes reasonable to speak of potential cure, provided the patient is in CR. Third, the data suggest that patients in the potentially cured cohort were not at risk of subsequent invasive cancer since, in our series, none of the patients developed subsequent malignancies. This finding contrasts with observations in survivors of other malignancies, who are at greatly increased risk of developing AML.

We conclude that a significant fraction of patients achieve long-term survival and seem to be cured of their disease. Overall, SCT is „curative" in more than 31% of ALL patients treated in first or further line of therapy. A minimum follow-up of 3 years is a reasonable predictor of long-term survival. Relatively few adverse events occur after 3–4 years in remission. These findings have implications regarding the need for and value of expensive and compulsive long-term follow-up of all adult ALL patients treated in clinical trials. Although the sample size is fairly large in this long-term follow-up study, we still cannot be completely confident about the incidence of unusual late, untoward events. Indeed, we could address the question of whether patients with ALL are at increased risk of secondary cancers. Nonetheless, these data are reassuring in that such events have not been observed in our series. Another question arises: How well do these patients do as citizens of the community? Indeed, the patients quality of life following a marrow transplant procedure is an important component of the overall success of the intervention.

Summary

Reports on outcomes of stem cell transplantation (SCT) in adult acute lymphoblastic leukemia (ALL) have rarely included results of long-term follow-up beyond 5 years. Of the 378 ALL patients referred to our hospital over the past 21-year period, 111 patients underwent SCT (allogeneic or autologous transplantation). We reviewed here long-term follow-up data among those patients. Because failure rates declined to relatively low levels after a first or later complete remission of more than 3-year duration, such patients comprised a „potentially cured“ cohort. Stem cell transplantation was then curative in more than 31% of ALL patients treated in first or further line of therapy.

References

1. Bennett JM, Catovsky D, Daniel MT, Flandrin G, Galton DAG, Gralnick HR, Sultan C. Proposals for the classification of acute leukaemias. Br J Haematol 33:451-458, 1976.
2. Blaise D, Gaspar MH, Stoppa AM, Michel G, Gastaut JA, Lepeu G, Tubiana N, Blanc AP, Rossi JF, Novakovitch G, Mannoni P, Mawas C, Maraninchi D, Carcassonne Y. Allogeneic or autologous bone marrow transplantation of acute lymphoblastic leukemia in first remission. Bone Marrow Transplant 5:7-12, 1990.
3. Blume KG, Schmidt GM, Chao NJ, Forman SJ. Bone Marrow transplantation from histocompatible sibling donors for patients with acute lymphoblastic leukemia. Haematol Blood Transfus 33:636-637, 1990.
4. Boucheix C, David B, Sebban C, Racadot E, Bené MC, Bernard A, Campos L, Jouault H, Sigaux F, Lepage E, Hervé P, Fiere D, for the French Group on Therapy for Adult Acute Lymphoblastic Leukemia. Immunophenotype of adult acute lymphoblastic leukemia, clinical parameters, and outcome: An analysis of a prospective trial including 562 tested patients (LALA87). Blood 84:1603-1612, 1994.
5. Charrin C, for the Groupe Français de Cytogénétique Hématologique. Cytogenetic abnormalities in adult acute lymphoblastic leukemia: Correlations with hematologic findings and outcome. A collaborative study of the Groupe Français de Cytogénétique Hématologique. Blood 87:3135-3142, 1996.
6. Dekker AW, van't Veer MB, Sizoo W, Haak HL, van der Lelie J, Ossenkoppele G, Huijgens PC, Schouten HC, Sonneveld P, Willemze R, Verdonck LF, van Putten WL, Löwenberg B. Intensive postremission chemotherapy without maintenance therapy in adults with acute lymphoblastic leukemia. Dutch Hemato-Oncology Research Group. J Clin Oncol 15:476-482, 1997.
7. De Witte T, Awwad B, Boezeman J, Schattenberg A, Muus P, Raemaekers J, Preijers F, Stijckmans P, Haanen C. Role of allogeneic bone marrow transplantation in adolescent or adult patients with acute lymphoblastic leukemia or lymphoblastic lymphoma in first remission. Bone Marrow Transplant 14:767-774, 1994.
8. Doney K, Fisher LD, Appelbaum FR, Buckner CD, Storb R, Singer J, Fefer A, Anasetti C, Beatty P, Bensinger W, Clift R, Hansen J, Hill R, Loughran TP, Martin P, Petersen FB, Sanders J, Sullivan KM, Stewart P, Weiden P, Witherspoon R, Thomas ED. Treatment of adult acute lymphoblastic leukemia with allogeneic bone marrow transplantation. Multivariate analysis of factors affecting acute graft-versus-host disease, relapse, and relapse-free survival. Bone Marrow Transplant 7:453-459, 1991.
9. Durrant IJ, Prentice HG, Richards SM. Intensification of treatment for adults with acute lymphoblastic leukaemia: results of U.K. Medical Research Council randomized trial UKALL XA. Medical Research Council Working Party on Leukaemia in Adults. Br J Haematol 99:84-92, 1997.
10. Ellison RR, Holland JF, Weil M, Jacquillat C, Boiron M, Bernard J, Sawitsky A, Rosner F, Gussoff B, Silver RT, Karanas A, Cuttner J, Spurr CL, Hayes DM, Bloom J, Leone LA, Haurani F, Kyle R, Hutchison JL, Forcier RJ, Moon JH. Arabinosyl cytosine: a useful agent in the treatment of acute leukemia in adults. Blood 32:507-523, 1968.

11. Fiere D, Lepage E, Sebban C, Boucheix C, Gisselbrecht C, Vernant JP, Varet B, Broustet A, Cahn JY, Rigal-Huguet F, Witz F, Michaux JL, Michallet M, Reiffers J, for the French Group on Therapy for Adult Acute Lymphoblastic Leukemia. Adult acute lymphoblastic leukemia: a multicentric randomized trial testing bone marrow transplantation as postremission therapy. J Clin Oncol 11:1990-2001, 1993.
12. Hoelzer D, Thiel E, Löffler H, Bodenstein H, Plaumann L, Büchner T, Urbanitz D, Koch P, Heimpel H, Engelhardt R, Müller U, Wendt FC, Sodomann H, Rühl H, Herrmann F, Kaboth W, Dietzfelbinger H, Pralle H, Lunscken C, Hellriegel KP, Spors S, Nowrousian RM, Fischer J, Frülle H, Mitrou PS, Pfreundschuh M, Görg C, Emmerich B, Queisser W, Meyer P, Labedzki L, Essers U, König H, Mainzer K, Herrmann R, Messerer D, Zwingers T. Intensified therapy in acute lymphoblastic and acute undifferentiated leukemia in adults. Blood 64:38-47, 1984.
13. Hoelzer D, Thiel E, Ludwig WD, Löffler H, Büchner T, Freund M, Heil G, Hiddemann W, Maschmeyer G, Völkers B, Gökbuget N, Aydemir U, for the German Adult ALL Study Group. Follow-up of the first two successive German multicentre trials for adult ALL (O1/81 and 02/84). Leukemia 7(suppl.2):S130-134, 1993.
14. Horowitz MM, Messerer D, Hoelzer D, Gale RP, Neiss A, Atkinson K, Barrett AJ, Büchner T, Freund M, Heil G, Hiddemann W, Kolb HJ, Löffler H, Marmont AM, Maschmeyer G, Rimm AA, Rozman C, Sobocinski KA, Speck B, Thiel E, Weisdorf DJ, Zwaan FE, Bortin MM. Chemotherapy compared with bone marrow transplantation for adults with acute lymphoblastic leukemia in first remission. Ann Intern Med 115:13-18, 1991.
15. Kaplan EL, Meier P. Nonparametric estimation form in complete observations. J Am Stat Assoc 53:457-481, 1958.
16. Larson RA, Dodge RK, Burns CP, Lee EJ, Stone RM, Schulman P, Duggan D, Davey FR, Sobol RE, Frankel SR, Hooberman AL, Westbrook CA, Arthur DC, George SL, Bloomfield CD, Schiffer CA. A five-drug remission induction regimen with intensive consolidation for adults with acute lymphoblastic leukemia: Cancer and Leukemia Group B study 8811. Blood 85:2025-2037, 1995.
17. Mandelli F, Annino L, Rotoli B, for the GIMEMA Cooperative Group. The GIMEMA ALL 0183 trial, analysis of 10-year follow-up. Br J Haematol 92:663-672, 1996.
18. Martin H, Atta J, Zumpe P, Eder M, Elsner S, Rode C, Wassmann B, Bruecher J, Hoelzer D. Purging of peripheral blood stem cells yields BCR-ABL-negative autografts in patients with BCR-ABL-positive acute lymphoblastic leukemia. Exp Hematol 23:1612-1618, 1995.
19. Michallet M, Tanguy ML, Socié G, Thiebaut A, Belhabri A, Milpied N, Reiffers J, Kuentz M, Cahn JY, Blaise D, Demeocq F, Jouet JP, Michallet AS, Ifrah N, Vilmer E, Molina L, Michel G, Lioure B, Cavazzana-Calvo M, Pico JL, Sadoun A, Guyotat D, Attal M, Curé H, Bordigoni P, Sutton L, Buzyn-Veil A, Tilly M, Leporrier M, Fegueux N, Dreyfus F, Rio B, Lutz P, Vernant JP. Second allogeneic haematopoietic stem cell transplantation in relapsed acute and chronic leukaemias for patients who underwent a first allogeneic bone marrow transplantation: a survey of the Société Française de Greffe de Moelle (SFGM). Br J Haematol 108:400-407, 2000.
20. Sebban C, Lepage E, Vernant JP, Gluckman E, Attal M, Reiffers J, Sutton L, Racadot E, Michallet M, Maraninchi S, Dreyfus F, Fiere D, for the French Group of Therapy of Adult Acute Lymphoblastic Leukemia. Allogeneic bone marrow transplantation in adult acute lymphoblastic leukemia in first complete remission: A comparative study. J Clin Oncol 12:2580-2587, 1994.
21. Wingard JR, Piantadosi S, Santos GW, Saral R, Vriesendorp HM, Yeager AM, Burns WH, Ambinder RF, Braine HG, Elfenbein G, Jones RJ, Kaizer H, May WS, Rowley SD, Sensenbrenner LL, Stuart RK, Titschka PJ, Vogelsang GB, Wagner JE, Beschorner WE, Brookmeyer R, Farmer ER. Allogeneic bone marrow transplantation for patients with high risk acute lymphoblastic leukemia. J Clin Oncol 8:820-830, 1990.

Clinical Transplantation – Solid Tumors

Autologous Transplantation in Breast Cancer in Europe and EBMT Data

G. Rosti, P. Ferrante, A. Cariello, G. Papiani, U. De Giorgi, P. Giovanis, C. Dazzi, and M. Marangolo

Department of Oncology and Hematology, AUSL Ravenna, Italy

Introduction

Breast carcinoma is still in the new milnennium a formidable challenge as for physicians and as for patients. Despite clear progress in early diagnosis and novel therapeutic strategies, still much has to be done as far as metastatic disease (which is an ultimately fatal disease for more than 95% of the patients) and high-risk or very high-risk operable carcinoma (i.e. patients with multiple axillary nodes).

From preclinical data (Frei and Canellos, 1980, Schabel et al,1984) we know that dose escalation of several antitumor drugs results in an increased cytotoxicity against breast cancer cells: moreover from hundreds of clinical trials in the past thirty years, breast cancer can be considered as a relatively chemosensitive disease (Henderson et al., 1988), with several active compounds available on the market or under evaluation in early clinical trials. A natural evolution from these assumptions is to try to increase the dose(s) of the drug(s) showing myelotoxicity as their major toxic effect. Bone marrow or more recently peripheral blood progenitors cells (PBPC) collected with leukapheresis may be used as a supportive tool in order to restore hematopoiesis. Early reports of high-dose chemotherapy published in the eighties have shown quite a high response rate in metastatic disease; the schedules employed consisted mainly of alkylators (Peters et al 1986, Antman et al 1987). In 1992 nearly 1500 patients have been collected worldwide (Antman et al 1992), 90% of them with metastatic disease. Response rate was as high as 50–70%, but most important was the fact that a cohort of patients experienced long-term disease-free survival in the range of 15–25% (Antman et al 1992). Several reports came out in the last decade and the worldwide interest for this promising strategy in breast carcinoma patients has considerably grown, leading to a number of publications on major journals (Zajewsky et al 1998, Montemurro et al 2000). Unfortunately the majority of these articles referred to phase II studies and the results can not easily compared to historical controls even from the same institution. This was true as for metastatic disease as for the adjuvant setting. This report will present the European Group for Blood and Marrow Transplantation Registry (EBMT) data as well as the European studies on autotransplantation for breast cancer.

The European activity

High-dose chemotherapy for breast carcinoma patients has been widely used in the past few years in Europe. According to the most recent surveys conducted by the EBMT (Gratwohl et al 1999) more than 2500 patients have been treated in 1997 even if a slight reduction in the following years has been observed (Gratwohl et al 2000) to the extent of about 10–15%. The vast majority of patients received PBPC, and ABMT has been nearly universally abandoned as a source of hematopoietic stem cell rescue. This type of survey allows us just to make demographic observations, but in order to evaluate results on big numbers, the only possible way is to look at Registries. The EBMT Solid Tumors Working Party set up in 1984 a Registry including patients grafted in Europe as well as in some non-European countries, which for geographical reasons refer to the EBMT 2000.

The EBMT Database

By February 2001, 7485 patients with breast carcinoma were registered (only 32 are male) The mean age at transplantation is 45 ± 8 years, median 45 year, with a range of 18–70 years. The majority of registered patients were treated for metastatic disease (3191 patients), whereas 2323 received high-dose as adjuvant therapy. Nine hundred and fifty-one patients were treated for inflammatory breast cancer.

Interestingly, 32% of patients were > 50 years old and 3% > 60 years at the time of graft among the ones treated in 1997–1998, while in the period 1992–1999 only 16% and 1% of the treated patients were older than 50 and 60 years of age respectively. As mentioned before, 95% of the patients received PBPC support, while ABMT was extremely rarely used; in Europe the combination of ABMT plus PBPC was employed only anecdotally because the shift towards peripheral cells was immediate around 1995 (Siena et al 1994, Rosti and Ferrante, 2000, Neymark and Rosti, 2000).

Toxic death rate

In the majority of papers published in the eighties, mortality death rate for high-dose chemotherapy was 10–15% and up, while in recent reports it has declined dramatically to 0–2%. The employed regimen seems to play an important role as probably does the status of disease and performance status (Peters et al 1999, Antman et al 1997, Rosti et al in press 2001). In the EBMT database toxic death rate for metastatic breast cancer is around 2%, while for adjuvant setting it is 0.9% (Fig. 1). These figures compare favourably with some issued in recent trials not employing BCNU at high doses.

Metastatic disease

Despite the fact that metastatic disease is nowadays a less chosen option for autografting compared with high-risk operable breast cancer patients in Europe,

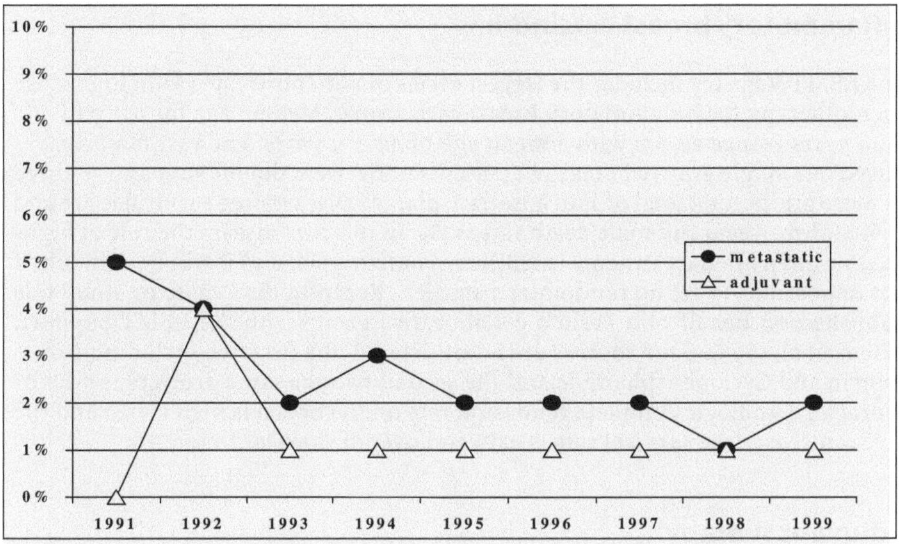

Fig. 1. Toxic death rates for metastatic and adjuvant patients . EBMT database

this disease is still widely accepted as a possible subject for high-dose treatment. The „ASCO 1999“ effect (i.e. the PBT-1 trial presentation) (Stadtmauer et al 2000) was incorrectly considered as „the last word“ on autografting for metastatic breast cancer by several medical oncologists worldwide has not yet shown its effects in Europe at the time of writing; however we are going to observe a steep decline in the number of patients treated for advanced disease in the next two years. From the EBMT breast cancer registry 428 patients with an adequate follow-up (i.e. treated until December 31st, 1996) receiving high-dose chemotherapy and hematopoietic stem cell rescue in first remission, show a highly significant progression-free survival when compared with those treated in other disease status (stable disease, partial remission, progression); median PFS is 25 months versus only 11 months. If we look at the data published by the ABMTR a similar curve has been presented (Rowlings et al 1999); moreover from one of the largest data base of patients treated with FAC standard chemotherapy (M.D. Anderson) (Greenberg et al., 1996), the proportion of patients in complete remission achieving a long-term disease-free progression has nearly reduced to half but, of course, apples cannot be compared with oranges, and the final word has to come out from phase III randomised studies. Unfortunately, the PBT-1 trial was unable to show any difference between STAMP V and prolonged CMF in patients in complete remission due to the small sample (Stadtmauer et al 2000). More recent results (Pecora et al 2000) clearly show that more active regimens do exists and that the results of the PBT-1 study may be significantly ameliorated if other strategies are employed.

Inflammatory breast carcinoma

The EBMT Registry includes the largest series of patients treated with high-dose chemotherapy for inflammatory breast carcinoma . Median age for 951 patients is 44 years (range 22-65) with a mean age of 44 ± 9 years. The vast majority received one single graft, whereas 144 patients underwent double shot and 36 three or more grafts, for a total of 1210 autotransplants.. Disease-free survival is around 40% at three years and toxic death rate is 1%. In this rare disease the role of high-dose or intensified treatments is still very controversial and it will be difficult, if not impossible, to set up randomized studies . Recently, the Pegase 02 study was published on behalf of a French collaborative group with the EBMT support. (Viens et al, 1999). Four courses are administered, the first two including Doxorubicin and Cyclophosphamide and the second two the same drugs plus 5-Fluorouracil . Pathologic complete remission rate on the breast is high (32%) and the 3-year disease-free survival rate is 45% and overall survival 70%.

Adjuvant therapy

As mentioned above, high-risk operable breast carcinoma has become the favourite option for high-dose chemotherapy in Europe overtaking advanced disease in the very recent past. The EBMT database includes 2323 patients receiving a total of grafts. Median age is 45 years (range 18–70) with a mean of 46 ± 9 years. Ninety-two percent of the patients received one single autotransplant while 8% had multiple grafts. The majority of adjuvant patients received PBPC transplantation and only 1% had the combination of ABMT and PBPC as hematopoietic support, slightly lower than in the North American Registry (Antman et al 1997).

Complete data set on 2231 patients is available and median disease-free survival is 72 months (Fig. 2). When stratifying for number of involved axillary nodes (i.e. < or > 9) no differences are present (data not shown). The data available in the literature on the possible benefit (randomised phase III studies) of high-dose treatment in breast cancer are limited. At the 1999 ASCO meeting, two major studies were presented (the South African one will not be taken into consideration due to clinical misconduct). The CALGB/SWOG/NCIC trial (Peters et al 1999) did not show any difference between high-dose (STAMP I) versus intermediate dose of Cisplatin, BCNU and Cyclophosphamide) except for a trend in the cohort of patients with a 3-year follow-up. Of course the trail will be represented in 2002 with adequate follow-up. The Interscandinavian study (Bergh et al., 2000) is a very difficult one, to be understood as patients with no disease and bone-marrow metastases have also been accrued and there was some concern about which was really the high-dose arm; in fact in the „non high-dose arm“ which consisted of a tailored escalated doses of FEC, patients received more anthracycline and 5-Fluorouracil and Cycloposphamide than the „high-dose arm“; moreover the risk of secondary leukaemia and myelodysplastic syndromes in the intensified and tailored FEC arm was not negligible (nine cases). At ASCO 2000 the first cohort of 284 patients of the Dutch National Trial were presented

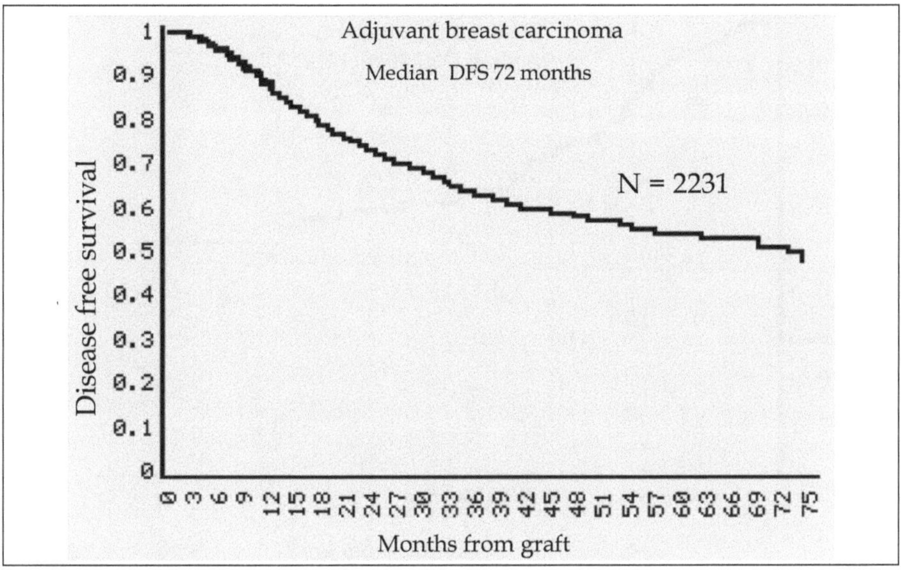

Fig. 2. Adjuvant high-dose chemotherapy : disease free survival.. EBMT database

(Rodenhuis et al. 2000) and with a follow-up of 3 years high-dose chemotherapy (STAMP V European version with double dose of Carboplatin) was significantly better than standard FEC as in terms of disease-free survival and overall survival. Of course we are waiting for the final presentation including all patients, which will be available in 2002. No data are available in the literature for patients with very high risk of relapse, i.e. those with massive axillary burden (>20 positive axillary nodes). The EBMT launched a retrospective Registry based analysis to evaluate the progression free survival for patients bearing such a dismal prognosis.

Seventy-five patients treated until December 1997 have been evaluated and those receiving primary chemotherapy excluded to avoid possible incorrect comparisons ; the vast majority received high-dose sequential chemotherapy as published by National Cancer Institute in Milan in 1997 (Gianni et al 1997).Toxic death rate was 0% and as disease free survival was 50 % at four years that suggests a possible role of high-dose chemotherapy in this particular cohort of patients. Figure 3 shows the disease-free survival for such patients. A preliminary analysis was conducted on a smaller number of patients regarding the possible benefit of post-surgery radiation therapy in this cohort and no difference were observed between patients undergoing such therapy or not (data not shown). In order to implement the number of patients and verify these data, in 2000 a retrospective study has been launched including patients from IBMTR (study BC #99-04), so we are in the position to have data on nearly 250 patients with > 20 positive axillary nodes at surgery shortly.

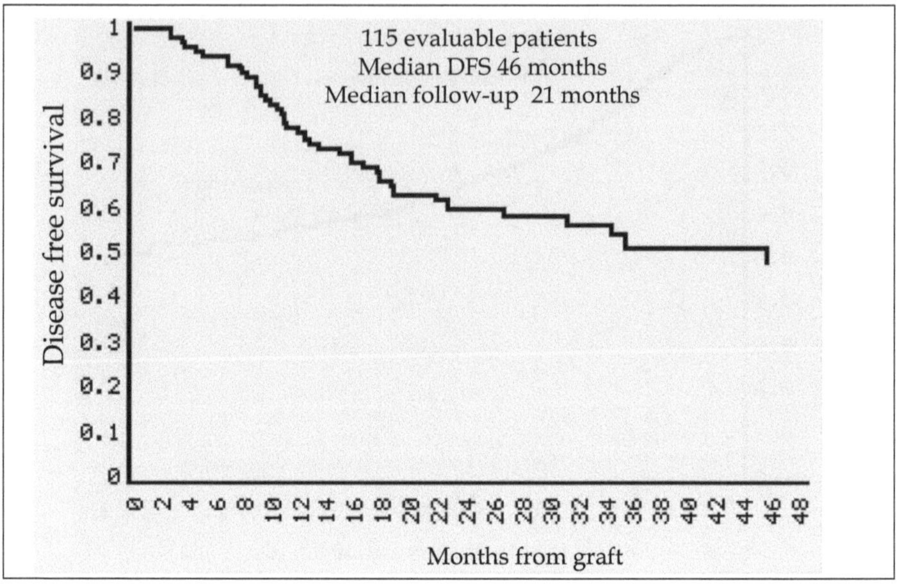

Fig. 3. Disease-free survival for patients with > 20 axillary lymphnodes treated with high-dose chemotherapy . EBMT database

Ongoing trials

Several ongoing studies are underway in Europe in the field of high-dose chemotherapy and hematopoietic support for breast cancer patients; some of them have just completed their accrual.

Dutch National Study: as mentioned before (Rodenhuis et al 2000) 885 patients with 4 or more axillary nodes have been randomized between standard FEC regimen for 5 courses versus four courses of FEC followed by one shot of modified STAMP V (Carboplatin at 1,600 mg/sqm). In the first cohort of 284 patients a clear significant benefit for the high-dose arm has been observed as in terms of overall and disease-free survival (detailed results are included in this book – see Rodehuis).

In 1999 at ASCO a small randomised study was presented by Dr Lotz on behalf of the PEGASE group, study Pegase 04 (Lotz et al., 1999). Patients with advanced disease, chemosensitive to first line therapy were randomized between CMA (high-dose Cyclophosphamide Mitoxantrone, and Melphalan), versus the pursuit of the same standard chemotherapy. The median progression-free survivals were 15.7 and 26.9 months in the standard and intensive groups (p= 0.04), whereas overall survival was not statistically different even if patients in the high-dose arm experienced a nearly double survival from randomization. The study likewise all the others from the Pegase Group, are undergoing a self requested audit before being published.

In Italy in August 1998 a phase III randomised study was closed comparing in 386 patients standard therapy (which in Italy is Epirubicin followed by CMF)

versus high-dose sequential chemotherapy, which is basically the same schedule as published by Gianni (Gianni et al 1997), but with the incorporation of two doses of Epirubicin and the exclusion of Cisplatin. No data are available at the time of writing and the first evaluation will be performed in early 2000.

The Anglo-Celtic study has just stopped its accrual with 610 patients with 4 or more positive axillary nodes randomized. Standard arm consists of Adriamycin for four courses followed by CMF, while the experimental one is Adriamycin as in the standard arm followed by Cyclophosphamide for PBPC collection and Cyclophosphamide and Thiotepa at high-doses.

At the present time no data are available yet. Another trial, PEGASE 01 was closed in December 1998 with 314 randomized patients: standard FEC with high-dose Epirubicin (100 mg/sqm) was compared to FEC followed by Cyclophosphamide, Mitoxantrone and Melphalan in patients with 8 or more positive lymphnodes. In January 2001 several trials are ongoing and we will refer about the major or more mature ones. In 1997 the EBMT Solid Tumors Working Party has launched in collaboration with the EBDIS Group a study called EDBIS1/EBMT in patients with naïve metastatic disease. The standard arm consists of Adriamycin and Docetaxel followed by CMF versus Adriamycin and Docetaxel and subsequently a tandem transplant with VIC (Etoposide, Ifosfamide and Carboplatin) and then CT (Cyclophosphamide and Thiotepa). At the time of writing 115 patients have been randomized. A similar study is ongoing in Germany with nearly 200 patients (GEBDIS study) which is nearly overimposable to the EBDIS/EBMT one, in terms of employed regimens and end points, and one in Italy on behalf of the Italian Group for Blood and Marrow Transplantation (GITMO) which compares Epirubicin and Docetaxel versus the same combination followed by a tandem shot of ICE and Thiotepa/Melphalan at high-doses. Recently the steering committee of the Italian randomised study preferred to close the trial due to slow accrual and possibly there will be a merging with the EBDIS1 study or the GEBDIS one.

A multi-institutional German study is comparing one course of STAMP V versus two courses of the same regimen in patients responding to standard upfront chemotherapy and more than 200 patients have been accrued so far.

In the scenario of high-dose therapy for operable breast cancer several studies are approaching the final accrual. A trial on behalf of the International Breast Cancer Study Group (IBCSG 15-95) has accrued nearly 300 patients ; it compares an anthracyclin base chemotherapy with an intensified therapy consisting of Epirubicin 200mg/sqm and Cyclophosphamide 4 g/sqm for three courses – each of them supported with PBPC: entry criteria request 8 or more nodes or 5 or more in case of T3 or negative receptor status.

In Germany a multi-institutional study is comparing standard chemotherapy (Epirubicin followed by CMF – i.e. EC -) versus EC followed by high-doses of Mitoxantrone, Thiotepa and Cyclophospamide. Three hundred and forty patients have already been included, and the trial should be completed by the end of 2001 with 400 cases.

All these major studies and several others not reported here will allow the scientific community to have data on homogeneous large groups of patients in the years to come, in order to try to answer the still unanswered question: is more better?

References

1. Gratwohl A, Passweg J, Baldomero H, Hermans J. Blood and marrow transplantation activity in 1997. European Group for Blood and Marrow Transplantation (EBMT). Bone Marrow Transplant 24 : 231-245.1999.
2. Rosti G, Ferrante P. The EBMT Solid Tumors Registry 2000 Report . C.E.L.I. Ed, Faenza, 2001.
3. Siena S, Bregni M, Di Nicola M, Ravagnani F, Peccatori F, Gandola L, Lombardi F, Tarella C, Bonadonna G, Gianni AM. Durability of hematopoiesis following autografting with peripheral blood progenitors. Ann Onc 5 : 935-941, 1994.
4. Rosti G, Ferrante P, Dazzi C, Ledermann L, Leyvraz S, Crown J, Ladenstein R, Koscelniak E, Marangolo M. High-dose chemotherapy in solid tumors : the EBMT database. Critical Rev Oncology/Hematology (in press 2001).
5. Peters W, Rosner G, Vredenburg J. Shpall E, Crump M, Richardson P, Marks L, Cirrincione C, Wood W, Henderson I, Hurd D, Norton L. A prospective, randomised comparison of two doses of combination alkylating agents as consoldation after CAF in high-risk primary breast cancer involving ten or more axillary lymph nodes: preliminary results of CALGB 9082/SWOG 9114/NCIC MA-13. Proc Am Soc Clin Oncol 18,1a, 1999
6. Antman KH, Rowlings PA, Vaughan WP, Pelz CJ, Fay JW, Fields KK, Freytes CO, Gale RP, Hillner BE, Holland HK, Kennedy MJ, Klein JP, Lazarus HM, McCarthy PL Jr, Saez R, Spitzer G, Stadtmauer EA, Williams SF, Wolff SN, Sobocinski KB, Armitage JO, Horowitz MM. High-dose chemotherapy with autologous hematopoietic stem-cell support for breast cancer in North America. J Clin Oncol 15 : 1870-1879, 1997.
7. Stadtmauer EA, O'Neill A, Goldstein LJ, Crilley PA, Mangan KF, Ingle JN, Brodsky I, Martino S, Lazarus HM, Erban JK, Sickles C, Glick JH . Conventional-dose chemotherapy compared with high-dose chemotherapy plus autologous hematopoietic stem-cell transplantation for metastatic breast cancer. Philadelphia Bone Marrow Transplant Group. N Engl J Med; 342: 1069-1076, 2000
8. Rowlings PA, Williams SF, Antman KH, Fields KK, Fay JW, Reed E, Pelz CJ, Klein JP, Sobocinski KB, Kennedy MJ, Freytes CO, McCarthy PL Jr, Herzig RH, Stadtmauer EA, Lazarus HM, Pecora AL, Bitran JD, Wolff SN, Gale RP, Vaughan WP, Spitzer G, Horowitz MM . Factors correlated with progression-free survival after high-dose chemotherapy and hematopoietic stem cell transplantation for metastatic breast cancer. JAMA: 282 : 1335-1343, 1999
9. Greenberg PA, Hortobagyi GN, Smith TL, Ziegler LD, Frye DK, Buzdar AU. Long-term follow-up of patients with complete remission following combination chemotherapy for metastatic breast cancer. J Clin Oncol 14 : 2197-2205, 1996.
10. Viens P, Palangié T, Janvier M., Fabbro M, Roché H, Delozier T, Labat JA, Linassier C, Audhuy B, Feuilhade F, Costa B, Delva B, Cure H, Rousseau F, Guillot A, Mousseau M, Ferrero JM, Barbou VJ, Jacquemier J, Puoillart P. First line high-dose chemotherapy with rG-CSF and repeated blood stem cell transplantation in untreated inflammatory breast cancer (Pegase 02 trial) Br J Cancer 81 : 449-456, 1999.
11. The Scandinavian Breast Cancer Study Group 9401 . Results from a randomized adjuvant breast cancer study with high dose chemotherapy with CTCb supported by autologous bone marrow stem cells versus escalated and tailored FEC therapy. Proc Am Soc Clin Oncol 18: 3a, 1999
12. Rodenhuis S, Bontenbal M, Beex L, van der Wall E Richel D, Noij M, Voest E, Hupperets P, Westermann A, Dalesio O, de Vries E. Randomized phase III study of high-dose chemotherapy with Cyclophosphamide,Thiotepa and Carboplatin in operable breast cancer with 4 or more axillary lymph nodes. Proc Soc Clin Oncol 19: 74a, 2000.
13. Gianni AM, Siena S, Bregni M, Di Nicola M, Orefice S, Cusumano F, Salvadori B, Luini A, Greco M, Zucali R, Rilke F, Zambetti M, Valagussa P, Bonadonna G. Efficacy, toxicity, and applicability of high-dose sequential chemotherapy as adjuvant treatment in operable breast cancer with 10 or more involved axillary nodes : five-year results. J Clin Oncol 15 : 2312-2321,1997.
14. Lotz JP, Curé H, Janvier M, Morvan F, Asselain B, Guillemont M, Laadem A, Maraninchi D, Gisselbrecht C, Roché H. High-dose chemotherapy (HD-CT) with hematopoietic stem cell transplantation (HSCT) for metastatic breast cancer (MBC) : results of the French protocol PEGASE 04. Proc Am Soc Clin Oncol 18, 43a,1999.

First-Line and Salvage High-Dose Chemotherapy in Patients with Germ-Cell Tumors

O. Rick[1], W. Siegert[1], and J. Beyer[2]

[1] Klinik für Innere Medizin m.S. Hämatologie/Onkologie, Universitätsklinikum Charité, Campus Virchow-Klinikum, Humboldt Universität, Berlin; [2] Klinik für Innere Medizin m.S. Hämatologie/Onkologie, Klinikum der Philipps Universität, Marburg

Introduction

Most patients with metastatic germ-cell tumors (GCT) will be cured by platin-based combination chemotherapy followed by surgical resection of residual masses [1]. The outcome is considerably worse for patients with poor prognostic features at initial diagnosis, such as large tumor burden, multiple sites, extrapulmonary visceral metastases and/or high levels of tumor markers. These patients have a chance of cure of less than 50% with standard first-line treatment and must therefore be classified as „poor-prognosis" patients [2]. Furthermore, patients with an inadequate response to first-line chemotherapy or relapse from prior complete remission have also a considerably less favorable outcome as compared to other patients with GCT. Conventional-dose salvage chemotherapy in combination with resection of residual masses will result in second complete remissions in only about 30–60% of patients. In addition, at least half of these patients will suffer further relapses and will ultimately die of their disease. Depending on the presence or absence of adverse prognostic factors, only about 15–30% of patients overall will become long-term survivors after conventional-dose salvage chemotherapy [3,4].

To improve the unfavorable outcome of patients with „poor-prognosis" at initial presentation and of patients with relapse or progressive disease after conventional-dose treatment, high-dose chemotherapy (HDCT) followed by autologous periperal blood progenitor-cell (APBPC) rescue has been explored as a therapeutic option [5, 6]. Due to increasing clinical experience in the management of side-effects, the use of peripheral blood progenitor cells, and the availability of hematopoietic growth factors, this HDCT has become relatively safe. Dose-escalations to about three to five times the conventional-dose can be achieved for most drugs active in GCT as hematologic toxicities no longer have to be considered. However, immediate and long-term non-hematologic organ toxicities such as neurotoxicity and renal impairment are substantial and limit further dose escalation. Furthermore, the long-term hematologic complications such as the incidence of secondary myelodysplasias or leukemias is increased even years after successful HDCT. This report reviews, the recent developments in respect to first-line and salvage HDCT strategies and discusses the role of prognostic factors for treatment outcome.

First-line chemotherapy in patients with „poor-prognosis" GCT

Conventional-dose chemotherapy

Since the late 1970s the use of cisplatin-based conventional-dose chemotherapy has dramatically improved the prognosis for patients with metastatic germ cell tumors and now cure rates exceed 80% even in patients with widely metastatic disease [7]. However, among patients with „advanced disease" according to Indiana University criteria or „poor prognosis" according to International Germ Cell Cancer Collaborative Group (IGCCCG) classification, long term survival rates range only between 45% and 55% after conventional-dose chemotherapy [2, 8]. Several investigators have attempted to improve the outcome of these patients with dose-intensified multi-drug regimens, including the alternating use of non-cross-resistant agents [9–12]. Yet, the current treatment standard still consists of four cycles of the three-drug combination of cisplatin, bleomycin, and etoposide (PEB) in conventional doses. In comparison with all other conventional-dose or dose-escalated regimens, PEB showed comparable results in respect to clinical outcome but with less toxicities [13]. Treatment strategies that explore HDCT as intensification of first-line treatment are nevertheless justified and improvement urgently needed given the unsatifactory results with four cycles PEB or other dose-intensified regimens in patients with „poor prognosis" GCT.

High-dose chemotherapy

One of the first trials that investigated HDCT followed by APBPC rescue was carried out by the French study group. One-hundred and fourteen patients were randomized to receive either conventional-dose treatment or conventional-dose treatment followed by intensification with HDCT. The trial showed no differences in complete remission (CR) rate and survival between the two study arms. However, this trial has been critizised for a number of methodologic problems and has never been fully published [14]. Investigators from Memorial Sloan-Kettering Cancer Center also demonstrated the feasibilty of first-line HDCT and, for the first time, observed an imrovement in survival in these patients as compared with historical controls [15]. Bokemeyer et al and the German Testicular Cancer Study Group investigated a strategy giving 3 to 4 sequential cycles of high-dose cisplatin, etoposide and ifosfamide (HD-PEI) followed by granulocyte-colony-stimulating-factor with or without APBPC rescue. The dosages of the regimen were escalated over seven dose levels. Among 238 patients with „advanced disease" 80% achieved a CR or a markernegative partial remission (PRm-). The overall and event-free survival was 80% and 72% after 3.2 years, respectively [16]. In a matched-pair analysis Bokemeyer et al subsequently compaired their results in 147 patients treated with first-line HD-PEI with 309 patients treated with conventional-dose chemotherapy. After a median follow up of nearly 22 month the overall and progession-free survival were significantly prolonged in HDCT patients with 82% versus 71% (p= .0184) and 75% versus 59% (p= .0056), respectively. Results of this trial indicated that an approximately 10% to 15% increase in cure rate is achievable in this high-risk patients with first-line HDCT. The investigators also postulated from their data, that the efficiency of salvage HDCT would be unable to compensate the survival benefit of first-line HDCT [5].

Prognostic factors

Since the early 1980'ies a large number of prognostic factors and several classifications using different prognostic factors have been reported [8,17–21]. This unsatisfactory situation has hindered the collaboration in randomized trials and has made the evaluation of nonrandomized studies impossible. Therefore, the IGCCCG initiated a multivariate analysis of 5,862 patients with metastatic seminomatous and nonseminomatous GCT. Based on these results a prognostic model was proposed that separated patients into three groups of „good-", „intermediate-" and „poor-prognosis" (Table 1). Currently, this classification is internationally accepted and recommended to be used in clinical practice [2].

Table 1. Prognostic classification for first-line treatment according to [2]

Good Prognosis	
Non-Seminoma	Seminoma
Testis/retroperitoneal primary and No non-pulmonary visceral metastases and Good markers AFP < 1000 ng/ml and HCG < 5000 U/l and LDH < 1.5 × upper limit of normal	Any primary site and No non-pulmonary visceral metastases and Normal AFP, any HCG, any LDH
Intermediate Prognosis	
Non-Seminoma	Seminoma
Testis/retroperitoneal primary and No non-pulmonary visceral metastases and Intermediate markers AFP ≥ 1000 and ≤ 10,000 ng/ml and HCG ≥ 5000 and ≤ 50,000 U/l or LDH ≥ 1.5 × N and ≤ 10 × N	Any primary site and Non-pulmonary visceral metastases and Normal AFP, any HCG, any LDH
Poor Prognosis	
Non-Seminoma	Seminoma
Mediastinal primary or Non-pulmonary visceral metastases *or* Poor markers AFP > 10,000 ng/ml or HCG > 50,000 U/l or LDH > 10 × upper limit of normal	No patients classified as poor prognosis

Salvage chemotherapy in patients with relapsed and/or refractory GCT

Conventional-dose chemotherapy

Overall, the rate of favorable responses after conventional-dose salvage in patients with relapsed and/or refractory GCT has been around 50%. Long-term remissions were obtained in about 15–30 % of patients. Successful regimens combined cisplatin with ifosfamide plus either etoposide or vinblastine (Table 2). Most recently paclitaxel was found to be active and has also been incorporated into salvage regimens [22–24]. However, at the present time no single salvage combination can be considered superior to others. Likewise, regimens that combine more than three drugs, that use escalated doses of cisplatin or intensive treatment schedules are probably more toxic, but do not conclusively result in better treatment outcomes [25]. The large variations in reponse rates and survival between these studies indicated that patients selection and prognostic factors are the most important indicator for treatment outcome and long-term survival.

Miller et al reported on 24 seminoma patients who relapsed or progressed after cisplatin-based chemotherapy [26]. With a long-term survival rate of 54 % the results with conventional-dose cisplatin, ifosfamide and vinblastine (VeIP) regimen were excellent and clearly superior to what would have been expected in nonseminoma patients. Loehrer et al. reported on 135 patients with seminoma or nonseminoma who had received conventional-dose VeIP after having failed one cisplatin-etoposide-based prior treatment [26]. The long-term event-free survival in the subgroup of nonseminoma patients was only 17%. Finally, Motzer et al. studied 30 seminoma and nonseminoma patients who relapsed after platinum-based first-line treatment and who all had favorable prognostic factors for response to salvage chemotherapy. In this highly selected group of patients 80%

Table 2. Commonly used conventional-dose first-line and salvage regimens

Drug combination		ref.	dosage and schedule	Duration of cycles	Number of cycles
Cisplatin Etoposide Bleomycin	**PEB**	[1]	20 mg/m² day 1-5 75-100 mg/m² day 1-5 30 mg day 2,9,16	21 days	4 cycles
Cisplatin Etoposide Ifosfamid	**PEI**	[4]	20 mg/m² day 1-5 75-100 mg/m² day 1-5 1.2 g/m² day 1-5	21 days	4 cycles
Cisplatin Vinblastine Ifosfamide	**VeIP**	[4]	20 mg/m² Tag 1-5 0.11 mg/kg Tag1+2 1.2 g/m² Tag 1-5	21 days	4 cycles
Paclitaxel Ifosfamide Cisplatin	**TIP**	[6, 22]	175 -250 mg/m² day 1 1.2 g/m² day 2-6 20 mg/m² day 2-6	21 days	4 cycles

ref. = reference

achieved a favorable response and 73% were living event-free with a median follow-up of 3 years [23]. These trials indicate that prognostic factors need to be considered in the interpretation of salvage data and might explain reported differences in response and survival between trials and study populations.

High-dose chemotherapy

In patients receiving second or subsequent salvage treatment investigators in the US and Europe still reported long-term remission rates of 15–25% using high-dose carboplatin and etoposide with or without the addition of an oxazaphosphorine as an alkylating drug [28].

More recently, three groups modified this initial schedule. The German Testicular Cancer Study Group explored a treatment strategy that combined intensive conventional-dose salvage with paclitaxel, ifosfamide and cisplatin followed by a single HDCT cycle with carboplatin, etoposide and thiotepa. The rationale for the trial was to optimize conventional-dose salvage treatment by using paclitaxel as well as by intensifying HDCT with thiotepa [6]. Motzer at al. investigated sequential dose-intensive paclitaxel and ifosfamide followed by three cycles of high-dose carboplatin and etoposide [24]. Rodenhuis et al. explored sequential dose-intensive treatment with etoposide and ifosfamide, followed by one cycle of high-dose carboplatin and etoposide and two cycles of high-dose carboplatin, cyclophosphamide and thiotepa [29].

These trials are encouraging that patients with second or subsequent relapses can still successfully be salvaged by HDCT. In addition, patients with poor prognostic features at the time of relapse or progression also seem to profit from early intensification of first salvage treatment. However, whereas side-effects differ between schedules, the results of these most recent trials indicate, that prognostic factors for treatment outcome after HDCT could be important than the use of a particular HDCT strategy or combination.

Prognostic factors

Several retrospective analyses have tried to identify prognostic factors for conventional-dose as well as for high-dose salvage chemotherapy. Primary mediastinal nonseminomatous tumors are usually incurable if first-line treatment fails. At least two large series did not find long-term survivors neither with conventional-dose treatment nor with HDCT [30, 31]. Although less well studied, the presence of brain metastases at the time of systemic relapse or progression might similarly pertend a poor prognosis for long-term survival.

Fossa et al. analyzed the results in 164 nonseminoma patients who progressed after cisplatin-based first-line chemotherapy and who received different conventional-dose regimens as first-salvage treatment [32]. Reponse to first-line treatment, response duration as defined by the progression-free interval as well as serum levels of human chorionic gonadotrophin (HCG) and alpha-fetoprotein prior salvage were identified as independent prognostic variables. Patients, who

Table 3. Prognostic model for conventional-dose salvage according to [32]

- no complete remission to first-line treatment
- progression-free interval < 2 years
- AFP > 100 kU/L or HCG > 100 U/L at initiation of salvage

	survival at 2 years (95% confidence intervals)
„good prognosis" one risk factor present #	74% (60%–88%)
„intermediate prognosis" any two risk factors present	45% (32%–58%)
„poor prognosis" all three risk factors present	7% (0%–15%)

either „no complete remission" or „AFP > 100 kU/L and/or HCG > 100 U/L"

progressed during cisplatin-based treatment had a particularly poor prognosis. Salvage treatment given prior to 1986, size of the treatment center and prognostic group according to a score of the British Medical Reserach Council were significant in univariate, but not in multivariate analysis. Based on these results a prognostic model was proposed (Table 3). Unfortunately, the impact of histology on prognosis could not be assessed as no seminoma patients were included. Other prognostic variables such as the presence or absence of primary mediastinal nonseminomatous tumors or brain metastases were not analyzed separately. Limited by its retrospective approach and the lack of a control group, this analysis cannot exclude the possibilty that the results of salvage chemotherapy might have even been superior had HDCT been used early in these patients. In an cooperative effort with other investigators in the US and Europe Beyer et al tried to identify prognostic variables in 383 patients treated with HDCT given as first or subsequent salvage treatment. Progressive disease at the time of HDCT, nonseminomatous mediastinal primary tumor, the degree of refractoriness to cisplatin and HCG levels prior HDCT were identified as prognostic variables for long-term survival [30].

Ongoing trials

First-line HDCT

Currently, large efforts are being made comparing HDCT to conventional-dose first-line treatment. A United States intergroup trial compares four cycles of PEB with two cycles of the same regimen plus two cycles of high-dose carboplatin, etoposide and cyclophosphamide followed by APBPC rescue. In Europe the genitourinary group of the European Organization for Research and Treatment of Cancer (EORTC) is taking a similar approach comparing four cycles of PEB to sequential HD-PEI in a prospective randomized trial.

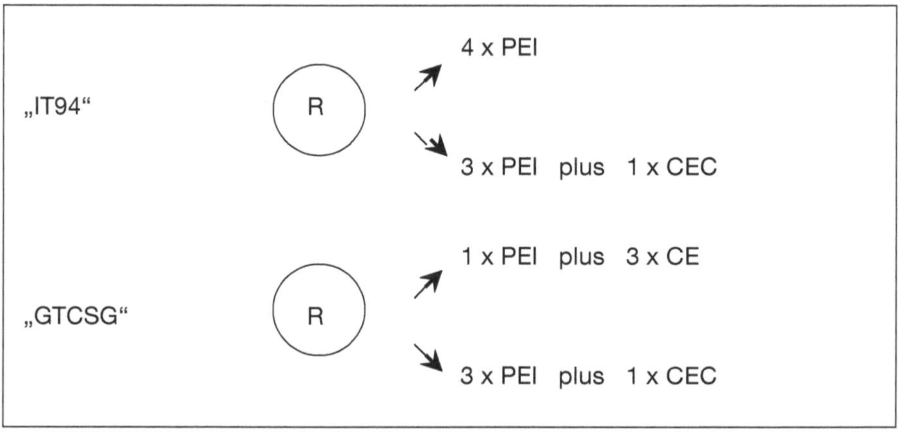

Fig. 1. Ongoing trials in Europe investigating HDCT as salvage treatment.
PEI = conventional-dose cisplatin, etoposide and ifosfamide; CEC = high-dose carbplatin, etoposide and cyclophosphamide; CE = high-dose carboplatin and etoposide; GTCSG = German Testicular Cancer Study Group

HDCT as salvage treatment

In the salvage situation two trials are actively recruiting. The multinational „IT94" trial randomizes patients with good prognostic features for first-salvage treatment with either four cycles of conventional-dose cisplatin, etoposide and ifosfamide or three cycles of the same regimen plus one cycle of high-dose carboplatin, etoposide and cyclophosphamide. In Germany, a prospective randomized trial is comparing single versus sequential HDCT in good or intermediate prognosis patients who require either first or subsequent salvage treatment (Fig. 1). The results of these trials should help to determine to role of HDCT particularly when given as intensification of first-salvage treatment.

Continuing problems

Still we do not know exactly how much HDCT can improve first-line or salvage treatment of patients with „poor-prognosis" at initial diagnosis or of patients with relapsed/refractory GCT. Is HDCT given as intensification of first-line chemotherapy really superior to HDCT given as first or subsequent salvage treatment? How do we avoid overtreatment with a potentially hazardous procedure? Does the addition of a new drug, such as paclitaxel to first-line HDCT improve efficacy? Can we identify patients who might profit from HDCT given as first-salvage treatment? A „risk adapted" stategy for first-salvage treatment using conventional-dose treatment in „good-prognosis" patients and high-dose treatment in „intermediate-" and „poor-prognosis" patients, as suggested by Motzer et al., is an attractive concept, but clearly needs to be further studied before it should be used in clinical practice [23]. And finally, how does salvage surgery fit in the multidisciplinary approach of treating GCT patients. Are there still curative options in patients who relapse after HDCT? How should we manage these patients? Is there a role for chemotherapy or should these patients be treated with agressive surgery alone?

Hemato-, neuro- and nephrotoxicity jeopardize the success HDCT impairing of the quality of life during and after treatment and giving rise to late treatment failures from secondary tumors. We investigated amifostine in a prospective randomized trial to see whether this drug would protect from treatment related myelosuppression, neurotoxicity and renal dysfunction during conventional-dose or high-dose chemotherapy. Unfortunately, amifostine given in the dose and combination studied seemed to provide only a small benefit for patients with GCT who receive cisplatin/paclitaxel-based conventional-dose treatment or HDCT [33]. Therefore, in the future new cytoprotective agents have to be developed.

Concluding remarks

In patients with „poor-prognosis" at initial diagnosis or in patients with relapsed/refractory disease, HDCT may be superior to conventional-dose treatment and can be curative for a substantial proportion of this patients. Strategies to intensify either first-line or salvage chemotherapy are currently being investigated. The results of salvage chemotherapy may further be improved if combined with salvage surgery in selected patients. In order to find rational approaches for rare clinical scenarios, cooperative multiinstitutional efforts are needed.

References

1. Bosl G, Motzer RJ (1997) Testicular germ-cell cancer. N Engl J Med 337:242-253.
2. International Germ Cell Cancer Collaborative Group (1997) International germ cell consensus classification: a prognostic factor-based staging system for metastatic germ cell cancers. J Clin Oncol 15:594-603.
3. Harstrick A, Schmoll HJ, Wilke H, et al. (1991) Cisplatin, etoposide, and ifosfamide salvage therapy for refractory or relapsing germ cell carcinoma. J Clin Oncol 9:1529-1535
4. Loehrer PJ, Lauer R, Roth BJ, et al. (1988) Salvage therapy in recurrent germ cell cancer: Ifosfamide and cisplatin plus either vinblastine or etoposide. Ann Intern Med 109:540-546
5. Bokemeyer C, Kollmannsberger C, Meisner C, et al. (1999) First-line high-dose chemotherapy compared with standard-dose PEB/VIP chemotherapy in patients with advanced germ cell tumors: a multivariate and matched-pair analysis. J Clin Oncol 17:3450-3456.
6. Rick O, Bokemeyer C, Beyer J, et al. (2001) Salvage treatment with paclitaxel, ifosfamide and cisplatin (TIP) plus high-dose carboplatin, etoposide and thiotepa (CET) followed by autologous stem cell rescue in patients with relapsed or refractory germ cell cancer. J Clin Oncol 19:81-88.
7. Einhorn LH (1990) Treatment of testicular cancer: a new and improved model. J Clin Oncol 8:1777-1781.
8. Birch R, Williams S, Cone A, et al. (1986) Prognostic factors for favorable outcome in disseminated germ cell tumors. J Clin Oncol 4:400-407.
9. Bower M, Newlands ES, Holden L, et al. (1997) Treatment of men with metastataic non-seminomatous germ cell tumours with cyclical POMB/ACE chemotherapy. Ann Oncol 8:477-483.
10. Kaye SB, Mead GM, Fossa SD, et al. (1998) Intensive induction sequential chemotherapy with BOP/VIP-B compared with treatment with BEP/EP for poor prognosis metastatic non-

seminomatous germ cell tumor: A randomized Medical Research Council/European Organization for Researche and Treatment of Cancer study. J Clin Oncol 16:692-701.
11. Culine S, Theodore C, Bekradda M et al. (1997) Experience with bleomycin, etoposide, cisplatin (BEP) an alternating cisplatin, cyclophosphamide, doxorubicin (CISCA(II))/vinblastine, bleomycine (VB (IV)) regimens of chemotherapy in poor-risk nonseminomatous germ cell tumors. Am J Clin Oncol 20:184-188.
12. de Wit R, Stoter G, Sleijfer DT, et al. (1995) Four cycles of BEP versus an alternating regimen and PVB and PEB in patients with poor prognosis metastatic testicular non-seminoma: A randomized study of the EORTC- Genitourinary Tract Cancer Cooperative Group. Br J Cancer 71:1311-1314.
13. Williams S, Birch R, Einhorn LH, et al. (1987). Treatment of disseminated germ cell tumors with cisplatin, bleomycin and either vinblastin or etoposid. New Engl J Med 316:1435-1440.
14. Chevreau C, Droz JP, Pico JL, et al. (1993). Early intensified chemotherapy with autologous bone marrow transplantation in first line treatment of poor risk non-seminomatous germ cell tumours: Preliminary results of a French randomized trial. Eur Urol 23:213-217.
15. Motzer RJ, Mazumdar M, Bajorin DF, et al. (1997). High-dose carboplatin, etoposide, and cyclophosphamide with autologous bone marrow transplantation in first-line therapy for patients with poor-risk germ cell tumors. J Clin Oncol 15:2546-2552.
16. Bokemeyer C, Harstrick A, Beyer J, et al. (1998). The use of dose-intensified chemotherapy in th treatment of metastatic nonseminomatous testicular germ cell tumors: German Testicular Cancer Study Group. Semin Oncol 25:24-32.
17. Bosl GJ, Geller NL, Cirrincione C, et al. (1983). Multivariate analysis of prognostic variables in patients with metastatic testicular cancer. Cancer Res 43:3403-3407.
18. Medical Research Council (1985). Prognostic factors in advanced non-seminomatous germ-cell testicular tumours: Results of a multicentre study. Lancet 1:8-12.
19. Stoter G, Sylvester R, Sleijfer DT, et al. (1987). Multivariate analysis of prognostic factors in patients with disseminated nonseminomatous testicular cancer: Results from an EORTC multiinstitutional phase III study. Cancer Res 47:2414-2418.
20. Droz JP, Kramer A, Ghosn M, et al. (1988). Prognostic factors in advanced nonseminomatous testicular cancer. Cancer 62:564-568.
21. Aass N, Klepp O, Stahl-Cavallin E, et al. (1991). Prognostic factors in unselected patients with nonseminomatous metastatic testicular cancer: A multicentre experience. J Clin Oncol 9:818-826.
22. Bokemeyer C, Beyer J, Metzner B, Rüther U, Harstrick A, Weissbach L, Köhrmann U, Verbeek W, Schmoll HJ (1996) Phase II study of paclitaxel in patients with relapsed or cisplatin-refractory testicular cancer. Ann Oncol 7:31-34.
23. Motzer RB, Sheinfeld J, Mazumdar M, et al. (2000) Paclitaxel, ifosfamide, and cisplatin second-line therapy for patients with relapsed testicular germ cell cancer. J Clin Oncol 18:2413-2418.
24. Motzer RJ, Mazumdar M, Sheinfeld J, Bajorin DF, Macapinlac HA, Bains M, Reich L, Flombaum C, Mariani T, Tong WP, Bosl GJ (2000) Sequential dose-intensive paclitaxel, ifosfamide, carboplatin and etoposide salvage therapy for germ cell tumor patients. J Clin Oncol 18:1173-1180.
25. Beyer J, Bokemeyer C, Schmoll HJ, Siegert W (1994) Treatment intensification in disseminated germ-cell tumors. World J Urol 12:207-213.
26. Miller KD, Loehrer PJ, Gonin R, Einhorn LH (1997) Salvage chemotherapy with vinblastine, ifosfamide, and cisplatin in recurrent seminoma. J Clin Oncol 15:1427-1431.
27. Loehrer PJ, Gonin R, Nichols CR, Weathers T, Einhorn LH (1998) Vinblastine plus ifosfamide plus cisplatin as initial salvage therapy in recurrent germ cell tumor. J Clin Oncol 16:2500-2504.
28. Rick O, Siegert W, Beyer J (1999) High-dose salvage chemotherapy. Germ-cell tumor treatment results in Germany. Int J Cancer 83:839-840.
29. Rodenhuis S, de Wit R, de Mulder PHM, Keizer HJ, Sleijfer DT, Lalisng RI, Bakker PJM, Mandjes I, Kooi M, de Vries EGE (1999) A multi-center prospective phase II study of high-dose chemotherapy in germ-cell cancer patients relapsing from complete remission. Ann Oncol 10:1467-1473.
30. Beyer J, Kramar A, Mandanas R, Linkesch W, Greinix A, Droz JP, Pico JL, Diehl A, Bokemeyer C, Schmoll HJ, Nichols CR, Einhorn LH, Siegert W (1996) High-dose chemotherapy as salvage treatment in germ cell tumors: a multivariate analysis of prognostic factors. J Clin Oncol 14:2638-2645.

31. Saxman SB, Nichols CR, Einhorn LH (1994) Salvage chemotherapy in patients with extragonadal nonseminomatous germ cell tumors: the Indiana University experience. J Clin Oncol 12:1390-1393.
32. Fossa SD, Stenning SP, Gerl A, Horwich A, Clark PI, Wilkinson PM, Jones WG, Williams MV, Oliver RT, Newlands ES, Mead GM, Cullen MH, Kaye SB, Rustin GJS, Cook PA (1999) Prognostic factors in patients progressing after platinum-based chemotherapy for malignant nonseminomatous germ cell tumours. Br J Cancer 80:1392-1399.
33. Rick O, Beyer J, Schwella N, et al. (2001). Amifostine as protection from chemotherapy-induced toxicities after conventional-dose and high-dose chemotherapy in patients with germ cell tumor. submitted

High Dose Chemotherapy in High-Risk Ewing Tumours: Results in 156 (EI)CESS Patients

B. Fröhlich[1], S. Ahrens[1], S. Burdach[2], A. Craft[3], R. Ladenstein[4], M. Paulussen[1], and H. Jürgens[1] on behalf of (EI)CESS and EURO-E.W.I.N.G. 99

[1] Dept. of Paediatric Haematology/Oncology, University of Münster, Germany, [2] Dept. of Paediatrics, University of Halle/Saale, Germany, [3]Dept. of Child Health, University of Newcastle-upon-Tyne, United Kingdom, [4]St. Anna Kinderspital, Vienna, Austria

Introduction

Primary metastases and relapse in Ewing tumours represent adverse risk factors leading to a poor prognosis for event free survival (EFS). Whereas patients with localised Ewing tumours have an EFS probability of 0.63 five years after diagnosis, five year-EFS is 0.22 in primary metastatic patients. Survival in patients with relapsed Ewing tumour correlates with the interval between diagnosis of the primary tumour and the relapse. Survival after two years is 0.32 in patients with an early relapse (≤ 24 months) and 0.07 in patients with a late relapse (>24 months) [1].

The poor outcome in high-risk Ewing tumour patients has prompted many attempts to improve the prognosis by the way of intensified treatment modalities like high-dose chemotherapy with stem cell rescue. In order to assess the potential benefit of high-dose chemotherapy in primary metastatic and relapsed Ewing tumour patients, the registry data on high-dose chemotherapy of the German/European Intergroup Cooperative Ewing's Sarcoma Studies ((EI)CESS) were analysed for outcome.

Patients and methods

Between January 1981 and December 1998, 93 patients with primary metastatic and 63 patients with relapsed Ewing tumours were registered in the German office of the (EI)CESS study.

Patients with primary metastatic Ewing tumours (n = 93)

In the primary metastatic group, 52 patients were male and 41 were female. The median age at diagnosis was 15 (0.3–42) years. The primary tumour was most often localised in the pelvis (n = 43, 46%). Other primary sites were rib (n = 14), spine (n = 8), scapula (n = 5), humerus (n = 4), tibia (n = 4), femur (n = 3), fibula (n = 3), soft tissue (n = 2), radius (n = 1), ulna (n = 1) and sternum (n = 1). In four cases information about the site of the primary tumour was unavailable. The

Table 1. Sites of primary metastases

	(n = 93)
bone/bone marrow (BM)	41 (44%)
lung/pleura	13 (14%)
bone/BM + lung/pleura	23 (25%)
bone/BM + others	2 (2%)
lung/pleura + others	3 (3%)
bone/BM + lung/pleura + others	6 (6%)
others	5 (5%)

sites of the primary metastases are listed in Table 1. For chemotherapy, most patients (n = 82, 88%) received VAIA (Vincristin, adriamycin, ifosfamide and d-actinomycin) or EVAIA (VAIA plus etoposide) according to the high risk arms of the (EI)CESS protocols. Nine patients were treated with modified (E)VAIA regimens and two patients received other chemotherapies. The length of induction chemotherapy varied between 2 and 14 courses. The local therapy consisted of either surgery (n = 3) or irradiation (n = 49) or both surgery and radiotherapy (n = 32). In five patients no local therapy was performed. Information about the mode of local therapy was missing in four patients.

After induction therapy 38/93 patients (41%) were in complete and 42/93 patients (45%) in partial remission. 5/93 patients (5%) received high-dose chemotherapy in progressive disease. Information about status at high dose therapy was unavailable in eight patients (9%).

Patients with relapsed Ewing tumours (n = 63)

Among patients with relapsed Ewing tumours, 35 had an early and 28 had a late relapse. 44 patients were male and 19 were female. The median age at relapse was 17.7 (1.7–35.4) years. The distribution of relapse sites is given in Table 2. In 21/63 patients reinduction chemotherapy consisted of carboplatinum, etoposide and ifosfamide according to the CESS/CWS-91 relapse protocol. 11/63 patients received cyclophosphamide plus etoposide according to the Rel-EICESS 96 pilot proto-

Table 2. Sites of relapse

	(n = 63)
bone/BM	21 (33%)
lung/pleura	21 (33%)
local	8 (13%)
bone/BM + lung/pleura	4 (6%)
bone/BM + lung/pleura + local	2 (3%)
lung + others	2 (5%)
others	5 (8%)

Table 3. Conditioning regimens in primary metastatic and relapsed patients (pts)

	primary metastatic pts (n = 93)	relapsed pts (n = 63)
ME(C)[1]	8 (9%)	13 (21%)
Hyper-ME(C)[2]	32 (34%)	23 (37%)
Double ME[3]	24 (26%)	11 (17%)
others	22 (24%)	13 (21%)
no information	7(8%)	3 (5%)

[1]ME(C): one course of melphalan and etoposide (± carboplatinum); [2]Hyper-ME(C): one course of melphalan and etoposide (± carboplatinum) plus total body irradiation; [3]Double ME: two courses of melphalan and etoposide

Table 4. Source of progenitor cells in primary metastatic and relapsed patients (pts)

	primary metastatic pts (n=93)	relapsed pts (n=63)
autologous PBSC[1]	72 (74%)	46 (76%)
autologous BM	9 (10%)	8 (13%)
allogeneic BM	7 (8%)	4 (6%)
syngeneic BM	1 (1%)	–
no information	4 (4%)	5 (8%)

col. Most patients (n = 27) had diverse treatment regimens, sometimes varying combination of cytostatic drugs. In four patients information about reinduction chemotherapy was not available. Local therapy was performed in 62/63 patients with relapsed Ewing tumours, and local therapy consisted of surgery (12/62), radiotherapy (9/62) or both surgery and irradiation (41/62). In one patient no local therapy was performed.

After reinduction therapy 28/63 patients (44%) with relapsed Ewing tumours were in complete and 24/63 patients (37%) were in partial remission. Two patients received high-dose chemotherapy in progressive disease. In nine patients (14%) no information about the status at high-dose chemotherapy was available.

Both, in primary metastatic and in relapsed Ewing tumours, modes of high-dose chemotherapy regimens varied. Mostly they consisted of melphalan and/or etoposide (90%) and were given as single or sequential course high dose chemotherapy, with or without total body irradiation. Conditioning regimens are detailed in Tables 3 and 4. As to the source of progenitor cells, autologous peripheral blood, autologous, allogeneic or syngeneic bone marrow was performed. For details see Table 4.

Event free and overall survival was calculated according to Kaplan and Meier [2].

Results

On 1 January 2000, 42/156 patients (27%) were in remission, whereas events were recorded in 114/156 patients (73%).

Patients with primary metastatic Ewing tumours (n = 93)

After a median time under study since stem cell rescue of 49 months, 24/93 patients (26%) were in complete remission. 56/93 patients (60%) had relapse or progressive disease. 8/93 patients (9%) died of complications (3/8 septicaemia, 1/8 bacterial pneumonia plus graft versus host disease (GvHD), 1/8 septicaemia, pneumonia plus GvHD, 1/8 capillary leakage syndrome, venoocclusive disease (VOD) plus multi-organ failure, 1/8 septicaemia, GvHD plus multi-organ failure, 1/8 pneumonia plus capillary leakage syndrome). 5/93 patients (5%) presented with secondary malignancies (2/5 myelodysplastic syndrome, 1/5 acute myelocytic leukemia, 1/5 acute lymphocytic leukemia, 1/5 liposarcoma).

There was no significant difference in the outcome of primary metastatic Ewing tumour patients between those who received high-dose chemotherapy and those who did not: Five-year EFS was 0.18 (+HDT) and 0.26 (-HDT), p=0.3627). Subgroup analysis demonstrated a benefit of high-dose chemotherapy only in patients with primary metastases to bone and lung (± other metastases): Five-year EFS was 0.22 in patients with high-dose chemotherapy and 0.03 in those without (p=0.0001). Neither patients with primary bone/bone marrow metastases (five-year EFS: 0.15 (+HDT) versus 0.19 (-HDT), p=0.7468) nor patients with primary lung metastases (three-year EFS: 0.46 (+HDT) versus 0.45 (-HDT), p=0.8435) showed a significantly better outcome when treated with high-dose chemotherapy.

Patients with relapsed Ewing tumours (n = 63)

After a median time under study since stem cell rescue of 49 months, 18/63 patients (29%) were in complete remission. 39/63 patients (62%) had relapse or progressive disease. 4/63 patients (6%) died of complications (1/4 septicaemia, 1/4 septicaemia plus multi-organ failure, 1/4 septicaemia, GvHD, VOD, capillary leakage syndrome plus multi-organ failure, 1/4 intraoperative pulmonary embolism). 2/63 patients (3%) presented with secondary malignancies (1/2 myelodysplastic syndrome, 1/2 carcinoma of the tongue).

In relapsed Ewing tumour patients, those treated with high-dose chemotherapy had a significant better outcome compared to patients treated with conventional chemotherapy regimens. EFS five years after diagnosis is 0.22 in patients with and 0.12 in patients without high-dose chemotherapy (p = 0.0001) (Fig. 1). Subgroup analyses show that both early and late relapsed Ewing tumour patients seem to benefit from high dose chemotherapy. Five-year EFS is 0.28 and 0.07 in patients with an early relapse (p = 0.0001), and 0.59 and 0.26 in patients with a late relapse (p = 0.0056).

Status at high-dose chemotherapy influences the outcome of patients with relapsed Ewing tumours (five-year EFS: 0.30 (complete remission) versus 0.10 (partial remission) versus 0.00 (progressive disease), p = 0.0001), but not in primary metastatic Ewing tumours (five-year EFS: 0.21 (complete remission) versus 0.24 (partial remission) versus 0.00 (progressive disease), p = 0.0867).

The given modalities of high-dose chemotherapy did not influence the outcome in primary metastatic Ewing (two-year EFS: 0.13 (ME(C)) versus 0.22

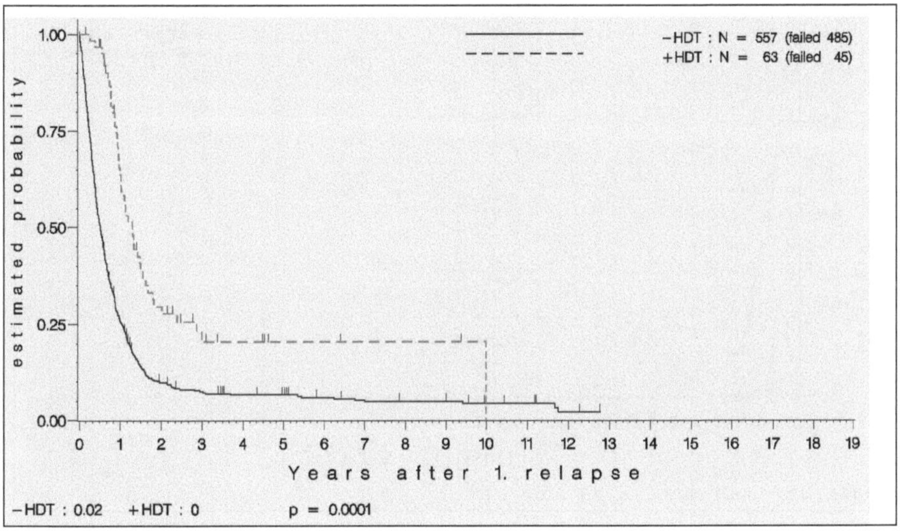

Fig. 1. Ewing tumour patients with relapse

(Hyper-ME(C)) versus 0.34 (Double ME), p = 0.4149) or in relapsed Ewing tumours (three-year EFS: 0.09 (ME(C)) versus 0.21 (Hyper-ME(C)) versus 0.57 (Double ME), p = 0.1804).

Discussion

High dose chemotherapy based on melphalan and/or etoposide (with or without total body irradiation) does not generally seem to improve outcome of high risk Ewing tumour patients. However, subgroup group analyses in patients with primary metastases show, that only those with primary metastases to bone and lung (± other metastases), who have the poorest prognosis under conventional chemotherapy appear to benefit from high-dose chemotherapy (Fig. 2). Outcome of patients with lung metastases, who have a better prognosis under conventional chemotherapy, and those with primary bone/bone marrow metastases were not improved with high-dose chemotherapy as given. In relapsed Ewing tumours, previous analyses had shown a benefit from high-dose chemotherapy only in patients with an early relapse [3[. However, the current analysis, which comprises a longer follow-up, shows that in both subgroups, in patients with early and late relapses, the outcome is significantly better in patients treated with high-dose chemotherapy than in those with conventional chemotherapy. The status at high-dose chemotherapy was of prognostic significance only in relapsed Ewing tumour patients (Fig. 3). In primary metastatic patients, there was no correlation between remission status at high-dose chemotherapy and outcome. However, all of those patients (n = 7), who received high-dose chemotherapy in progressive disease died within months after stem cell rescue.

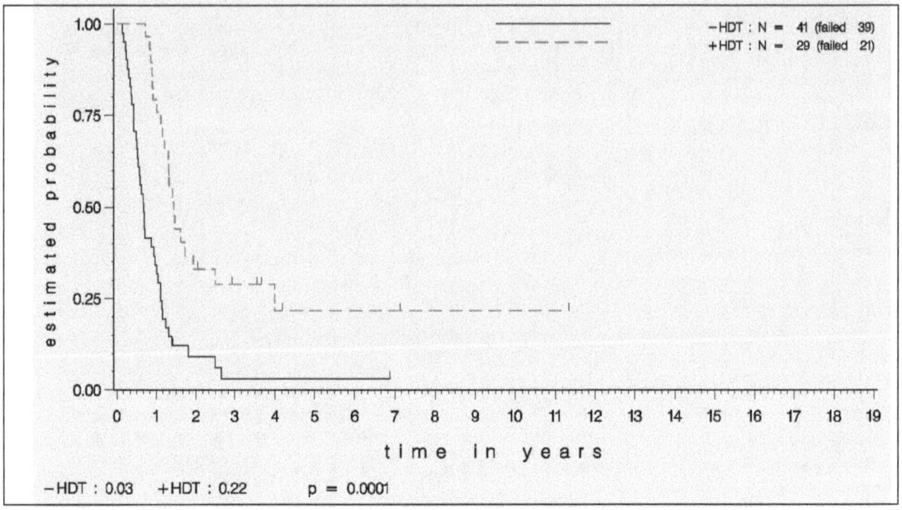

Fig. 2. Ewing tumour patients with primary bone and lung (± other) metastases

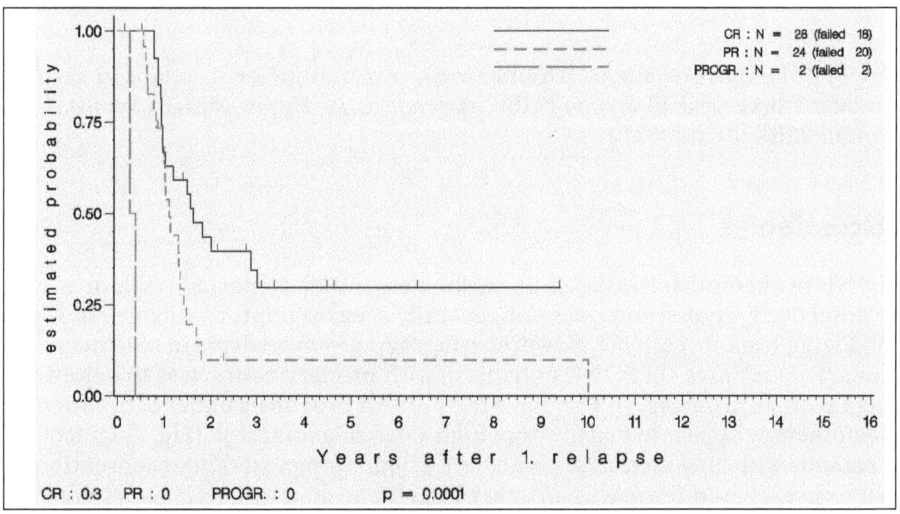

Fig. 3. Status at high dose chemotherapy in relapsed Ewing tumour patients

The present analysis failed to identify a melphalan and/or etoposide-based high-dose chemotherapy regimen, that was superior to other regimens. There was no significant difference between patients who additionally received total body irradiation and those who had a single course regimen or a sequential course regimen. However, studies on busulfan-containing high-dose chemotherapies, demonstrated a superior outcome of patients who received high-dose chemotherapy based on busulfan compared to those treated with other high-dose chemotherapy regimens, especially high-dose chemotherapy with total body irradiation [4–7].

So far, all studies on high-dose chemotherapy in high-risk Ewing tumour patients have been based on retrospective analyses. In order to verify the potential benefit of high-dose chemotherapy prospective, randomised trials are warranted. The recently activated EURO-E.W.I.N.G. 99 protocol is the first Ewing tumour treatment protocol, where busulfan high-dose chemotherapy is compared to conventional therapy in high-risk Ewing tumour patients in a randomised design.

References

1. Craft AW, Cotterill SJ, Malcolm AJ, et al. (1998) Ifosfamide containing chemotherapy in Ewing's sarcoma: The second UKCCSG/MRC Ewing's Toumors Study (ET-2). J Clin Oncol 16: 3628-3633
2. Kaplan El, Meier P. (1958) Nonparametric estimation from incomplete observations. J Am Stat Assoc 53: 457-481 (abstract)
3. Fröhlich B, Ahrens S, Burdach S, et al. (1999) Hochdosistherapie bei primär metastasiertem und rezidiviertem Ewing-Sarkom. Klin Pädiatr 211 284-290
4. Ladenstein R, Gadner H, Hartmann O et al. (1995) Europäische Erfahrung mit Megatherapie und autologer Knochenmarktransplantation bei soliden Tumoren mit ungünstiger Prognose (Ewing-Sarkom, Keimzelltumoren und Hirntumoren). Wien Med Wschr 145: 55-57
5. Ladenstein R, Lasset C, Pinkerton R, et al. (1995) Impact of megatherapy in children with high-risk Ewing's tumours in complete remission: a report from the EBMT Solid Tumour Registry. Bone Marrow Transplant 15: 697-705
6. Ladenstein R, Hartmann O, Pinkerton R, et al. for the EBMT Solid Tumour Pediatric Working Party (1998) A multivariate and matched pair analysis on high-risk Ewing tumour patients undergoing MGT/SCR in Europe. Bone Marrow Transplant 21: 227-227 (abstract)
7. Atra A, Whelan JS, Calvagna V, et al. (1997) High-dose busulphan/melphalan with autologous stem cell rescue in Ewing's sarcoma. Bone Marrow Transplant 20: 843-846

Rapid Sequence Tandem Transplant in Children with High-Risk Neuroblastoma

S. A. Grupp[1], J. W. Stern[1], N. Bunin[1], D. von Allmen[2], G. Pierson[1], Ch. Nancarrow[3], R. Adams[4], G. Griffin[5], and L. Diller[3]

[1]Department of Pediatrics, Division of Oncology; [2]Pediatric Surgery, Children's Hospital of Philadelphia, University of Pennsylvania, School of Medicine, Philadelphia, PA; [3]Department of Pediatric Oncology, Dana-Farber Cancer Institute and Department of Medicine, Children's Hospital, Boston, MA; [4]Pediatric Oncology, Primary Children's Hospital, Salt Lake City, UT; [5]Department of Pediatrics, A.I. Dupont Hospital, Wilmington, DE

Abstract

The majority of patients with high risk neuroblastoma (NB) still relapse. We have designed a Phase II trial for children with advanced NB utilizing a program of induction chemotherapy followed by tandem high-dose, myeloablative treatments with stem cell rescue (HDT/SCR) in rapid sequence. The study has completed accrual and, in the most recent update of the data, 62 patients are evaluable. 107 cycles of HDT/SCR have been completed. Pheresis has been possible for every case, despite the young age of these patients, with an average of 7.2×10^6 $CD34^+$ cells/kg/cycle available. Engraftment has been rapid, with median time to neutrophil engraftment of 11 days. Seven patients who completed the first HDT course did not complete the second, and there were five toxic deaths. With a median follow-up of 24 months from diagnosis, the 3 year point estimate of EFS is 63%. Some of the patients received stem cells purged by CD34 selection and the engraftment and EFS of these patients are similar to the overall group. This work demonstrates that a tandem HDT/SCR regimen for high-risk NB is feasible in children and may improve disease-free survival.

Introduction

Despite improvements in treatment and supportive care, most patients with high-risk neuroblastoma (NB) recur. The addition of high dose chemotherapy with

---

This research was supported in part by the University of Pennsylvania Cancer Center (SG), by the Benacerraf /Frei Clinical Investigator Award, Dana-Farber Cancer Institute (LD) and the Fiftieth Anniversary Program for Scholars in Medicine, Harvard Medical School (LD).

The abbreviations used are: ANC, absolute neutrophil count; EFS, event-free survival; HDC, high-dose chemoradiotherapy; ICC, immunocytochemistry; NB, neuroblastoma; PBPC, peripheral blood progenitor cells; platelet transfusion independence, PTI; SCR, stem cell rescue; VOD, hepatic veno-occlusive disease.

bone marrow support has recently shown to improve event-free survival (EFS) in a randomized study by the Children's Cancer Group [1]. The survival advantage for patients treated most aggressively was further improved upon by the addition of cis-retinoic acid in the setting of minimal residual disease. Among patients randomized to both high dose chemotherapy with autologous bone marrow rescue and cis-retinoic acid, EFS from diagnosis was estimated to be 40%. In order to explore whether further intensification of consolidation therapy might further improve EFS in this group of patients we have designed a study of tandem high dose chemoradiotherapy supported by peripheral blood progenitor cells (PBPC). In designing this regimen, we utilized the following design criteria:

1. induction therapy with standard agents in conventional doses,
2. use of PBPC as a stem cell source,
3. collection of PBPC relatively early in induction and as soon as disease was documented to have cleared from the marrow,
4. CD34 selection of PBPC to assess engraftment and test this strategy to purge contaminating NB,
5. two cycles of high dose chemoradiotherapy with PBPC rescue utilizing non-crossreactive conditioning regimens.

Adequate stem/progenitor cells collected from adults have been shown to support patients through tandem transplant courses [2, 3]. PBPC support of children through single transplant has also been explored [4, 5] and shown to provide rapid engraftment [6], but there are no published tandem transplant trials using PBPC in pediatrics. Here, we report on the feasibility of tandem transplantation in young children with NB and promising preliminary EFS results in this group of high-risk patients.

Patients and Methods

Eligibility criteria

Patients with high-risk NB over one year of age who had not received prior therapy were eligible for this trial. This included patients with INSS [7] Stage 4 disease or INSS Stage 3 disease with either unfavorable histology or *MYCN* amplification. Diagnosis of NB was determined by biopsy of the primary lesion or a metastatic lesion or by documentation of tumor cells in a bone marrow aspirate accompanied by increased urinary catecholamine levels. Patients were initially staged by a computed tomography scan of the primary tumor site plus the chest as well as a ^{99}Tc bone scan, bilateral bone marrow aspirates and biopsies and, where available, a ^{125}I-metaiodobenzylguanidine (MIBG) scan. For assignment of risk stratification, *MYCN* amplification was determined by fluorescence in situ hybridization or Southern blotting, and specimens were reviewed for Shimada classification.

Protocols and consent forms were approved by each participation hospital's Institutional Review Board. Informed consent was obtained from the parents of each child after confirmation of diagnosis. The hospitals participating in these studies included the Dana Farber Cancer Institute, Boston, MA (DFCI), Children's Hospital of Philadelphia, PA (CHOP), Emory University, Atlanta, GA, and Primary Children's Hospital, Salt Lake City, UT. Each consecutive eligible patient presenting to the participating institutions was offered enrollment onto the protocol during the study period.

Treatments

After confirmation of diagnosis patients were begun on protocol induction therapy. For patients whose risk status was confirmed only by the finding of *MYCN* amplification after one cycle of chemotherapy, entry onto the protocol could occur at the second cycle. Bone marrow specimens were obtained at intervals during induction therapy to confirm remission of disease in the bone marrow. This was determined by both morphologic examination using Wright-Giemsa stain and NB immunocytochemistry (ICC; performed by Impath/BIS Laboratories, Reseda, CA). PBPC were collected after recovery the third cycle of chemotherapy only if ICC revealed less than 5% neuroblasts in the bone marrow. If sufficient cells were not collected after third cycle of chemotherapy, there was the option to collect further PBPC after the fourth cycle of chemotherapy. If marrow did not clear adequately after the third cycle of chemotherapy, delay of one cycle for PBPC collection was permissible. If adequate marrow clearing was not documented after the fourth cycle of chemotherapy, the patient was taken off study. After the fourth or fifth cycle of induction therapy each patient underwent resection of the primary tumor. Determination of the existence and extent of residual disease was made in conjunction with the surgeon, radiotherapist, and pathologist.

Drug doses during induction therapy are detailed in the initial report of this trial [8] and the overall treatment plan is summarized in Figure 1. Patients received daily subcutaneous human granulocyte colony stimulating factor (G-CSF) after each cycle of chemotherapy. The dose of G-CSF was 5 µg/kg during non-pheresis cycles and was increased to 10 µg/kg during pheresis cycles. The chemotherapy courses were scheduled to be 21 days apart but delays were permissible to allow recovery of the ANC to >750/µl and platelet count >75,000/µl. With the infrequent exception of patients who had a surgical and pathologic complete resection, the pre-surgical extent of primary tumor received local radiotherapy of 10.8–24 cGy before the patient proceeded to the consolidation phase of the treatment.

PBPC collections

After confirmation of adequate clearing of disease from bone marrow, patients underwent PBPC pheresis at the point when the ANC exceeded 1000/µl after the nadir. G-CSF was continued during pheresis until pheresis was complete. The pheresis plan mandated collection of three separate products. Two products were collected with a goal of 4×10^6 $CD34^+$ cells/kg (minimum 1×10^6 CD34+/kg) for each cycle of tandem HDC/SCR. Additionally, a backup product was collected with

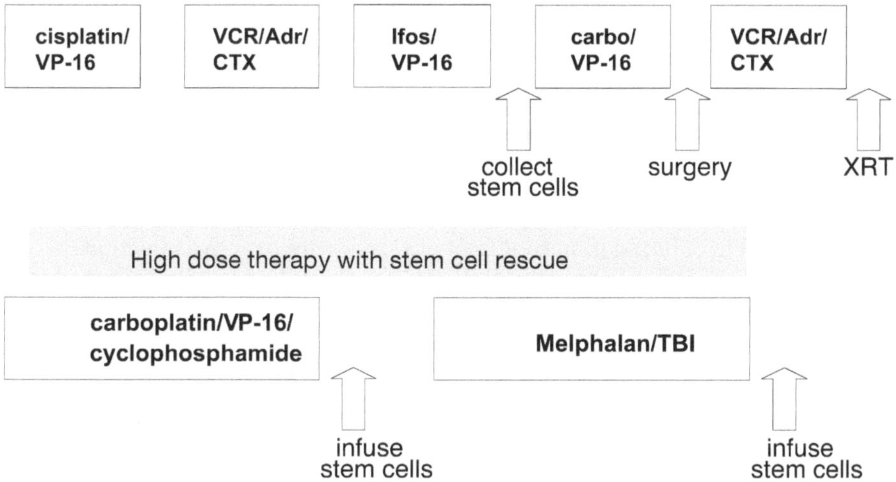

Fig. 1. Summary of induction therapy and tandem transplant protocol. VAdrC, vincristine, doxorubicin, cyclophosphamide; Ifos/VP, ifosfamide, etoposide; carbo/VP, carboplatinum, etoposide; cisplatin/VP, cisplatin, etoposide; TBI, total body irradiation; XRT, local radiotherapy.

the goal of 2 x 10^6 CD34+ cells/kg (minimum 1x10^6 $CD34^+$ cells/kg) for separate cryopreservation. In an initial feasibility phase of the protocol, the collected PBPCs were cryopreserved without further processing. After completion of this initial feasibility phase, subsequent patients at two of the institutions (DFCI and CHOP) received CD34 selected PBPC. To allow for collection of adequate numbers of $CD34^+$ cells a first day's pheresis product was held overnight and then pooled with the second day's collection. This pooled product was then CD34 selected. Initially, products underwent CD34 selection using Ceprate SC device (Cellpro, Bothell, WA). Later on in the study both stem cell laboratories switched to using the Isolex 300i device (Nexell, Irvine, CA). These devices purify $CD34^+$ stem, and progneitor cells from PBPC collections. They allow for 2–3 log depletion of CD34- cells, a population that may include possible contaminating tumor [9]. The pre-CD34 selected product was subjected to ICC and samples were also cryopreserved both pre- and post-CD34 selection for RT-PCR assessment of contaminating tumor [10]. In the earliest phase of the study some patients also had bone marrow harvested as the stem cell backup instead of PBPC. In the latter phases of the study the investigators were given the option of using unselected PBPC as the backup instead.

Consolidation HDC/SCR

After completion of induction therapy patients then went on to consolidation therapy with tandem HDC/SCR. See Figure 1 for drugs used in the conditioning regimens. Engraftment data was recorded after HDC/SCR. Neutrophil engraftment was considered to have occurred on the day post-transplant when the ANC was >500/µl. The first post-transplant day on which platelet transfusion was not required for the subsequent week was considered the day of platelet transfusion independence (PTI). The diagnosis of veno-occlusive disease (VOD) was made using standard clinical criteria [11]. In order to be eligible for HDC/SCR patients had to have had adequate clearing of bone marrow disease and collection of acceptable numbers of PBPC. There could be no evidence of disease progression (patients were fully restaged prior to consolidation). Organ function including adequate renal, cardiac and pulmonary function was assessed before HDC/SCR and patients who proceeded to consolidation could not have evidence of active infection.

In order to proceed to the second HDC/SCR patients had to have tolerated the first HDC/SCR without evidence of life threatening organ toxicity or severe VOD (VOD was considered to be severe when the total bilirubin level during transplant was greater than 10 mg/dl). The back up stem cell product had to be available for the patient to continue to the second HDC/SCR. Restaging of disease between the first and the second HDC took place only if the patient had clinical indicators of progressive disease. If they had evidence of progressive disease, they were to be removed from the study, although this did not occur. The protocol required the patients be ready for the second HDC/SCR six weeks after the first HDC/SCR, although the actual interval was sometimes up to ten days longer for scheduling reasons or to permit the completion of antibiotic treatment. Our intent was to proceed with the second HDC/SCR rapidly. The short interval between treatments was chosen to allow maximum treatment intensity. There was also the concern that any patient who had not adequately recovered within the six week interval might not be a good candidate for a second HDC procedure.

Statistical considerations

EFS was measured from the time of diagnosis to the day of relapse or progression, the day of death, in remission, or the last date upon which the patient in remission was known to be alive. The method of Kaplan and Meier [12] for incomplete data was used to estimate the EFS curves.

Results

The experience of the first 39 patients treated on this protocol has been reported [8] and the protocol has completed accrual. 62 patients were enrolled and are assessable for their response. The median age of these patients at diagnosis was 3.4 years (range 12 months to 18 years). 91% had Stage 4 disease, 42% had amplification of *MYCN* and 76% had bone metastases. Five patients with stage 3 disease were enrolled, three with *MYCN* amplification and 2 with unfavorable histology by Shimada criteria. One of the principal feasibility concerns was the ability to pherese small patients to collect stem cells. PBPC collection was successfully completed in all eligible patients. Intravenous access for pheresis in most patients was accomplished using an 8 French double lumen tunneled pheresis catheter (MedComp, Harleysville, PA). Only one patient required femoral line placement.

In some of the patients weighing less than 12 kg, long-term placement of a tunneled pheresis catheter was thought to be infeasible and a temporary pheresis catheter was placed, generally on the opposite side from the patient's tunneled double lumen catheter. Collection of $CD34^+$ cells was not age-dependent. In patients under three years 7.4×10^6 $CD34^+$ cells/kg were collected while in patients over three years we collected 7.0×10^6 $CD34^+$ cells/kg.

Figure 2 summarizes the progression of patients through the protocol. Our second feasibility concern was the ability to deliver tandem cycles of HDC/SCR in these young patients. Of the 62 patients on study, 58 were evaluable for transplant toxicity having completed at least one cycle of HDC/SCR. One patient did not experience adequate clearing of marrow disease prior to the fourth cycle of chemotherapy and was taken off study, one was taken off study prior to HDC/SCR at parental request, and 2 experienced disease progression during induction. Of these 58 patients, 51 completed both cycles of HDC/SCR. Five patients were taken off study between HDC cycles at patient or parental request and two patients developed liver toxicity that raised the concern of potential VOD on the second HDC/SCR and were taken off study.

All patients experienced expected transplant-related toxicities including mucositis and pancytopenia. One patient experienced reversible congestive heart failure and another patient developed a clinical sepsis syndrome during his conditioning during the first HDC and did not proceed to the second cycle. We were particularly concerned about the potential for VOD on the second cycle of HDC/SCR. For this reason we monitored patients closely for any evidence of VOD or other hepatic injury. Four patients experienced VOD during treatment. One patient had a mild elevation of bilirubin during the first cycle with minimal fluid retention and then had severe and ultimately fatal VOD during the second cycle.

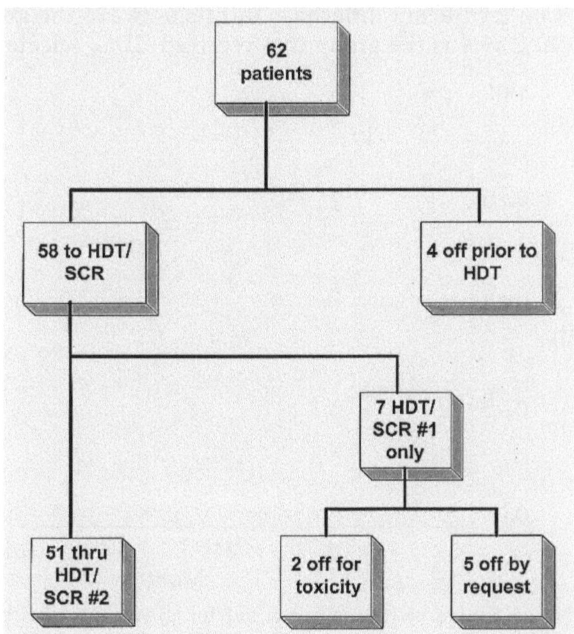

Fig. 2. Summary of patient flow through the tandem transplant protocol.

Three patients had VOD only during the second HDC/SCR. These patients were treated supportively and two of these patients received investigational defibrotide therapy. A final patient developed elevated transaminase levels during the first HDC/SCR, although there was no evidence of VOD or hyperbilirubinemia. Viral cultures revealed adenovirus infection and the transaminase levels normalized without further clinical sequelae. However, this patient did not meet the criteria needed to proceed to the second transplant. Treatment-related mortality occurred in five patients. In addition to the death from VOD described above, four deaths occurred after the second transplant procedure and after engraftment of neutrophils. One patient had an episode of Enterobacter sepsis proceeding to multiorgan system failure. A second patient developed VOD at day 14 s/p the second HDC/SCR. In the setting of improving VOD the patient then developed fatal respiratory compromise. CMV infection was noted at autopsy. The third patient experienced adenovirus sepsis and subsequently died of severe myocardial dysfunction. Finally, the fourth patient died after engraftment of rapidly progressive Epstein Barr virus lymphoproliferative disease.

Engraftment was rapid in these PBPC-supported transplants. The median day to ANC over 500/μl was 11. Platelet transfusion independence occurred at a median of 29 days. CD34 selection did not change the speed of engraftment. One patient required infusion of his back up stem cell product when he had not shown signs of hematopoietic recovery on day 28 following his second HDC. This was despite rapid engraftment during his first HDC. He then received the back up stem cell product on day +31 after which engraftment occurred on day +55.

The median follow up of these patients is 24 months. 42 of 62 patients have no evaluable disease, there have been five toxic deaths and 15 patients have experienced relapse or progressive disease. Three-year EFS is 63% (90% ci 50-74%) (Fig. 3a). There is no significant difference in EFS between the group that received unselected PBPC versus the group that received CD34 selected PBPC (Fig. 3b), or between

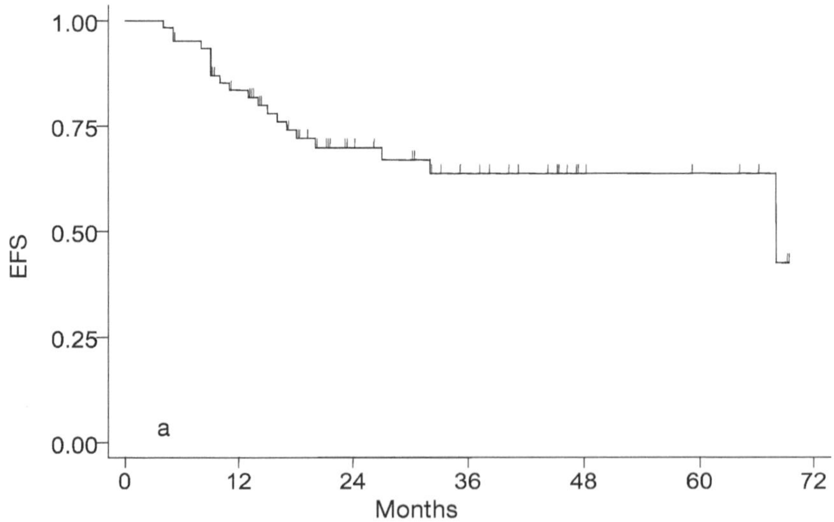

Fig. 3a. Kaplan-Meier analysis of EFS for all 62 patients with high-risk NB

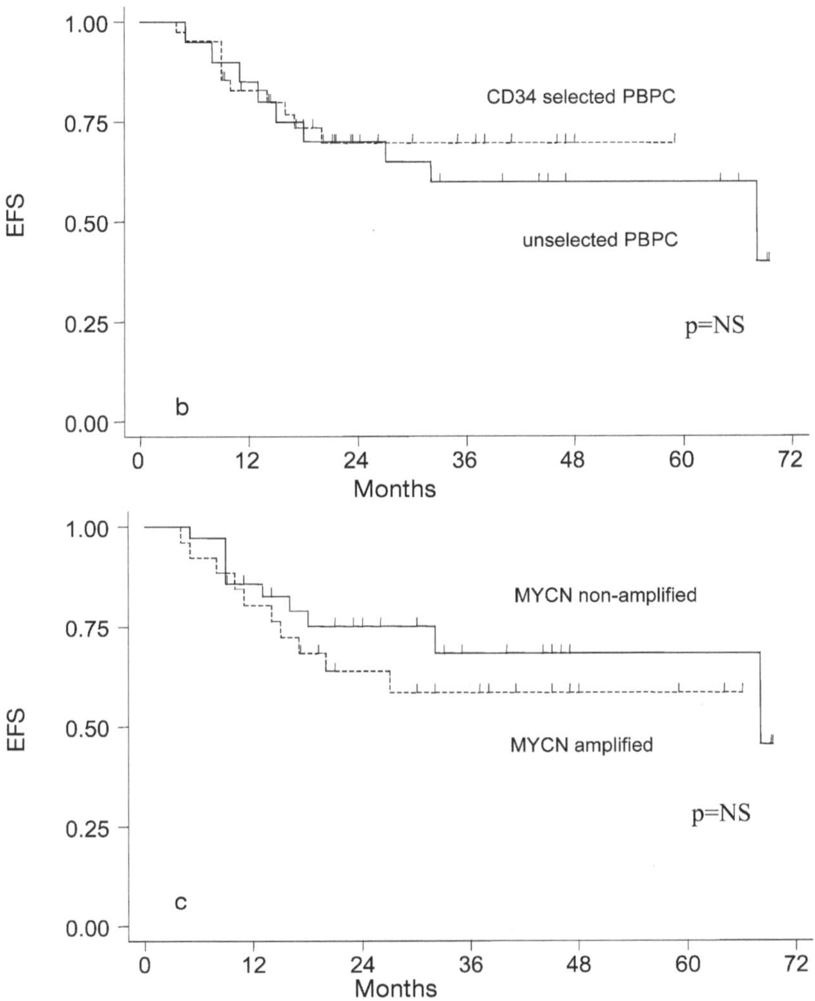

Fig. 3b, c. *b* Kaplan-Meier analysis of EFS for patients supported with unselected PBPC (solid line, N = 20) or CD34+ selected PBPC (dashed line, N = 42). Patients with events prior to transplant are included in these curves according to intent to treat; *c* Kaplan-Meier analysis of EFS for patients with MYCN amplified tumors (dashed line, N = 26) or MYCN non-amplified tumors (solid line, N = 36).

patients with *MYCN* amplification or no amplification (4 patients with unknown *MYCN* status are included in the latter group; Fig. 3c).

Discussion

Here, we update the first major experience with PBPC supported tandem transplantation in children. We have found this treatment approached to be feasible even in small children, with sufficient PBPC collected to support tandem courses of HDC/SCR. Toxicities of the regimen have been as expected with one death from VOD. Overall treatment related mortality on this study was 8% which is similar to prior single transplant studies [1].

Experience with autologous transplantation largely using bone marrow as a stem cell source has been variable. The Children's Cancer Group has used bone marrow transplantation with purged bone marrow support in patients with advanced stage NB and survival among the patients who received bone marrow transplantation (38%) was better than expected from historical controls [13,14]. Use of allogeneic bone marrow transplantation in this setting provided no survival advantage. More recently, the CCG 3891 study demonstrated a superior event-free survival rate in the patients treated with autologous bone marrow transplantation compared to continuation chemotherapy. This study also demonstrated improved survival in patients receiving cis-retinoic acid after completion of their chemotherapy, with an estimated EFS of 40% in the best arm of the study [1]. Others have explored the use of PBPC as stem cell support instead of marrow in high-risk NB, with variable results but generally improved toxicity and more rapid engraftment [15-19]. Our experience in this limited institution pilot study compares favorably to these results. The use of peripheral blood progenitor cells to support HDC has allowed the design of a feasible tandem transplant regimen. Prior experience with tandem transplantation using bone marrow as a stem cell source was infeasible because of high transplant-related mortality rate [20]. Another aspect of the study described here was the use of CD34 selection in order to purge tumor from stem cell products. The results of analyses of tumor depletion using this technique are described in the accompanying report by Ash et al.

In summary, we have shown the feasibility of treating patients with high-risk NB with intensive induction chemotherapy followed by tandem HDC/SCR in rapid sequence. Further followup in this group of patients will be needed to determine whether this approach has an impact on long term event-free survival, however, early results are encouraging. In an attempt to determine the impact of tandem stem cell transplantation on patients with high-risk NB, the Children's Oncology Group is planning a randomized trial comparing single and tandem HDC/SCR in these patients.

References

1. Matthay KK, Villablanca JG, Seeger RC, Stram DO, Harris RE, Ramsay NK, Swift P, Shimada H, Black CT, Brodeur GM, Gerbing RB, Reynolds CP. Treatment of high-risk neuroblastoma with intensive chemotherapy, radiotherapy, autologous bone marrow transplantation, and 13-cis-retinoic acid. N Engl J Med. 1999;341:1165-1173
2. Broun ER, Sridhara R, Sledge GW, Loesch D, Kneebone PH, Hanna M, Hromas R, Cornetta K, Einhorn LH. Tandem autotransplantation for the treatment of metastatic breast cancer. J Clin Oncol. 1995;13:2050-2055
3. Lotz JP, Bouleuc C, Andre T, Touboul E, Macovei C, Hannoun L, Lefranc JP, Houry S, Uzan S, Izrael V. Tandem high-dose chemotherapy with ifosfamide, carboplatin, and teniposide with autologous bone marrow transplantation for the treatment of poor prognosis common epithelial ovarian carcinoma. Cancer. 1996;77:2250-2259

4. Cohn SL, Moss TJ, Hoover M, Katzenstein HM, Haut PR, Morgan ER, Green AA, Kletzel M. Treatment of poor-risk neuroblastoma patients with high-dose chemotherapy and autologous peripheral stem cell rescue. Bone Marrow Transplant. 1997;20:543-551
5. Haut PR, Cohn S, Morgan E, Hubbell M, Danner-Koptik K, Olszewski M, Schaff M, Kletzel M. Efficacy of autologous peripheral blood stem cell (PBSC) harvest and engraftment after ablative chemotherapy in pediatric patients. Biol Blood Marrow Transplant. 1998;4:38-42
6. Diaz MA, Villa M, Madero L, Benito A, Alegre A, Fernandez-Ranada JM. Analysis of engraftment kinetics in pediatric patients undergoing autologous PBPC transplantation. J Hematother. 1998;7:367-373
7. Brodeur GM, Pritchard J, Berthold F, Carlsen NLT, Castel V, Castleberry RP, De Bernardi B, Evans AE, Favrot M, Hedborg F, Kaneko M, Kemshead J, Lampert F, Lee REJ, Look AT, Pearson ADJ, Philip T, Roald B, Sawada T, Seeger RC, Tsuchida Y, Voute PA. Revisions of the international criteria for neuroblastoma diagnosis, staging, and response to treatment. J Clin Oncol. 1993;11:1466-1477
8. Grupp SA, Stern JW, Bunin N, Nancarrow C, Ross AA, Mogul M, Adams R, Grier HE, Gorlin JB, Shamberger R, Marcus K, Neuberg D, Weinstein HJ, Diller L. Tandem high dose therapy in rapid sequence for children with high-risk neuroblastoma. J Clin Onc. 2000;18:2567-2575
9. Shpall EJ, Jones RB, Bearman SI, Franklin WA, Archer PG, Curiel T, Bitter M, Claman HN, Stemmer SM, Purdy M, Myers SE, Hami L, Taffs S, Heimfeld S, Hallagan J, Berenson RJ. Transplantation of enriched CD34-positive autologous marrow into breast cancer patients following high-dose chemotherapy: influence of CD34-positive peripheral-blood progenitors and growth factors on engraftment. J Clin Oncol. 1994;12:28-36
10. Donovan J, Temel J, Zuckerman A, Gribben J, Fang J, Pierson G, Ross A, Diller L, Grupp SA. CD34 selection as a stem cell purging strategy for neuroblastoma: pre-clinical and clinical studies. Med. Ped. Oncol. 2000;in press
11. Bearman SI, Anderson GL, Mori M, Hinds MS, Shulman HM, McDonald GB. Venoocclusive disease of the liver: development of a model for predicting fatal outcome after marrow transplantation. J Clin Oncol. 1993;11:1729-1736
12. Kaplan EL, Meier P. Nonparametric estimation from incomplete observations. J Am Stat Assoc. 1958;53:457-481
13. Matthay KK, Harris R, Reynolds CP, Shimada H, Black T, Stram DO, Seeger RC. Improved event-free survival for autologous bone marrow transplantation vs chemotherapy in neuroblastoma: a Childrens Cancer Group study. Med Pediatr Oncol. 1998;31:191, O-197
14. Matthay KK. Impact of myeloablative therapy with bone marrow transplantation in advanced neuroblastoma. Bone Marrow Transplant. 1996;18:S21-24
15. Kletzel M, Longino R, Danner K, Olszewski M, Moss T. Peripheral blood stem cell rescue in children with advanced stage neuroblastoma. Prog Clin Biol Res. 1994;389:513-519
16. Kletzel M, Abella EM, Sandler ES, Williams LL, Ogden AK, Pollock BH, Wall DA. Thiotepa and cyclophosphamide with stem cell rescue for consolidation therapy for children with high-risk neuroblastoma: a phase I/II study of the Pediatric Blood and Marrow Transplant Consortium. J Pediatr Hematol Oncol. 1998;20:49-54
17. Handgretinger R, Greil J, Schurmann U, Lang P, Gonzalez-Ramella O, Schmidt I, Fuhrer R, Niethammer D, Klingebiel T. Positive selection and transplantation of peripheral $CD34^+$ progenitor cells: feasibility and purging efficacy in pediatric patients with neuroblastoma. J Hematother. 1997;6:235-242
18. Kanold J, Yakouben K, Tchirkov A, Carret A-S, Vannier J-P, LeGall E, Bordigoni P, Demeocq F. Long-term results of $CD34^+$ cell transplantation in children with neuroblastoma. Med Pediatr Oncol. 2000;35:1-7
19. Kanold J, Yakouben K, Tchirkov A, Halle P, Carret AS, Berger M, Rapatel C, deLumley L, Vannier JP, Plantaz D, LeGall E, Lutz P, Mechinaud F, Rialland X, Combaret V, Bordigoni P, Deméocq F. Long-term follow-up after $CD34^+$ cell transplantation in children with neuroblastoma. Blood. 1998;92:445a (abstr 1842)
20. Philip T, Ladenstein R, Zucker JM, Pinkerton R, Bouffet E, Louis D, Siegert W, Bernard JL, Frappaz D, Coze C. Double megatherapy and autologous bone marrow transplantation for advanced neuroblastoma: the LMCE2 Study. Br J Cancer. 1993;67:119-127

Anti-Angiogenesis

Angiogenesis Inhibitor TNP-470 During Bone Marrow Transplant and in Minimal Residual Disease

J. Fang[1], J. W. Stern[1], S. Shusterman[1], K. Alcorn, G. Pierson[1], R. Barr[1], B. Pawel[2], L. Diller[3], J. M. Maris[1], and S. A. Grupp[1]

[1]Division of Oncology; [2]Division of Pathology, Department of Pediatrics, Children's Hospital of Philadelphia, University of Pennsylvania School of Medicine, Philadelphia, PA; [3]Pediatric Oncology, Dana Farber Cancer Institute, Boston, MA

Abstract

High-dose therapy with stem cell rescue is a treatment option for patients with advanced solid tumors. Although this approach has promise for some pediatric cancers, especially neuroblastoma, it is limited by the risk of relapse post transplant, as well as concern about possible reinfused tumor cells in autologous stem cell products. Anti-angiogenic agents given during and after recovery from high-dose therapy with stem cell rescue may decrease the risk of relapse. Additionally, such agents may have their greatest therapeutic effect when administered at a point of minimal residual disease, rather than to treat bulky tumor. TNP-470 is an anti-angiogenic agent now in clinical trials. We have tested TNP-470 in the treatment of neuroblastoma in a mouse xenograft model, and demonstrate that it is most effective when given at lowest disease burden. Additionally, and to assess the feasibility of using anti-angiogenic agents during the period of post-transplant hematopoietic recovery, we have developed a model of stem cell transplant in mice. Mice were treated with TNP-470 and assessed for survival and engraftment. Both treated and control mice demonstrated reliable multilineage engraftment as well as normal lymphoid maturation with no excess mortality in the treated group. This indicates that inhibitors of angiogenesis do not adversely impact engraftment after stem cell transplantation and suggests a clinical study design in which such agents might best be employed in the immediate after stem cell transplant.

Introduction

Intensified chemotherapy has improved survival rates for some patients with high-risk solid tumors, including patients with relapsed Hodgkin's disease and neuroblastoma [1, 2]. Increases in dose-intensification have been rendered feasible by improved supportive care, use of hematopoietic growth factors and use of peripheral blood progenitor cells (or „stem cells") to allow rapid return of marrow function after myeloablative chemotherapy. This approach has been

---

Supported by: WW Smith Charitable Trust (SG), University of Pennsylvania Cancer Center (SG), K12 Clinical Oncology Research Career Development Award (SS) and a Joseph Stokes Research Institute High Risk/High Impact Grant (JMM).

termed megatherapy or high-dose chemotherapy with stem cell rescue. However, even the most dose-intensified approaches are still limited by the risk of relapse after the procedure.

One major risk factor for relapse after high-dose chemotherapy with stem cell rescue is presence of bulk disease prior to the stem cell procedure. Even for patients who are in complete remission, however, relapse is still a concern. For these patients, relapse may arise from minimal residual disease within the patient or tumor inadvertently collected with the stem cell product and later reinfused. There is indirect evidence suggesting that reinfused tumor may contribute to relapse. In neuroblastoma, gene-marked tumor cells infused with bone marrow used to support high-dose chemotherapy can be detected at sites of subsequent relapse [3, 4]. In patients with lymphoma who undergo stem cell transplantation, molecular detection of tumor in the stem cell product is a predictor for relapse [5]. However, no trial has shown an advantage for patients who receive tumor-purged stem cell products.

In order to translate increase rates of complete remission provided by intensified chemotherapy into further improvements in survival, complementary approaches are needed. The anti-angiogenic agents may represent one such approach. Anti-angiogenic therapy has shown promising results in animal studies [6–10] and has been relatively nontoxic in early human clinical trials. Although phase I development has focused on treatment of relapsed patients with bulk disease, the angiogenesis inhibitors may prove to have greatest efficacy when given in the state of minimal residual disease, after achieving the best result possible with chemotherapy. Because these drugs have their effect at the level of normal endothelium [11], clonal evolution or induced chemotherapy resistance within the tumor should not affect response to anti-angiogenic agents [10]. Given post stem cell infusion in the setting of high-dose chemotherapy with stem cell rescue, anti-angiogenic agents have potential to lessen the risk of relapse from minimal residual disease, whether within the patient or infused with the stem cell support.

There are several reasons why neuroblastoma is a particularly attractive target for anti-angiogenic treatment after stem cell transplant. First, neuroblastoma is a highly vascular solid tumor and the vascularity is correlated with advanced disease features and poor outcome [21]. Second, on a molecular level, increased expression of the angiogenic factors VEGF, bFGF, and PDGF as well as the endothelial integrins $\alpha_v\beta_3$ and $\alpha_v\beta_3$ are also associated with advanced disease features [28,29]. Last, antiangiogenic drugs have low potential for toxicity and resistance because they specifically target endothelial cells and would theoretically not add to treatment-related morbidity [10].

In order to explore the feasibility and efficacy of a strategy employing angiogenesis inhibitors post-transplant in minimal residual disease, we have employed mouse xenograft and stem cell transplant models. The angiogenesis inhibitor used in these studies, TNP-470, is currently in clinical trials [24, 25]. TNP-470 is active in mouse xenograft models in bulk disease, with even greater efficacy apparent in the setting of minimal residual disease [12–14].

Materials and Methods

Donors, recipients and preparative regimen

Transgenic mice expressing a human IgM transgene (Tg[1]) in the FVB background were used as the donor source of bone marrow stem cells for transplantation. Marrow was collected from Tg+ mice from femurs flushed with sterile PBS. Recipients were FVB mice (Jax, Bar Harbor, ME) or Tg negative littermates of the Tg positive donors, treated in groups of 5–8 animals/intervention. Recipients received total body irradiation (TBI) in an M38-1 Irradiator (Isomedix) at a dose rate of 2.7 Gy/min in a mixed/split fashion with a 3 hour interfraction interval to allow a higher dose of radiation without significant gastrointestinal toxicity. After completion of TBI, mice received stem cells via tail vein injection. The mice were maintained in a humidity and temperature controlled area in autoclaved microisolator cages and fed ad libitum and provided acidified water. Mice were assessed three times weekly after stem cell infusion. All studies were approved by the Animal Care and Use Committee of the Children's Hospital of Philadelphia.

Xenografting

Four to six week old athymic (nu/nu) mice (National Cancer Institute, Frederick, MD) were used. 10^7 tumor cells were suspended in 0.2 ml of Matrigel (Collaborative Biomedical Products, Bedford, MA). Cell suspensions were injected SQ into the right flank of nude mice. Tumor growth was observed within 10–14 days following inoculation in 95% of animals. Tumor measurements were made by Vernier caliper three times a week and tumor volumes were calculated using the ellipsoid formula: length x width x height x 0.52 [27]. Mice were examined daily for signs of progressive disease and weights were followed three times weekly.

Drugs and Treatments

TNP-470 was provided by TAP Pharmaceuticals (Deerfield, IL) and stored in the dark at 4°C. Prior to use, TNP-470 was reconstituted in sterile saline and stored in daily aliquots at -80°C. TNP-470 was used at a dose of 20-100 mg/kg given SQ three times per week or at a dose of 20, 30, or 40 mg/kg/week given by continuous IP infusion using an Alzet infusion pump (Alza Co., Palo Alto, CA). For the stem cell transplant experiments, the continuous TNP-470 infusion began on the day prior to transplant to allow for pump implantation (see below).

For xenograft experiments, TNP-470 treatment was continued until the tumors of the control animals exceeded 3.0 cm^3 when all mice were sacrificed and a representative sample was autopsied. Randomization to TNP-470 or control was

[1] Abbreviations used: bone marrow, BM; bone marrow transplant, BMT; intraperitoneal, IP; subcutaneously, SQ; total body irradiation, TBI; transgene, Tg.

balanced according to tumor size and/or mouse weight at treatment initiation. Cyclophosphamide (Mead Johnson, New Jersey) was reconstituted with sterile water (20 mg/ml) and stored at 4°C. The dose of cyclophosphamide was 450 mg/kg divided into 3 doses over 6 days, given by intraperitoneal injection. Dexamethasone (1 mg/kg) (American Pharmaceutical Partners Inc., Los Angeles, CA) and ondansetron (3 mg/kg) (Glaxo Wellcome Inc., Research Triangle Park, NC) were given subcutaneously 30 minutes prior to cyclophosphamide administration for gastric protection. Ketamine (Fort Dodge Animal Health, Fort Dodge, IO) at a dose of 150 mg/kg and Xylazine (Bayer Co., Shawnee Mission, KS) at a dose of 8 mg/kg were used for sedation and analgesia during Alzet infusion pump placement.

Alzet infusion pump placement

Using sterile technique following anesthesia, a 1 cm midline abdominal incision was made and 14 day Alzet micro-osmotic pumps (0.25µl/hr, model 1002) containing either TNP-470 or saline were placed intraperitoneally. The peritoneum and skin were then secured separately using 4–0 vicryl suture. The animals were allowed to recover overnight and then subjected to xenografting the same day or TBI and stem cell infusion on the following day.

Cell and Bone marrow culture

Light density cells separated by density gradient centrifugation (Lymphocyte Separation Medium, ICN Pharmaceutical, Costa Mesa, CA) from normal human BM donors were plated in methylcellulose medium with recombinant cytokines. This medium, MethoCult GF (Stem Cell Technologies, Vancouver, Canada), contains stem cell factor, GM-CSF, IL-3 and erythropoietin. 5×10^4 BM cells/dish were cultured with TNP-470 at concentrations ranging from 1 µg/ml to 1 mg/ml, with duplicate cultures at each dose. The plates were scored after 14 days of culture, enumerating colony-forming unit granulocyte/macrophage (CFU-GM), CFU-mix, CFU-erythrocyte and burst-forming unit erythrocyte (CFU-E and BFU-E). The CHP-134 cell line was derived from the primary tumor of a patient with high-risk neuroblastoma [26]. The cells were grown in RPMI-1640 containing 10% fetal bovine serum and L-glutamine, 1% penicillin and streptomycin, and 0.05% gentamicin.

Analysis of engraftment

Engraftment of donor stem cells was demonstrated by both flow cytometry and by polymerase chain reaction (PCR). Following cervical dislocation, BM and splenocytes were collected from recipient mice. Analysis was performed after red cell lysis by NH_4Cl. For flow cytometric analysis of lymphoid engraftment, Tg IgM expressed only in B cells derived from the donor was detected by antibodies recognizing human IgM (RAHM; Jackson ImmunoResearch, West Grove, PA) and mouse CD45R (B220, Pharmingen, Torreyana, CA) in a two-color protocol on a FACS Caliber cytometer (Becton-Dickinson, Franklin Lakes, NJ). Splenocytes from untransplanted Tg- and Tg+ mice provided negative and positive controls, respectively. Lymphoid engraftment was defined as the percentage of lymphoid cells in spleen and BM that were B220/RAHM positive. In addition to flow cytometry, genomic DNA from tail snips, blood, BM and splenocytes was analyzed by polymerase chain reaction for the presence of the transgene, using a procedure and primers previously reported [15]. The transgene is detectable by PCR in all donor-derived cells in the recipient, while the tail snips of Tg- mice provided a negative control. Genomic DNA was also isolated from splenic and peripheral blood T cells. Splenic T cells were isolated using the Cellect T isolation column (Biotex, Edmonton, Canada) according to the manufacturer's protocol.

Peripheral blood T cells were sorted on the FACS Vantage (Becton-Dickson) after staining with antibodies recognizing mouse CD3 (Pharmingen). Recovery of peripheral blood counts was also analyzed. Blood was collected from cardiac puncture and placed in EDTA tubes. Analysis was then performed using a HemeVet instrument using mouse-specific parameters. Hemoglobin was measured and white blood cells (WBC) and platelets were enumerated.

Results

Effect of TNP-470 on neuroblastoma xenograft growth

Initial experiments assessed the effect of TNP-470 given by intermittent SQ injection. This treatment was initiated when the mean xenografted (CHP-134 cells) tumor volume reached 0.17 cm^3. There was a significant difference in tumor growth rate between the mice receiving TNP-470 and the mice receiving saline (data not shown) with a T/C on day 16 of 0.3. A second cohort of mice received either TNP-470 or saline by continuous IP infusion when the mean tumor volume reached 0.17 cm^3. TNP-470 was given at 3 doses (20, 30, and 40 mg/kg/week). Mice receiving the highest dose of TNP-470 became severely cachectic shortly after the initiation of treatment and died by treatment day 16. Mice receiving TNP-470 at 30 mg/kg/week had marked inhibition of tumor growth but also had severe weight loss (mean = 21% of body weight). Mice receiving TNP-470 at a dose of 20 mg/kg/week had a significant inhibition of tumor growth compared to saline-treated mice (data not shown) with a T/C on day 16 of 0.4. These mice had mild weight loss (mean = 12% of body weight) but no other signs of acute toxicity.

In subsequent experiments, we focused on subclinical tumors, in an attempt to model minimal residual disease. Two approaches were used. First, mice with mean tumor volumes of 0.35 cm^3 were treated with cyclophosphamide (day 0). On day 10 following cyclophosphamide when tumors were inapparent or difficult to palpate, the mice were randomly assigned to receive either subcutaneous TNP-470 or saline. There was a significant inhibition of tumor growth in mice receiving TNP-470 compared to saline (Fig. 1a; $P < 0.001$) with a T/C at day 30 of 0.1. Second, mice were randomly distributed to receive either TNP-470 or saline

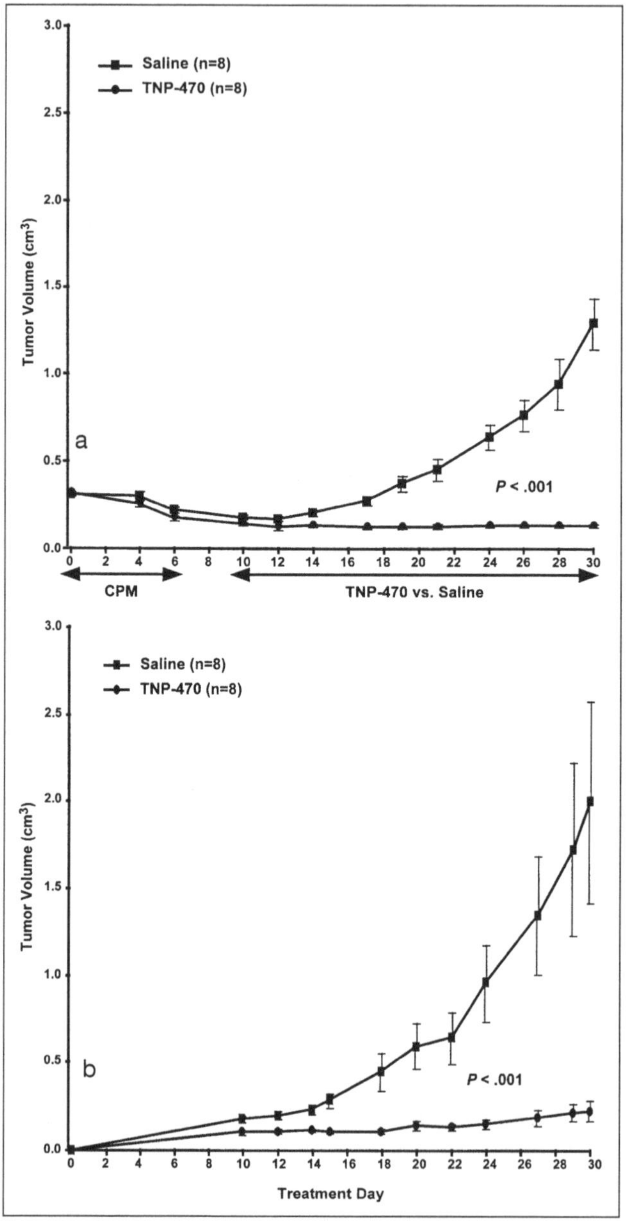

Fig. 1a, b. Effect of TNP-470 on subclinical disease. *a* Mean tumor volumes of mice receiving cyclophosphamide (CPM) followed by either TNP-470 or saline. Cyclophosphamide was started on day 0 at a dose of 450 mg/kg divided into 3 doses over 6 days. Mice were randomized to receive TNP-470 (100 mg/kg/dose subcutaneously 3 times weekly) or saline at day 10. The T/C at day 30 was 0.1. *b* Mean tumor volume of mice receiving TNP-470 (100 mg/kg/dose subcutaneously 3 times weekly) or saline 12 hours following xenograft inoculation (T/C at day 30 = 0.1).

12 hours following placement of CHP-134 xenografts. The mice receiving saline had rapid tumor growth, while those receiving TNP-470 formed small tumors with markedly reduced growth velocity (Fig. 1b; $p < 0.001$). The T/C at day 30 was 0.1. The only toxicity seen in this experiment was local skin irritation in mice receiving TNP-470.

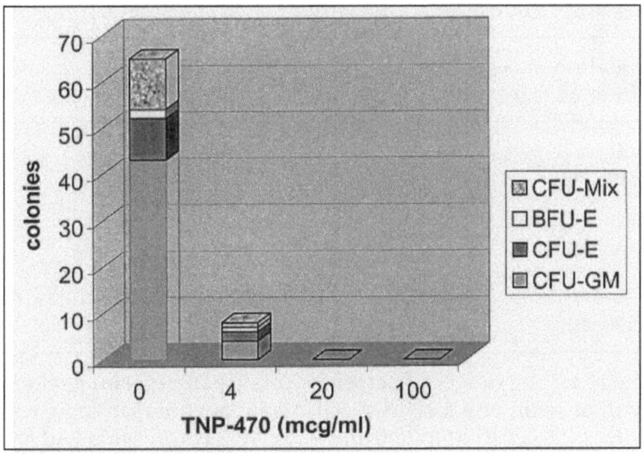

Fig. 2. TNP-470 at high concentrations is inhibitory for in-vitro colony formation from BM hematopoietic progenitors. BM cells were cultured in duplicate in standard methylcellulose medium supplemented with growth factors with the indicated concentrations of TNP-470. These results are representative of three experiments.

Effect of TNP-470 on bone marrow colony-forming cells

Although hematologic toxicity has not been described in the TNP-470 phase I trials [24, 25], there is one report of *in-vitro* evidence of BM toxicity [16]. In order to confirm this finding, we investigated the effect of relatively high concentrations of TNP-470 (0–100 µg/ml) on growth of human hematopoietic progenitors in standard methylcellulose culture. As shown in Figure 2, inhibition of colony formation in the presence of TNP-470 was observed both for myeloid and erythroid colonies. 4 µg/ml of TNP-470 caused >80% inhibition of colony formation and higher doses caused complete inhibition of colony-forming cells. Although this assay is not necessarily predictive of *in-vivo* BM toxicity, the result emphasizes the need to develop a pre-clinical model of stem cell transplantation to assess the effect of anti-angiogenic agents on engraftment.

Validating the stem cell transplant model

Our goal in developing a model of stem cell transplant in which to test the effects of angiogenesis inhibitors on engraftment was to define a dose of TBI that was lethal without stem cell rescue, followed by defining a threshold stem cell dose that reliably provided engraftment. The lethal dose of radiation was determined by tail vein injection of 0 or 5 x 10^6 BM cells after varying doses of TBI. As shown in Table 1, mortality with and without marrow support was investigated at TBI doses levels of 500 cGy (300 cGy followed by 200 cGy), 700 cGy (400/300) and 900 cGy (500/400). Mice given 900 cGy had 80-100% mortality when no stem cell support was given and only 0–12.5% mortality when 5 x 10^6 BM cells were infused.

Having chosen the TBI dose of 900 cGy for further studies, we then sought a minimum stem cell dose that would reliably provide engraftment in most recipients. Choosing such a threshold stem cell dose would increase the likelihood of demonstrating a small effect of TNP-470 on engraftment. For these experiments, engraftment was defined as >5% Tg+ B cells in the spleen or BM as de-

Table 1. TBI dose with and without stem cell support

TBI dose in cGy (fraction size)	Mortality – no support	Mortality – marrow support
500 (300, 200)	10–25%	0
700 (400, 300)	50–60%	10%
900 (500, 400)	100%	0-12.5%

Data indicate ranges of percent mortality in experimental groups given the indicated TBI dose with or without 5 x 10^6 BM cells to support hematologic recovery. 8–10 recipient mice/group with 2 (500 cGy) or 3 (700 and 900 cGy) groups evaluated at each dose.

Table 2. Relationship of BM cell dose to engraftment and mortality

BM dose (x10^6 cells)	Mortality	Engraftment
0	100%	NA
0.5	60–80%	0–20%
1	40%	100%
2	8–37.5%	75–100%
3	0–17%	100%
5	0–20%	80–100%

Data indicate ranges of percent mortality in experimental groups given 900 cGy TBI followed by the indicated dose of BM cells. 5-8 recipient mice/group with 2-3 groups evaluated at each dose. NA = not applicable.

tected by flow cytometry on d+28 post stem cell infusion (d+28). Lethally irradiated mice were injected with BM doses ranging from 0 to 5 x 10^6 cells in 1 x 10^6 dose intervals. Mortality was determined by observation and engraftment of B cells was determined at each dose level by flow cytometry (Table 2). A cell dose of 2–3 x 10^6 stem cells per mouse was found to have a 8-40% mortality with 75–100% rate of BM engraftment thus assuring consistent engraftment at a minimum cell dose. The radiation and cell doses established a baseline that was used in TNP-470 experiments.

Effect of TNP-470 on engraftment

Several dose levels of TNP-470 were explored to assess any effect on BM engraftment and engraftment kinetics. These dosing regimens are summarized in Table 3. Immediately following lethal irradiation and tail vein injection of Tg+ BM cells, recipient mice were given either TNP-470 or saline starting on d0. Dose schedules were also varied from a single dose at the time of stem cell infusion to an initial dose

Table 3. TNP-470 Dose Levels

Dose Level	Dose on Day 0	Subsequent dose and schedule
1	20 mg/kg	20 mg/kg q M, W, F
2	100 mg/kg	none
3	100 mg/kg	20 mg/kg q M, W, F
4	100 mg/kg	100 mg/kg q M, W, F
Continuous infusion	10 mg/kg/week starting on d-1	

on d0 followed by administration of TNP-470 or saline 3 times a week (Table 3). Mice were initially sacrificed on d+28–32 at all dose levels. Comparative kinetics were then further analyzed by sacrificing groups of mice at d+21, +24, and +28 at dose level 3.

Overall survival at all dose levels was 73% for mice treated with placebo and 66% for TNP-470 treated animals (Fig. 3). When analysis was completed at dose level 1 (20 mg/kg on do and then thrice weekly) survival among treated mice was 57% and 64% for controls. Furthermore, for dose level 2, (100 mg/kg on do only) 71% of treated mice survived to experiment completion while 76% of con-

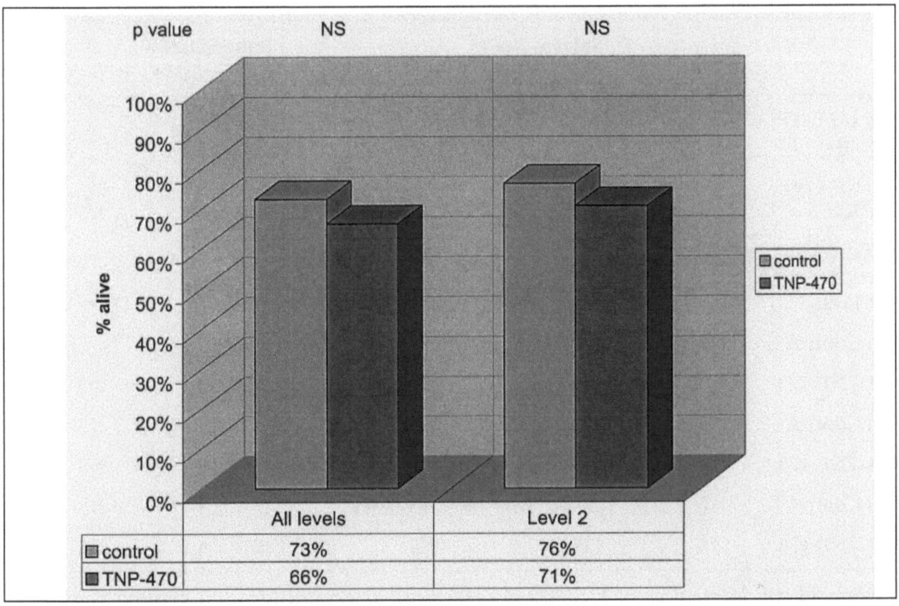

Fig. 3. Survival after stem cell transplant in TNP-470-treated and control mice. Overall survival after stem cell rescue at all dose levels (see Table 3 for details of dosing) is indicated on the right. Survival after stem cell rescue at dose level 2 (a single dose of TNP-470 on the day of stem cell rescue) is also separately indicated. These data represent the average lymphoid engraftment of at least 3 experiments per dose level, with 5–8 mice per group. The differences between treatment and control are not statistically significant.

trol mice were alive at d+28–32, statistically not significant. At the doses tested, these data provide no indication of a dose-dependent effect of TNP-470 on post-bone marrow transplant (BMT) survival. Toxicities overall were minimal, although the treated mice at dose level 4 (100 mg/kg 3 x/week) experienced greater weight loss than the control animals and showed evidence of skin irritation at the injection sites.

Lymphocyte engraftment was not affected by treatment with TNP-470. When analyzed by flow cytometry to determine the percentage of B lymphocytes expressing the donor-origin transgenic IgM (B220+/IgM+), TNP-470 treated and control transplanted mice expressed similar percentages of Tg IgM+ cells in spleen and BM (Table 4).

Engraftment kinetics were then explored at dose level 3 (100 mg/kg on d0, followed by 20 mg/kg 3 times/wk). Splenic reconstitution in treated animals at d+21, +24 and +28 was comparable to control. BM engraftment for TNP-470 exposed mice was significantly better than controls at d+21, though this difference disappeared at d+24 and +28 (Table 4).

We also performed PCR on various cell populations to detect cells that carry the Tg. The transgene is detectable in any cell derived from the graft, regardless of lineage (B cells or non-B cells). In Figure 4a, DNA from BM and splenocytes

Table 4. Lymphoid engraftment after stem cell rescue[1].

	N=	Spleen B220+/IgM+	p=	Bone Marrow B220+/IgM+	p=
D 28 s/p BMT Control	54	11% ± 1.2[2]		20% ± 1.4	
All TNP-470 dose levels	54	14% ± 1.4	**NS**	22% ± 1.8	NS
Engraftment kinetics, dose level 3					
D 21 Control	8	12% ± 4.2		15% ± 2.5	
D 21 TNP-470	5	13% ± 2.8	NS	**27% ± 4.1**	**.03**
D 24 Control	6	22% ± 5.3	NS	28% + 4.8	NS
D 24 TNP-470	6	31% ± 5.4	NS	25% ± 2.7	NS
D 28 Control	10	9% ± 1.1	NS	23% ± 4.1	NS
D 28 TNP-470	14	11% ± 2.0	NS	28% ± 4.2	NS

[1] Lymphoid engraftment at all TNP-470 dose levels as determined by flow cytometry is indicated in the upper half of the table. Engraftment kinetics at dose level 3 are indicated in the lower half of the table. Bone marrow and splenic reconstitution with donor-derived cells were measured at d+21, +24 and +28 post BMT.

[2] Mean ± SEM. Only the value indicated in bold is significantly different from control. Recipient mice were assayed for engraftment by detection of the IgM transgene derived from donor stem cells. Percentage of B220+/Tg IgM+ cells in the lymphoid size/granularity gate are indicated.

from transplanted mice treated with TNP-470 or saline were analyzed for the presence of the transgene by PCR. The transgene was detected in all samples analyzed, regardless of treatment with TNP-470. Tail DNA from a Tg- animal provided a negative control, and BM and spleen from a Tg+ animal was used as a positive control. As seen in Figure 4b, T cells were isolated from spleen and peripheral blood of transplanted animals one month after transplant and subjected

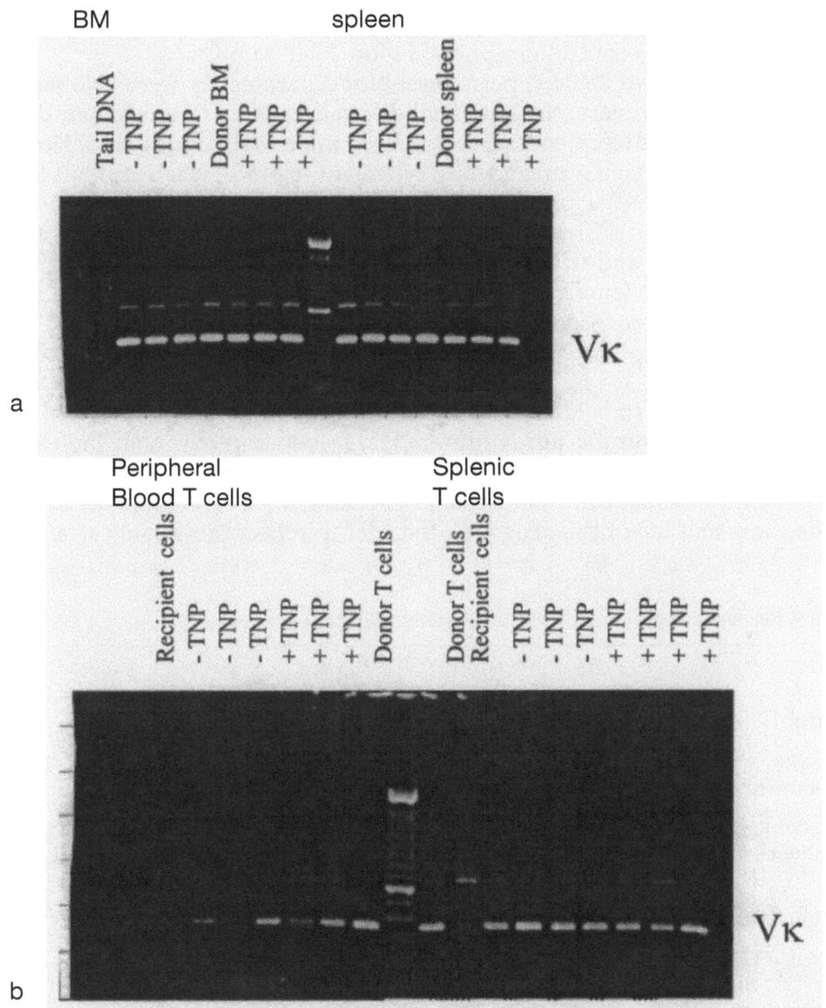

Fig. 4a,b. PCR analysis of Tg expression in BM, spleen and peripheral blood. *a* Genomic DNA was made from BM cells and splenocytes depleted of red blood cells. The transgene was then detected by PCR (Vk). *b* T cells were flow sorted from peripheral blood or column purified from spleen and then subjected to PCR to detect the transgene. Tail DNA from the Tg- recipient pro vided the negative control, while BM, spleen and splenic T cells from a Tg+ donor provided positive controls for expression of the transgene.

to PCR detection of the Tg. For peripheral blood, T cells were isolated after Ficoll separation of the mononuclear cell fraction using the FACS Vantage cell sorter to sort $CD3^+$ cells. For splenocytes, T cells were isolated using a mouse T cell isolation column. Cytometric analysis of the splenic T cells showed that the T cells were 92–95% $CD3^+$ after column isolation (data not shown). Post-sort analysis of peripheral blood T cells was not possible because of the extremely small number of cells isolated. Again, repopulation of the T cell lineage with donor-derived cells was seen in both TNP-470-treated and control animals, with the Tg detected in all splenic T cell samples, 3/3 TNP-470-treated peripheral blood T cell samples, and 2/3 control peripheral blood T cell samples.

As summarized in Table 5, peripheral blood parameters were also assessed for hematologic recovery. No statistical differences were found in hemoglobin or platelet count between control and treated mice (data not shown). However, control mice had a higher mean white cell count (6700/µl) than animals treated with intermittent TNP-470 (3600/µl) that was statistically significant ($p<0.04$). Despite the statistical difference, the post-BMT white cell count reached by treated mice was adequate and within the normal range. Bone marrow cellularity was also assessed in the femurs of transplanted animals. At d+28 after dose level 3, there was no difference in marrow cellularity between TNP-470-treated transplanted mice, transplanted control mice, or untransplanted control mice (data not shown).

Although TNP-470 is effective in mouse xenograft models in treating established and early neuroblastoma tumors [12, 14] when given in an intermittent schedule, the current human clinical trials are including a continuous infusion component (personal communication, D. Milkowski) to overcome the concerns of the short half life of the drug [25]. In order to reflect this dosing strategy, we

Table 5. Recovery of peripheral WBC after stem cell rescue

	N=	WBC[1]	p=
Control	12	6.3 ± 0.7[2]	
TNP-470 intermittent dosing[3]	10	**3.6 ± 0.7**	**.04**
TNP-470 continuous infusion[4]	10	6.3 ± 0.4	NS
PBS continuous infusion	10	**4.6 ± 0.3**	**.03**
Untreated FVB mice	10	7.1 ± 0.7	NS

[1] White blood cell count in $10^3/\mu L$. WBC counts at d+28 post BMT in control animals and animals treated with TNP-470, continuous phosphate-buffered saline, as well as untransplanted untreated mice as a normal reference (FVB).
[2] Mean ± SEM. Only the values indicated in bold are significantly different from control.
[3] These animals received TNP-470 at dose level 3, SQ three times/wk, d 0 through d 28.
[4] These animals received TNP-470 IP via Alzet pump at 10 mg/kg/wk.

used peritoneally implanted Alzet osmotic pumps to deliver TNP-470 continuously over 14 days. In other studies, we have shown that significantly lower total doses provide similar anti-tumor effects and are tolerated in the continuous infusion setting (data not shown and [14]). Thus, we chose a dose of 10 mg/kg/week given continuously as the highest dose that did not cause cachexia in transplanted and xenografted animals. In these experiments, pumps were implanted on d-1 prior to BMT. TBI and stem cell infusion occurred on d0, and the animals were sacrificed on d+28. Lymphoid engraftment was assessed in these animals as above, and no differences were observed between TNP-470-treated animals, saline treated animals (both by continuous infusion), or transplanted animals with no pump implanted (data not shown). As with the bolus dosing, we saw no significant differences in hemoglobin or platelet recovery between TNP-470-treated and control animals. However, in distinction to the bolus-dosed animals, we observed no differences in WBC recovery in the animals given TNP-470 by continuous infusion (Table 5) compared to animals that had been transplanted but had no pump implanted or normal (untreated and untransplanted) recipient mice. Among these animals, we did see lower WBC in the saline-treated animals (WBC=6300/µl in the TNP-470-treated mice vs. 4600/µl in the saline controls, $p<0.03$). Again, this difference, though statistically significant, is likely not clinically significant.

Discussion

Relapse after maximal dose-intensity therapy may in part result from contamination of the stem cell product with tumor cells [3, 4]. Whether relapse results from reinfused tumor cells or cells remaining in the patient, most patients are in a state of minimal residual disease after transplant. This provides a clinical situation in which the use of angiogenesis inhibitors may be most effective. It is of importance, therefore, to establish that angiogenesis inhibitors such as TNP-470 do not inhibit engraftment of normal BM cells and that full immune and hematologic reconstitution proceeds uninterrupted. We show here that a reliable system for stem cell transplant can be developed in a mouse model using stem cells from donor mice that express a transgene that is detected by flow cytometry and PCR, transplanted into lethally irradiated recipients. TNP-470 can be administered in this setting, starting on d0 of transplantation, with minimal toxicity and no excess mortality in the TNP-470-treated group, whether the drug was administered as a bolus dose or as continuous infusion. Both treated and control mice demonstrated reliable multilineage engraftment as well as normal B cell maturation. Furthermore, engraftment kinetics were not slowed by treatment with TNP-470 immediately following infusion of donor stem cells. There was evidence of decreased WBC in the bolus TNP-470 group compared to controls at d+28, but the opposite effect was seen in animals given continuously administered TNP-470, where saline-treated mice showed slightly lower WBC than TNP-470-treated or normal mice.

Metastatic solid tumors of childhood have been historically difficult to treat, especially high-risk neuroblastoma. Surgery plus conventional chemoradiotherapy has provided only 20% survival at best [17]. Addition of autologous BMT and biotherapy with 13-cis-retinoic acid improved 3 year event-free survival to approximately 40% in a Children's Cancer Group Phase III randomized trial [2]. Further dose-intensification with tandem transplantation and use of peripheral blood progenitor cells as stem cell support has provided evidence of further improvement in event-free survival [18, 19], but this approach has not yet been validated in a Phase III study. Despite these relative improvements in outcome, the majority of children with high-risk neuroblastoma still experience relapse. Chemotherapy dose-intensification has reached its limit; novel agents and approaches are needed.

Folkman first reported that analogues of fumagillin are potent inhibitors of endothelial cell proliferation, leading to the discovery of TNP-470 [20]. Cohn and associates reported that increased vascularity in neuroblastoma is associated with aggressive disease and poor outcome [21] suggesting that there may be a role for angiogenesis inhibitors in the treatment of advanced disease. Since that time, several studies have explored the use of TNP-470 in animal models of malignant tumors. Our first observations in this study confirm that TNP-470 effectively inhibits neuroblastoma xenograft growth when administered as a single agent. We then demonstrated enhanced efficacy in models of minimal residual disease. First, we showed that TNP-470 clearly stabilized tumor regression following treatment with cyclophosphamide. Second, in a prevention model designed to mimic a state of minimal residual disease at the primary tumor site, we showed that TNP-470 very effectively reduced the rate of tumor growth.

Thus, TNP-470 seems to be most effective when used in the setting of minimal disease burden [12], especially when used prior to objective evidence of disease establishment [14]. Other studies have found that TNP-470 first administered 10 days after inoculation of mice with two different neuroblastoma cell lines decreased both the primary tumor volume and the size and number of lymph node and liver metastases [22]. Similar results have been seen with other xenograft models using malignant human cell lines such as choriocarcinoma, ovarian cancer and endometrial cancer [23].

The stem cell transplant data presented here show that TNP-470 does not adversely impact engraftment after stem cell infusion and may provide a complimentary approach to the treatment of advanced pediatric solid tumors. Taken together with the xenograft model experience and the sense that angiogenesis inhibitors may work best when disease burden is at its least, our data point to a potential study design where anti-angiogenic agents are given in the post-transplant period in attempt to consolidate a remission and possibly increase the likelihood of long-term disease control.

References

1. Matthay, K. K., Harris, R., Reynolds, C. P., Shimada, H., Black, T., Stram, D. O., and Seeger, R. C. Improved event-free survival for autologous bone marrow transplantation vs chemotherapy in neuroblastoma: a Childrens Cancer Group study, Med Pediatr Oncol. *31:* 191, O-7, 1998.

2. Matthay, K. K., Villablanca, J. G., Seeger, R. C., Stram, D. O., Harris, R. E., Ramsay, N. K., Swift, P., Shimada, H., Black, C. T., Brodeur, G. M., Gerbing, R. B., and Reynolds, C. P. Treatment of high-risk neuroblastoma with intensive chemotherapy, radiotherapy, autologous bone marrow transplantation, and 13-cis-retinoic acid, N Engl J Med. *341:* 1165-1173, 1999.
3. Rill, D. R., Santana, V. M., Roberts, W. M., Nilson, T., Bowman, L. C., Krance, R. A., Heslop, H. E., Moen, R. C., Ihle, J. N., and Brenner, M. K. Direct demonstration that autologous bone marrow transplantation for solid tumors can return a multiplicity of tumorigenic cells, Blood. *84:* 380-383, 1994.
4. Brenner, M., Rill, D., Moen, R., Krance, R., Mirro, J., Anderson, W., and Ihle, J. Gene-marking to trace origin of relapse after autologous bone-marrow transplantation, Lancet. *341:* 85-86, 1993.
5. Freedman, A. S., Neuberg, D., Mauch, P., Soiffer, R. J., Anderson, K. C., Fisher, D. C., Schlossman, R., Alyea, E. P., Takvorian, T., Jallow, H., Kuhlman, C., Ritz, J., Nadler, L. M., and Gribben, J. G. Long-term follow-up of autologous bone marrow transplantation in patients with relapsed follicular lymphoma, Blood. *94:* 3325-3333, 1999.
6. O'Reilly, M. S., Holmgren, L., Shing, Y., Chen, C., Rosenthal, R. A., Moses, M., Lane, W. S., Cao, Y., Sage, E. H., and Folkman, J. Angiostatin: a novel angiogenesis inhibitor that mediates the suppression of metastases by a Lewis lung carcinoma, Cell. *79:* 315-328, 1994.
7. Folkman, J. Fighting cancer by attacking its blood supply, Sci Am. *275:* 150-154, 1996.
8. Folkman, J. Addressing tumor blood vessels, Nat Biotechnol. *15:* 510, 1997.
9. Parangi, S., O'Reilly, M., Christofori, G., Homgren, L., Grosfeld, J., Folkman, J., and Hanahan, D. Antiangiogenic therapy of transgenic mice impairs de novo tumor growth, Proc Natl Acad Sci U S A. *93:* 2002-2007, 1996.
10. Boehm, T., Folkman, J., Browder, T., and O'Reilly, M. S. Antiangiogenic therapy of experimental cancer does not induce acquired drug resistance, Nature. *390:* 404-407, 1997.
11. Kusaka, M., Sudo, K., Matsutani, E., Kozai, Y., Marui, S., Fujita, T., Ingber, D., and Folkman, J. Cytostatic inhibition of endothelial cell growth by the angiogenesis inhibitor TNP-470 (AGM-1470), Br J Cancer. *69:* 212-216, 1994.
12. Katzenstein, H. M., Rademaker, A. W., Senger, C., Salwen, H. R., Nguyen, N. N., Thorner, P. S., Litsas, L., and Cohn, S. L. Effectiveness of the angiogenesis inhibitor TNP-470 in reducing the growth of human neuroblastoma in nude mice inversely correlates with tumor burden, Clin Cancer Res. *5:* 4273-4278, 1999.
13. Wassberg, E., Pahlman, S., Westlin, J. E., and Christofferson, R. The angiogenesis inhibitor TNP-470 reduces the growth rate of human neuroblastoma in nude rats, Pediatr Res. *41:* 327-333, 1997.
14. Shusterman, S., Grupp, S. A., and Maris, J. M. Inhibition of tumor growth in a human neuroblastoma xenograft model with TNP-470, Med Ped Oncol. *35:511-673-676*, 2000.
15. Cronin, F. E., Jiang, M., Abbas, A. K., and Grupp, S. A. Role of mu heavy chain in B cell development. I. Blocked B cell maturation but complete allelic exclusion in the absence of Ig alpha/beta, J Immunol. *161:* 252-259, 1998.
16. Hasuike, T., Hino, M., Yamane, T., Nishizawa, Y., Morii, H., and Tatsumi, N. Effects of TNP-470, a potent angiogenesis inhibitor, on growth of hematopoietic progenitors, Eur J Haematol. *58:* 293-294, 1997.
17. Matthay, K. K., O'Leary, M. C., Ramsay, N. K., Villablanca, J., Reynolds, C. P., Atkinson, J. B., Haase, G. M., Stram, D. O., and Seeger, R. C. Role of myeloablative therapy in improved outcome for high risk neuroblastoma: review of recent Children's Cancer Group results, Eur J Cancer. *31A:* 572-575, 1995.
18. Grupp, S. A., Stern, J. W., Bunin, N., Nancarrow, C., Ross, A. A., Mogul, M., Adams, R., Grier, H. E., Gorlin, J. B., Shamberger, R., Marcus, K., Neuberg, D., Weinstein, H. J., and Diller, L. Tandem high dose therapy in rapid sequence for children with high-risk neuroblastoma, J Clin Onc. *18:* 2567-2575, 2000.
19. Grupp, S. A., Stern, J. W., Bunin, N., Nancarrow, C., Adams, R., Gorlin, J. B., Griffin, G., and Diller, L. Rapid sequence tandem stem cell transplant for children with high-risk neuroblastoma, Med Pediatr Oncol. 35:*696-700*, 2000.
20. Ingber, D., Fujita, T., Kishimoto, S., Sudo, K., Kanamaru, T., Brem, H., and Folkman, J. Synthetic analogues of fumagillin that inhibit angiogenesis and suppress tumour growth, Nature. *348:* 555-557, 1990.

21. Meitar, D., Crawford, S. E., Rademaker, A. W., and Cohn, S. L. Tumor angiogenesis correlates with metastatic disease, N-myc amplification, and poor outcome in human neuroblastoma, J Clin Oncol. *14:* 405-414, 1996.
22. Nagabuchi, E., VanderKolk, W. Y., Une, Y., and Ziegler, M. M. TNP-470 antiangiogenic therapy for advanced murine neuroblastoma, J Pediatr Surg. *32:* 287-293, 1997.
23. Yanase, T., Tamura, M., Fujita, K., Kodama, S., and Tanaka, K. Inhibitory effect of angiogenesis inhibitor TNP-470 on tumor growth and metastasis of human cell lines in vitro and in vivo, Cancer Res. *53:* 2566-2570, 1993.
24. Milkowski, D.M. and Weiss, R.A. TNP-470. *In:* Antiangiogenic Agents in Cancer Therapy, pp. 385-398. Teicher, B.A., ed. Humana Press, Totawa, N.J., 2000.
25. Bhargava, P., Marshall, J,L., Rizvi, N., Dahut, W., Yoe, J., Figuera, M., Phipps, K., Ong, V.S., Kato, A. and Hawkins, M.J. A phase I and pharmacokinetic study of TNP-470 administered weekly to patients with advanced cancer. Clinical Cancer Research. 5:1989-95, 1999.
26. Schlesinger, H.R., Gerson, J.M., Moorhead, P.S., Maguire, H., and Hummeler, K. Establishment and characterization of human neuroblastoma cell lines, Cancer Research. *36:* 3094-100, 1976.
27. Tomayko, M. M. and Reynolds, C. P. Determination of subcutaneous tumor size in athymic (nude) mice, Cancer Chemotherapy & Pharmacology. *24:* 148-54, 1989.
28. Erdreich-Epstein, A., Shimada, H., Groshen, S., Liu, M., Metelitsa, L. S., Kim, K. S., Stins, M. F., Seeger, R. C., and Durden, D. L. Integrins alpha(v)beta3 and alpha(v)beta5 are expressed by endothelium of high-risk neuroblastoma and their inhibition is associated with increased endogenous ceramide, Cancer Research. *60:* 712-21, 2000.
29. Eggert, A., Ikegaki, N., Kwiatkowski, J., Zhao, H., Brodeur, G. M., and Himelstein, B. P. High-level expression of angiogenic factors is associated with advanced tumor stage in human neuroblastomas, Clinical Cancer Research. *6:* 1900-1908, 2000.

Challenges in the Treatment of Fungal Infections

Prophylaxis of Fungal Infections in Neutropenic Patients with Hematologic Malignancies

F. KROSCHINSKY, and U. SCHULER

Medizinische Klinik und Poliklinik I, Fetscherstrasse 74, D-01307 Dresden, Germany

Prophylaxis against invasive fungal infection (IFI) in neutropenic patients remains a cornerstone of antifungal strategies mainly because diagnosis of fungal infections remains fraught with problems and the therapy of clinically overt infection, especially with molds, remains associated with high mortality. For most hematological diseases, the current therapeutic strategy relies on repetitive courses of chemotherapy. After an episode of IFI the risk of recurrence of the infections in a new episode of neutropenia is substantial. Therefore case-fatality rates of IFI do not reflect the entire prognostic impact of these infections, as the further therapy of the respective underlying disease may be hampered, delayed or entirely impossible. Overall mortality rates of IFI have been reported in the range of 47–64% [1]. [2]Subgroups of patients with e.g. allogeneic transplants, graft versus host disease (GVHD) and concurrent infections (CMV) my do substantially worse, with case fatality rates of 85–100% [3].

Prophylactic strategies are based on risk factors and should be distinguished from both preemptive and empirical treatment strategies. This has recently been confounded in a meta-analysis [4], criticized by Kribbler et al. [5]. In our opinion the term ‚empirical therapy‘ should be used in a patient with obvious signs of infection of unclear etiology, whereas the term ‚preemptive‘ would apply (in transferring the use of the term in CMV infection) e.g. to a patient with not yet evident infection, but the combination of a high-risk situation and demonstration of a potential pathogen. Prophylaxis would be defined as the use of antimycotic drugs in patients with a sufficiently high risk for infection. This review concentrates on newer developments in this field, especially on the potential role of itraconazole oral solution.

Fungi commonly involved in infection

Prophylactic strategies have to be directed against the most common pathogens in the respective circumstances. IFIs are most commonly caused by *Candida spp.* and *Aspergillus spp.*. Other fungi (mucorales, *Fusarium spp.*, cryptococcus) are rare in this context and therefore not primary targets of prophylaxis.

The widespread introduction of azoles (e.g. fluconazole) led to a shift in the species involved, with a clear reduction in both colonization and invasive infection with *Candida albicans*. For yeasts there is evidence for both endogenous (long term colonisation) and exogenous (clusters of identical strains, transmission by staff) infection. The dominant mode of transmission with molds is airborne, with the lung as primary target, therefore high-efficiency particulate air (HEPA) filtered rooms are commonly employed in the nursing of patients of the highest risk groups.

Risk factors for IFI

In patients with chemotherapy, the main factors affecting the risk of IFI are neutropenia and mucosal damage. Additionally the risk is related to the underlying disease, the chemotherapeutic agents employed and the patient's age (higher in the extremes of age). Within the neutropenic population, the risk is related to severity (lower risk 0.1–0·5 × 109/l, high risk <0.1 × 109/l)and duration (low < 7 days, high >21 days of profound neutropenia [6]. Therefore most chemotherapy regimens employed for solid tumors are below the threshold of risk, that warrants drug prophylaxis.

Among hematological malignancies acute myeloid leukemia (AML) may be associated with the highest risk for aspergillosis [2]. This is explained most likely by a reduction in the absolute numbers of neutrophils at the onset of treatment and the more intensive chemotherapy required for the treatment of this malignancy. In the setting of allogeneic stem cell transplantation the occurrence of GVHD and the use of corticosteroids (either as GVHD-prophylaxis or treatment) is closely related the risk of IFI [7–9]. Accordingly, the risk for IFI is associated with the risk for GVHD, being higher in HLA-mismatched or unrelated transplants compared to a HLA-matched sibling transplants [10]. In the context if GVHD IFI, especially aspergillosis is not necessarily associated with neutropenia. Colonization frequently precedes invasive disease [11, 12], especially if several sites are involved [13, 14], or *Candida tropicalis* is detected.

The risk of altered gastrointestinal flora and ensuing infection may further depend on the administration of broad spectrum antibiotics and the use of high-dose Ara-C plus etoposide [9].

Prophylaxis with azoles

There have been numerous studies evaluating azoles in comparison to plazebo or polyenes (e.g. [15–21]). While most studies with fluconazole were able to show a reduction in the overall incidence of fungal infections, this was mainly due to the reduction of superficial infections. Other secondary endpoints, such as the incidence of empiric amphotericin B or the time to use of i.v. amphotericin B were also positively affected [19, 20]. Only the two studies done in BMT-patients [17, 18] showed a substantial reduction in invasive infections and even improved survival of patients [18].

For several years, itraconazole was available as a capsule formulation only. This was associated with poor bioavailability of the drug, especially in patients with mucosal damage. More recently, an oral solution of an itraconazole-cyclodextrin complex has resulted in improved pharmacokinetics after oral intake. Today, levels

Table 1. Trough levels of itraconazole in neutropenic patients

	Cmin values	Patients
Prentice et al. (1995) [22]	1468 ± 306 ng/ml at day 15	chemotherapy
Prentice et al. (1994) [23]	845 ± 221 ng/ml at day 15	autograft recipients
Michallet et al. (1998) [24]	300 ± 90 ng/ml at day 7	allograft recipients

of 500 ng/ml (as determined by HPLC) are regarded as necessary for the treatment or prevention of mold infections. Results of pharmacokinetic studies with this solution are shown in Table 1.

Slightly more than twice these values can be expected for the major metabolite (hydroxyitraconazole), which is also antimycotically active. Due to the large volume of distribution of the drug, it seems advisable in some circumstances to use loading doses (e.g. 4 x 200 mg/day orally for 2–3 days), in order to reach effective drug levels more quickly.

Three large randomized studies used the itraconazole solution in the prophylactic setting. Itraconazole was dosed at 400 mg/day. The design and results are summarized in Table 2.

In one study [25] cyclodextrin was used as the placebo and there was an unexpected, but not significant, excess of proven deep *Aspergillus spp.* infections with itraconazole use (1 vs. 4). The second study [26] compared itraconazole solution to fluconazole solution (100 mg/d) and included both chemotherapy- and transplant- patients (both autograft and allografts). No Aspergillus infection was seen with itraconazole, with only one *C. albicans* proven fungaemia and no fungal deaths. With fluconazole, there were seven fungal deaths (proven: five *Aspergillus spp.*, one *C. tropicalis*; probable: one *Aspergillus spp.*, P = 0·024). The third study used amphotericin B capsules (2 g/day) as a comparator [27]. Despite favorable trends for itraconazole (fewer proven IFI [8 vs. 13], fewer proven *Aspergil-*

Table 2. Studies evaluating itraconazole oral solution as antifungal prophylaxis in neutropenic patients

	Treatment-groups	n	Empirical amphotericin B	Invasive aspergillosis	Fungal deaths
Menichetti et al. (1999) [25]	ITRA solution	201	43*	4	1
	Placebo	204	59	1	5
Morgenstern et al. (1999) [26]	ITRA solution	288	39*	0	0*
	FLU solution	293	58	4	7
Harousseau et al. (1999) [27]	ITRA solution	281	90	5	1
	AMB capsules	276	102	9	5

* P=<0.05

lus spp. [5 vs. 9] and fewer fungal deaths [1 vs. 5]) none of the differences proved to be statistically significant. In these prophylaxis studies, compliance with the oral solution was a problem in a substantial proportion of patients, because of cyclodextrin gastrointestinal toxicity.

Both azoles used in the prophylactic setting show a number of drug interactions, mainly related to substrates metabolized by the cytochrome CYP3A4. Of importance is the delayed elimination of midazolam and the increased toxicity of vinca-alkaloids (described for itraconazole)[28]. Increased drug levels of cyclosporin A and tacrolimus during azole treatment require close monitoring and dose adjustments [29].

The meta-analysis of Bow et al. [30], published only in abstract form, analyzed studies with antifungal prophylaxis in neutropenia and unlike the analysis by Gotzsche [4] did not include studies on empiric therapy. There was a highly significant reduction of the need of empirical antifungal therapy (OR 0.56; C.I. 0.47–0.67). The azoles showed a significant reduction in IFI (OR 0.43; C.I. 0.33–0.59). In this meta-analysis, decreased fungal mortality could however only be shown in patients undergoing stem cell transplantation, an effect on overall mortality could not be demonstrated.

Secondary prophylaxis

During subsequent episodes of neutropenia there is high risk of recurrence for patients with previous episodes of IFI, especially with aspergillosis. Therefore secondary prophylaxis was addressed in several retrospective analyses. In BMT-patients, Karp et al. used i.v. amphotericin B as secondary prophylaxis. Only two of nine patients suffered relapse of invasive aspergillosis compared with a 50% incidence in an historical cohort [31].

Other approaches

There have been several studies on the prophylactic use of low dose amphotericin B or even liposomal amphotericin. Evidence for the former is mainly from retrospective studies (e.g. [8]), while use of the latter is prohibitive because of its high cost. Aerosolized amphotericin seems an attractive approach to disrupt the primary route of infection for moulds. It was therefore used in several settings, but a recent randomized study failed to show a benefit for this strategy [32].

General measures, such as hand washing may help to reduce exogenous infections with yeast, which in some cases could be traced to transmission by staff. Prevention of Aspergillus infection by the airborne route may be achieved by High-efficiency particulate air (HEPA) filtration [33-35]. However, in allogeneic transplant patients, the risk of infection shows a bimodal distribution over time. While it is possible to nurse patients during the initial phase of neutropenia and mucositis in a protective environment, there is a second peak of incidence associated with late GVHD, at a time, when the majority of patients has already left the hospital.

Summary

There is clear evidence for a benefit of fluconazole prophylaxis in BMT patients. The lack of activity of fluconazole in aspergillosis makes prophylaxis with itraconazole an interesting alternative. Evidence from studies in non-transplant patients is less convincing. Itraconazole has been tested mainly in this group, a study in a transplant only cohort of patients is not yet available.

References

1. Bow EJ, Loewen R, Cheang MS, Shore TB, Rubinger M, Schacter B (1997) Cytotoxic therapy-induced D-xylose malabsorption and invasive infection during remission-induction therapy for acute myeloid leukemia in adults. J Clin Oncol. 15:2254-2261
2. Denning DW, Marinus A, Cohen J, Spence D, Herbrecht R, Pagano L, Kibbler C, Kcrmery V, Offner F, Cordonnier C, Jehn U, Ellis M, Collette L, Sylvester R (1998) An EORTC multicentre prospective survey of invasive aspergillosis in haematological patients: diagnosis and therapeutic outcome. EORTC Invasive Fungal Infections Cooperative Group. J Infect. 37:173-180
3. Meyers JD (1990) Fungal infections in bone marrow transplant patients. Semin.Oncol. 17:10-13
4. Gotzsche PC, Johansen HK (1997) Meta-analysis of prophylactic or empirical antifungal treatment versus placebo or no treatment in patients with cancer complicated by neutropenia. BMJ. 314:1238-1244
5. Kibbler CC, Manuel R, Prentice HG (1997) Prophylactic and empirical antifungal treatment in cancer complicated by neutropenia. Combining different antifungal strategies in same systematic review is inappropriate. BMJ. 315:488-489
6. Gerson SL, Talbot GH, Hurwitz S, Strom BL, Lusk EJ, Cassileth PA (1984) Prolonged granulocytopenia: the major risk factor for invasive pulmonary aspergillosis in patients with acute leukemia. Ann.Intern.Med 100:345-351
7. Sayer HG, Longton G, Bowden R, Pepe M, Storb R (1994) Increased risk of infection in marrow transplant patients receiving methylprednisolone for graft-versus-host disease prevention. Blood 84:1328-1332
8. O'Donnell MR, Schmidt GM, Tegtmeier BR, Faucett C, Fahey JL, Ito J, Nademanee A, Niland J, Parker P, Smith EP (1994) Prediction of systemic fungal infection in allogeneic marrow recipients: impact of amphotericin prophylaxis in high-risk patients. J Clin Oncol. 12:827-834
9. Bow EJ, Loewen R, Cheang MS, Schacter B (1995) Invasive fungal disease in adults undergoing remission-induction therapy for acute myeloid leukemia: the pathogenetic role of the antileukemic regimen. Clin Infect.Dis. 21:361-369
10. Jantunen E, Ruutu P, Niskanen L, Volin L, Parkkali T, Koukila-Kahkola P, Ruutu T (1997) Incidence and risk factors for invasive fungal infections in allogeneic BMT recipients. Bone Marrow Transplant. 19:801-808
11. Sandford GR, Merz WG, Wingard JR, Charache P, Saral R (1980) The value of fungal surveillance cultures as predictors of systemic fungal infections. J Infect.Dis. 142:503-509
12. Schwartz RS, Mackintosh FR, Schrier SL, Greenberg PL (1984) Multivariate analysis of factors associated with invasive fungal disease during remission induction therapy for acute myelogenous leukemia. Cancer 53:411-419
13. Guiot HF, Fibbe WE, van 't Wout (1994) Risk factors for fungal infection in patients with malignant hematologic disorders: implications for empirical therapy and prophylaxis. Clin Infect.Dis. 18:525-532
14. Martino P, Girmenia C, Micozzi A, De Bernardis F, Boccanera M, Cassone A (1994) Prospective study of Candida colonization, use of empiric amphotericin B and development of invasive mycosis in neutropenic patients. Eur.J Clin Microbiol.Infect.Dis. 13:797-804
15. Philpott-Howard JN, Wade JJ, Mufti GJ, Brammer KW, Ehninger G (1993) Randomized comparison of oral fluconazole versus oral polyenes for the prevention of fungal infection in patients at risk of neutropenia. Multicentre Study Group. J Antimicrob.Chemother. 31:973-984

16. Menichetti F, Del Favero A, Martino P, Bucaneve G, Micozzi A, D'Antonio D, Ricci P, Carotenuto M, Liso V, Nosari AM (1994) Preventing fungal infection in neutropenic patients with acute leukemia: fluconazole compared with oral amphotericin B. The GIMEMA Infection Program. Ann.Intern.Med 120:913-918
17. Goodman JL, Winston DJ, Greenfield RA, Chandrasekar PH, Fox B, Kaizer H, Shadduck RK, Shea TC, Stiff P, Friedman DJ (1992) A controlled trial of fluconazole to prevent fungal infections in patients undergoing bone marrow transplantation. N.Engl.J.Med. 326:845-851
18. Slavin MA, Osborne B, Adams R, Levenstein MJ, Schoch HG, Feldman AR, Meyers JD, Bowden RA (1995) Efficacy and safety of fluconazole prophylaxis for fungal infections after marrow transplantation—a prospective, randomized, double-blind study. J.Infect.Dis. 171:1545-1552
19. Schaffner A, Schaffner M (1995) Effect of prophylactic fluconazole on the frequency of fungal infections, amphotericin B use, and health care costs in patients undergoing intensive chemotherapy for hematologic neoplasias. J Infect.Dis. 172:1035-1041
20. Winston DJ, Chandrasekar PH, Lazarus HM, Goodman JL, Silber JL, Horowitz H, Shadduck RK, Rosenfeld CS, Ho WG, Islam MZ (1993) Fluconazole prophylaxis of fungal infections in patients with acute leukemia. Results of a randomized placebo-controlled, double-blind, multicenter trial [see comments]. Ann.Intern.Med. 118:495-503
21. Ninane J (1994) A multicentre study of fluconazole versus oral polyenes in the prevention of fungal infection in children with hematological or oncological malignancies. Multicentre Study Group. Eur.J Clin Microbiol.Infect.Dis. 13:330-337
22. Prentice AG, Warnock DW, Johnson SA, Taylor PC, Oliver DA (1995) Multiple dose pharmacokinetics of an oral solution of itraconazole in patients receiving chemotherapy for acute myeloid leukaemia. J.Antimicrob.Chemother. 36:657-663
23. Prentice AG, Warnock DW, Johnson SA, Phillips MJ, Oliver DA (1994) Multiple dose pharmacokinetics of an oral solution of itraconazole in autologous bone marrow transplant recipients. J.Antimicrob.Chemother. 34:247-252
24. Michallet M, Persat F, Kranzhofer N, Levron JC, Prat C, Belhabri A, Chwetzoff E, Le Moing JP, Fiere D, Piens MA (1998) Pharmacokinetics of itraconazole oral solution in allogeneic bone marrow transplant patients receiving total body irradiation. Bone Marrow Transplant. 21:1239-1243
25. Menichetti F, Del Favero A, Martino P, Bucaneve G, Micozzi A, Girmenia C, Barbabietola G, Pagano L, Leoni P, Specchia G, Caiozzo A, Raimondi R, Mandelli F (1999) Itraconazole oral solution as prophylaxis for fungal infections in neutropenic patients with hematologic malignancies: a randomized, placebo-controlled, double-blind, multicenter trial. GIMEMA Infection Program. Gruppo Italiano Malattie Ematologiche dell'Adulto. Clin.Infect.Dis. 28:250-255
26. Morgenstern GR, Prentice AG, Prentice HG, Ropner JE, Schey SA, Warnock DW (1999) A randomized controlled trial of itraconazole versus fluconazole for the prevention of fungal infections in patients with haematological malignancies. U.K. Multicentre Antifungal Prophylaxis Study Group [In Process Citation]. Br.J.Haematol. 105:901-911
27. Harousseau JL, Dekker AW, Stamatoullas-Bastard A, Fassas A, Linkesch W, Gouveia J, De Bock R, Rovira M, Seifert WF, Joosen H, Peeters M, De Beule K (Itraconazole oral solution for primary prophylaxis of fungal infections in patients with hematological malignancy and profound neutropenia: a randomized, double-blind, double-placebo, multicenter trial comparing itraconazole and amphotericin B. Antimicrob.Agents Chemother.2000.Jul.;44.(7.):1887.-93. 44:1887-1893
28. Chan JD (1998) Pharmacokinetic drug interactions of vinca alkaloids: summary of case reports. Pharmacotherapy. 18:1304-1307
29. McLachlan AJ, Tett SE (1998) Effect of metabolic inhibitors on cyclosporine pharmacokinetics using a population approach. Ther.Drug Monit. 20:390-395
30. Bow EJ, Laverdiere M, Luurila H, et al (2001) Anti-fungal prophylaxis in neutropenic cancer patients ± a meta-analysis of randomised controlled trials. Blood 94 suppl 1:339a(Abstract)
31. Karp JE, Burch PA, Merz WG (1988) An approach to intensive antileukemia therapy in patients with previous invasive aspergillosis. Am J Med 85:203-206
32. Schwartz S, Behre G, Heinemann V, Wandt H, Schilling E, Arning M, Trittin A, Kern WV, Boenisch O, Bosse D, Lenz K, Ludwig WD, Hiddemann W, Siegert W, Beyer J (1999) Aerosolized amphotericin B inhalations as prophylaxis of invasive aspergillus infections during prolonged neutropenia: results of a prospective randomized multicenter trial. Blood 93:3654-3661

33. McWhinney PH, Kibbler CC, Hamon MD, Smith OP, Gandhi L, Berger LA, Walesby RK, Hoffbrand AV, Prentice HG (1993) Progress in the diagnosis and management of aspergillosis in bone marrow transplantation: 13 years' experience. Clin Infect.Dis. 17:397-404
34. Passweg JR, Rowlings PA, Atkinson KA, Barrett AJ, Gale RP, Gratwohl A, Jacobsen N, Klein JP, Ljungman P, Russell JA, Schaefer UW, Sobocinski KA, Vossen JM, Zhang MJ, Horowitz MM (1998) Influence of protective isolation on outcome of allogeneic bone marrow transplantation for leukemia. Bone Marrow Transplant. 21:1231-1238
35. Wald A, Leisenring W, van-Burik JA, Bowden RA (1997) Epidemiology of Aspergillus infections in a large cohort of patients undergoing bone marrow transplantation. J.Infect.Dis. 175:1459-1466

Subject Index

Printing: Strauss GmbH, Mörlenbach
Binding: Schäffer, Grünstadt

MIX
Papier aus verantwortungsvollen Quellen
Paper from responsible sources
FSC® C105338

If you have any concerns about our products,
you can contact us on
ProductSafety@springernature.com

In case Publisher is established outside the EU,
the EU authorized representative is:
Springer Nature Customer Service Center GmbH
Europaplatz 3, 69115 Heidelberg, Germany

Printed by Libri Plureos GmbH
in Hamburg, Germany